Advances in Urology®
Volume 6

Advances in Urology®

Radiology of Impotence, *by Ronald W. Lewis, B.G. Parulkar, C. Michael Johnson, and W. Eugene Miller*
Nerve-Sparing Modifications of Retroperitoneal Lymphadenectomy, *by Jerome P. Richie*

Volume 4

Bacillus Calmette-Guerin Immunotherapy in Bladder Cancer, *by Angelo S. Paola and Donald L. Lamm*
Treatment of Invasive Bladder Cancer, *by James E. Montie*
Endocrine Management of Prostate Cancer, *by Fritz H. Schröder and Claus G. Röhrbom*
Cavitron Resection (Ultrasonic Aspiration) of the Prostate, *by Terrence R. Malloy*
Balloon Dilatation of the Prostate, *by Lester A. Klein*
Indications for the Use of Drugs in the Male Reproductive System, *by Carol M. Proudfit*
Medical Management of Renal Stone Disease, *by Fredric L. Coe and Joan Parks*
The Pathophysiology of Incontinence in the Elderly, *by Pat D. O'Donnell*
The Diagnosis of Renal Hypertension, *by Mark C. Saddler and Henry R. Black*
Advances in Genitourinary Laparoscopy, *by David A. Bloom and Kurt Semm*
Endocrine Abnormalities in Children Associated with Ambiguous Genitalia: Diagnosis and Management, *by Bruce Blyth*

Volume 5

Partial Nephrectomy for Renal Cell Carcinoma, *by Eric A. Klein and Andrew C. Novick*
Flow Cytometry in Urologic Practice, *by Ihn Seong Whang and Mitchell C. Benson*
The Management of Stage T1 Grade 3 Transitional Cell Carcinoma of the Bladder, *by Mark J. Waples and Edward M. Messing*
Management of Urinary Tract Infections, *by Anthony J. Schaeffer*
The Use of Flexible Ureteropyeloscopy, *by Demetrius H. Bagley*
The Unstable Bladder: The Clinical Relevance of a Urodynamic Diagnosis, *by Edward J. McGuire*
Operative Repair of Rectocele, Enterocele, and Cystocele, *by Shlomo Raz, Deborah R. Erickson, and Ernest M. Sussman*
Use of Collagen Injections for Treatment of Incontinence and Reflux, *by Rodney A. Appell*
Urethral Strictures: Current Management, *by George D. Webster and Joseph M. Khoury*

Advances in Urology®

Volume 6 · 1993

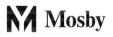 Mosby

St. Louis Baltimore Boston Chicago London Philadelphia Sydney Toronto

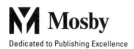

Dedicated to Publishing Excellence

Sponsoring Editor: Cora R. Williams
Project Manager: Denise Dungey
Project Supervisor: Maria Nevinger
Production Editor: Laura Pelehach
Staff Support Administrator: Barbara M. Kelly

Editorial Office:
Mosby–Year Book, Inc.
200 North LaSalle St.
Chicago, IL 60601

International Standard Serial Number: 0894-4385
International Standard Book Number: 0-8151-5694-4

Contributors

Richard B. Alexander, M.D.
Senior Investigator, Division of Urologic Oncology, Surgery Branch, National Cancer Institute, Bethesda, Maryland

Michael J. Barry, M.D.
Director, Health Services Research, Henry J. Kaiser Family Foundation Faculty Scholar in General Internal Medicine, Department of Medicine, Harvard Medical School; Medical Practices Evaluation Center, Massachusetts General Hospital, Boston, Massachusetts

David A. Bloom, M.D.
Professor of Surgery, Section of Urology, University of Michigan, Ann Arbor, Michigan

Floyd J. Fowler, Jr., Ph.D.
Senior Research Scientist, Center for Survey Research, University of Massachusetts, Boston, Massachusetts

Andrew L. Freedman, M.D.
Resident, Department of Surgery/Urology, University of California, Los Angeles School of Medicine, Los Angeles, California

M'Liss A. Hudson, M.D.
Assistant Professor, Division of Urologic Surgery, Washington University, School of Medicine, St. Louis, Missouri

Louis J. Ignarro, Ph.D.
Professor of Pharmacology, University of California, Los Angeles School of Medicine, Los Angeles, California

Peter M. Knapp, M.D.
Methodist Hospital of Indiana; Assistant Clinical Professor, Department of Urology, Indiana University School of Medicine, Indianapolis, Indiana

John W. Konnak, M.D.
Professor, Surgery-Urology, The University of Michigan Medical Center, Ann Arbor, Michigan

W. Marston Linehan, M.D.
Chief, Division of Urologic Oncology, Surgery Branch, National Cancer Institute, Bethesda, Maryland

Malcolm Moore, M.D.
Assistant Professor, Department of Medicine and Pharmacology, Princess Margaret Hospital and University of Toronto, Toronto, Ontario, Canada

David F. Paulson, M.D.

Professor and Chief, Division of Urologic Surgery, Duke University Medical Center, Durham, North Carolina

Samuel J. Peretsman, M.D.

Vice-Chairman, Department of Urology, Wilford Hall United States Air Force Medical Center, San Antonio, Texas

Jacob Rajfer, M.D.

Professor of Surgery/Urology, University of California, Los Angeles School of Medicine, Los Angeles, California; Chief, Division of Urology, Habor-University of California, Los Angeles Medical Center, Torrance, California

Steven A. Rosenberg, M.D., Ph.D

Chief, Surgery Branch, National Cancer Institute, Bethesda, Maryland

Jill K. Sanvordenker, R.N.

Nurse Clinician, Department of Pediatrics, Section of Urology, University of Michigan, Ann Arbor, Michigan

Yoram I. Siegel, M.D.

Research Fellow, Methodist Hospital of Indiana; Institute for Kidney Stone Disease, Indianapolis, Indiana

Mark Sigman, M.D.

Assistant Professor of Urology, Division of Urology, Brown University; Department of Urology, Rhode Island Hospital, Providence, Rhode Island

Ian Tannock, M.D., Ph.D.

Professor and Chairman, Department of Medicine, Princess Margaret Hospital and University of Toronto, Toronto, Ontario, Canada

Ian M. Thompson, M.D.

Chief, Urology Service, Brooke Army Medical Center, San Antonio, Texas

McClellan M. Walther, M.D.

Senior Investigator, Division of Urologic Oncology, Surgery Branch, National Cancer Institute, Bethesda, Maryland

Preface

This sixth volume of *Advances in Urology*® continues to provide a comprehensive review of some of the more recent innovations and changes in the clinical practice of urology. Two subjects are included that reflect our increasing concern with certain important social issues that are of particular interest to the urologist. The opening chapter by David Bloom, M.D., and Jill Sanvordenker, R.N., is both informative and thoughtful and should be of great help to the clinician who has to deal with a case of child abuse. This has been the subject of much discourse in the past 10 years and is a topic with which all practicing physicians need to be familiar. The chapter on the methodology of evaluating the subjective outcome of treatment for benign prostatic hypertrophy by Drs. Michael Barry and Floyd Fowler concerns the very important issue of how we, as surgeons, assess the effects of our treatment, particularly when the outcome is concerned with the quality of life and relief of symptoms rather than with survival rates. The increasing use of public funds in payment for medical care will generate a greater need for these kinds of evaluation. This timely, well-presented paper provides some insight into the problems of both the design and assessment of studies to determine outcomes. While there may not be universal agreement about the methods employed, they provide a very good indication of ways to approach these questions. The authors point how some of the parameters that we have traditionally used to evaluate our results are not always reliable indicators when they are subjected to careful analysis.

There are three chapters that deal with the current problems of potency and reproduction. The excellent review of the recent progress that has been made in the understanding of the physiology of erection is by Drs. Freedman, Ignarro and Rajfer from the University of California in Los Angeles. They indicate how investigation of the pharmacodynamics of tumescence will lead to improved methods of medical therapy for impotence. In his chapter, Dr. Konnak describes the present indications for and the results of vasovasostomy and vasoepididymostomy, and discusses the significance of sperm antibodies that are commonly found in these patients. Dr. Mark Sigman has written a very lucid account of the embryology and resulting anatomic changes that occur in congenital absence of the vas. Microepididymal aspiration of sperm can now be successfully performed in these patients, and used for in vitro fertilization. Dr. Sigman includes an up-to-date account of the current methods of sperm enhancement and in vitro fertilization techniques providing the urologist with a clear conception of the present role and efficacy of these new modalities in the treatment of male infertility.

There have been many attempts to explore the non–self immunogenic expression of renal cell cancers for therapeutic purposes. The group of surgical investigators at the National Cancer Institute, under the leadership of

Dr. Rosenberg, are the leaders in the field. Drs. Alexander, Walther, Linehan, and Rosenberg describe their extensive experience with immunotherapy for renal cancer. There is an excellent account of the theoretic and immunologic concepts and experimental data that support the use of this form of treatment for cancer. This should enable the practicing urologist to evaluate the role of this relatively new form of treatment for those cases of renal cell carcinoma that cannot be successfully treated by surgical extirpation alone.

Drs. Moore and Tannock have written a very well considered and comprehensive evaluation of the role of combination chemotherapy for bladder cancer. They critically examine the results of adjuvant treatment given at different times in relation to surgery and radiation. The review comes at a time when there is enough preliminary experience with these agents to be able to determine how they may be used in the future.

The next three chapters review three important aspects of prostate carcinoma that have attracted attention recently, namely diagnosis, expectant treatment, and hormonal manipulation. Serum prostatic specific antigen determination is relatively new, but there is already sufficient information for guidelines to be formulated to improve our ability to make the diagnosis and determine the prognosis of prostate cancer. Dr. Hudson's informative and well-written review of the recent and voluminous data concerning PSA should be a valuable help to any clinician who cares for these patients. The thoughtful and wide-ranging discussion of the available evidence supporting expectant management of carcinoma of the prostate by Drs. Thompson and Peretsman summarizes an important point of view in the management of this disease at a time when there is generally a very aggressive approach to therapy. As the authors point out, despite a number of helpful indicators, no one has as yet a biologic crystal ball that provides a sound basis to decide on the best treatment of this complex disease in a particular patient. Dr. Paulson has written an in-depth review of the present status of the theoretic considerations and clinical application of hormonal manipulation in patients with advanced prostate cancer. There is an excellent account of the biologic mechanisms involved with the use of the various agents. He concludes with a balanced account of the recent controversy regarding androgen deprivation as an adjunct to radical prostatectomy in patients in whom the cancer is clinically confined to the gland, but who have metastatic disease in the lymph nodes.

The concluding chapter on the use of local hyperthermia in the treatment of a number of diseases of the prostate by Drs. Knapp and Siegel reviews the published information on this new treatment together with an account of their own experience. It should help the urologist to reach his own conclusions as to the efficacy of this much-publicized form of therapy. I am sure that anyone who reads these essays will find them both instructive and interesting.

Bernard Lytton, M.B., F.R.C.S.

Contents

Hormonal Therapy in Prostate Cancer.
By David F. Paulson **225**

Hyperthermia for Prostate Disease.
By Peter M. Knapp and Yoram I. Siegel **263**

Genitourinary Manifestations of Sexual Abuse in Children*

David A. Bloom, M.D.

Professor of Surgery, Section of Urology, University of Michigan, Ann Arbor,
Michigan

Jill K. Sanvordenker, R.N.

Nurse Clinician, Department of Pediatrics, Section of Urology, University of
Michigan, Ann Arbor, Michigan

Child abuse in general and sexual abuse in particular have accompanied humankind throughout history, although propriety accounts for the scarce descriptions of these events. Homicide inquests in London between 1673 and 1782 included suffocation, strangling, clubbing, drowning, and rape among the causes of death of children.[1] Child abuse, and sexual abuse especially, remained outside the bounds of proper medical discourse, let alone public discussion. In 1946, Caffey's report of multiple long bone injury in infants as evidence for child abuse was an important milestone,[2] but Kempe's paper on the "Battered Child Syndrome" in 1962 put child abuse on the medical agenda and an explosion of interest followed[3] (Fig 1). A useful definition of child abuse is "an interaction or lack of interaction which results in non-accidental harm to the individual's physical and/or developmental states."[4] Most nations and localities have specific legal definitions. State laws in the United States require that health professionals report suspected child abuse.[5] Child abuse may involve 1.5% of all children and account for 5,000 deaths per year in the United States.[6] There is no good evidence that other countries have substantially better records, if one accounts for variabilities in reporting. What appears to be an increase in incidence probably is only an increase in reporting resulting from social attitudinal changes and legal mandates to report suspected abuse.[7]

Sexual abuse as one form of child abuse may comprise 10% of overall abuse, although any data are likely to underrepresent the true incidence.[8] A retrospective recall survey of 2,019 adults in England in 1984 suggested that some type of sexual abuse had occurred in 10%.[9] Similar surveys in the United States revealed incidences of 27% to 38% in women and 16% in men.[10] We define sexual abuse in children as exploitation of a child for gratification or profit and emphasize that abuse comprises a spectrum that

*Supported in part by the Babock Urological Endowment Fund.

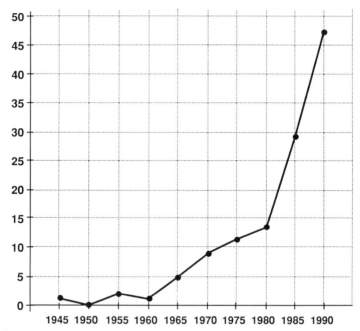

FIG 1.
Medical publications related to sexual abuse of children in *JAMA*, *Pediatrics*, and the *Am J Dis Child* (1945–1990).

includes exhibitionism, pornography, fondling, and penetration. For a given child, there may be progression over time from noninvasive to invasive forms of abuse. Sexual abuse usually is difficult to detect and, even after various forms of intercourse, there may be no physical evidence of abuse. Marshall and Davidson showed that 71% of abused children had no physical evidence of abuse and that 48% of children who had been sexually penetrated had no physical findings.[11] DeJong and Rose found that physical evidence was present in only 23% of cases that resulted in felony conviction for sexual abuse.[12] Furthermore, children typically are reticent to reveal either single incidents or prolonged courses of abuse. Nonetheless, sexual abuse does take a physical and emotional toll, and sometimes leaves a few clues behind. Most physicians have limited knowledge of sexual abuse and may fail to recognize even the more flagrant clues.[13, 14] The domain of the urologist provides a unique opportunity to unmask childhood sexual abuse by recognition of symptoms, signs, and vulnerable family and social situations. In some instances, the genitourinary manifestations of sexual abuse create a presenting complaint, but more commonly, genitourinary signs or symptoms are subtle, if they are present at all. In an active pediatric urologic practice, we suspect or uncover one new case of sexual abuse every 1 to 3 months, and these instances most likely are the tip of the iceberg. We reviewed recent sexual abuse evaluations at the University of Michigan, looking for genitourinary manifestations of abuse, and were able to draw some useful conclusions.

Clues to Abuse in the Medical History

Physicians need to be precise in eliciting historical data and recording physical findings. In many instances, poor documentation "does not matter," but in children who may have been abused, observational skills and clerical details matter greatly, especially in a court of law. We submit that any child with urinary infection or voiding dysfunction, much less a child suspected of being abused, needs to undergo a careful and well-detailed evaluation. Problems in infancy must be elicited. The age of toilet training and the degree of success should be established. For some children, this point in time marks the start of recognizable urinary trouble, but for others, incontinence and infections begin after a period of quiescence. One must establish when voiding dysfunction or infection began and ascertain if this coincided with a change in the child's life, schooling, or supervision. The problem should be defined quantitatively. For example, the number of infections per year, wet nights per week, wet days per week, and clothes changes per day, and the frequency of pad changes should be determined. A bowel history needs to be obtained, looking for fecal soiling, constipation, days between bowel movements, and so forth. The degree of soiling must be explained: Is it a "skid mark," a larger smudge, or a bulky fecal mass? Is this a daily event, or how often does it occur in a month? Has there been a recent change in voiding or bowel habits? The historical presence of sexually transmitted diseases, vaginal bleeding, or discharges must be ascertained and, in pubertal girls, menstrual activity, pregnancy, and the use of oral contraceptives must be queried. The examiner must evaluate the family and social situation carefully: With whom does the child live? Is the school situation and performance satisfactory? Have these changed? What about the peer group? What is the after school and weekend supervision? The interviewer should look for behavioral problems, depression, and experience with drugs or alcohol. Normal elimination parameters have not received much attention in the literature, although a few recent studies have helped fill this void.[15] The specific details of sexual activity take care and sensitivity to elicit. An experienced and skilled interviewer frequently can ascertain the type and sites of abuse through the use of anatomically correct dolls.[16]

Physical Examination in Sexual Abuse

Physical examination begins with a first impression of the family and child. Poor hygiene, unusual behavior, and hostile interactions in the examining room should be documented, as these sometimes are clues to neglect and abuse. It is important to create a supportive, nonthreatening atmosphere for the examination. Time invested in gaining rapport and trust is well spent. In both sexes, a complete physical examination is important. The oral cavity should not be overlooked. Poor dentition may be evidence of overall neglect. Oral injuries may result from penetration and oral swabs may show semen or be positive for alkaline phosphatase in addition to sexually transmitted bacteria. Another important dental aspect of sexual abuse is the presence of bite marks. Human bite marks are distinct from animal bites, and the dimensions are evidence of the age of the offender.[17]

Evaluation of acute abuse has its own particular mandates and such abuse is unlikely to present initially in the pediatric urology clinic. Most emergency room facilities are well equipped to deal with female rape, the most visible example of child sexual abuse.[18] Examination and treatment of the acutely abused male victim has specific requirements.[19] In the clinic it is more likely that chronic abuse will be discovered. Careful genital examination is important if it can be performed with the assent of the child. Some children are more comfortable being examined while on their parent's lap. Examination is largely worthless and psychologically damaging in a child who is not relaxed. In addition to the physical examination, clothing (including underwear) should be inspected for urine, stool, blood, other secretions, and general cleanliness. The presence of sperm or acid phosphatase on a child or her clothing can be detected by ultraviolet light (Wood's lamp). Dr. Koop and others advocate testing for sexually transmitted diseases, including syphilis and the human immunodeficiency virus.[20-22]

A single, careful examination by someone experienced in matters of child abuse is preferred to repetitive examinations by persons with ascending levels of expertise. When a child is reluctant, we avoid a forced examination. We also generally avoid digital or instrumental examination in an awake child. In occasional circumstances, examination under anesthesia is a good alternative. Furthermore, this allows assembly of all relevant personal and photographic documentation of any findings without humiliation of the patient. Ricci provides an excellent primer of photographic techniques.[23] Physical examination of a child additionally should include a description of the stage of sexual development. The staging systems described by Marshall and Tanner are useful for this purpose[24, 25] (Tables 1 and 2). Any time a child is anesthetized for a genitourinary procedure, a careful genital inspection should be performed and documented. Anatomic landmarks and important measurements can be ascertained at no emotional expense to the child and, occasionally, significant abnormalities will be detected unexpectedly. Condyloma accuminata may be evidence of abuse, although this also can be transmitted to infants innocently during routine care.

The anal examination is important in both sexes. Buttocks are parted gently while the patient is in a decubitus position and are inspected for skin trauma, discoloration, chronic inflammation, fissures, skin tags, hemorrhoids, anal wink, and perianal laxity. Supine and knee-chest inspection may reveal additional findings. Contusions, lacerations, and the presence

TABLE 1.
Pubertal Stages in Girls*

Breast stages
   1. Preadolescent, elevation of papilla
      only
   2. Breast bud
   3. Further enlargement of breast and
      areola; no separation of contours
   4. Areola and papilla form secondary
      mound
   5. Mature stage; recession of areola
Pubic hair stages
   1. No pubic hair
   2. Sparse growth of long, downy hair
   3. Darker, coarser, curled hair; sparsely
      spread
   4. Adult-type hair, but still less than in
      adults
   5. Adult type and quantity of hair

*Data from Marshall WA, Tanner JM: *Arch Dis
Child* 1969; 44:291–303.

of semen are obvious evidence of acute abuse. Foreign bodies and recto-sigmoid injury proximal to the anus also must be considered. Chronic abuse, however, may be very difficult to detect on physical examination and may leave no physical evidence. Only recently has much attention been paid to normal anogenital anatomy. McCann and colleagues evaluated the perianal area in a group of nonabused prepubertal children consisting of 161 girls and 106 boys (ranging from 2 months to 11 years in age). Typical physical findings consisted of venous engorgement after 2 minutes in the knee-chest position (52%), erythema (41%), increased pigmentation (30%), and wedge-shaped smooth areas anterior or posterior to the midline (26%). Anterior anal skin tags or folds were found in 11%, but only in the girls. They also observed that anal dilation occurred in 49% of the children and, in 62%, the anus opened and closed intermittently during examination.[26] Although it is not pathognomonic, as McCann et al. demonstrated, the phenomenon of reflex anal dilation has received great attention as a possible sign of abuse. This sign occurs a few moments after the buttocks have been spread gently with the patient in a decubitus posture. When the sign is present, the anus relaxes and one can visualize the anal canal and rectal mucosa as though a door had opened. Hobbs and Wynne observed that anal intercourse was a common form of abuse in fe-

TABLE 2.
Pubertal Stages in Boys*

Genital stages in boys
  1. Preadolescent
  2. Scrotum and testes have enlarged; change in scrotal texture
  3. Penile growth, length more than breadth; further testis and scrotum growth
  4. Further penile growth with glans development; scrotal darkening
  5. Adult size and shape of genitalia
Pubic hair stages in boys
  1. Preadolescent
  2. Sparse, long, slightly pigmented hair at base of penis
  3. Darker, coarser, more pigmented hair; spread over pubic symphysis
  4. Adult-type hair, but restricted distribution
  5. Adult type and quantity of hair; inverse triangle with spread to medial thigh
  6. Spread beyond the inverse triangle occurs in 80% of men by mid-20s

*Data from Marshall WA, Tanner JM: *Arch Dis Child* 1970; 45:13–23.

males under 5 years of age and in males, and investigated this sign in a group of abused children.[9] Flaherty and Weiss found that 44% of abused and neglected children had concurrent medical problems including anemia, otitis, sexually transmitted diseases, and lead poisoning. They concluded that all children evaluated for abuse or neglect should have complete medical evaluations.[27]

Girls

Whereas we generally inspect the female genitalia in a frog-leg posture, others prefer the knee-chest position. The transverse vaginal diameter varies with examination position and tends to enlarge with age, but generally remains 4 to 7 mm in the prepubertal girl.[28] Excessive labial traction may exaggerate the measurement. In the frog-leg examination position, the labia majora are pulled outward gently to allow the introitus to gape open. In the knee-chest position, the labia can be spread aside gently. McCann et al. compared findings from three genital examination techniques in prepubertal girls (supine with labial separation, supine with labial traction, and knee-chest) to colposcopic photographs, and found the supine separation method to be inferior. Nevertheless, they suggested using multiple methods during examination to take advantage of the strengths of each.[29] One must identify all landmarks and measure the horizontal vaginal diameter (Fig 2). A cotton applicator may be used to move hymenal folds gently in order to visualize the complete introital aperture; these folds may conceal scars. Nonetheless, Emans estimated that only 7% of sexually abused girls have abnormal measurements.[30] Berenson et al. found that the hymen in newborn girls is predominantly annular or fimbriated with variants consisting of ridges and bands. Appearances may change postnatally as the effect of maternal estrogen is withdrawn.[31] Berenson and coworkers also evaluated the introitus in 211 normal prepubertal girls and recognized that the normal variants include bumps and notches on the anterior half of the hymenal aperture; posterior (4- to 8-o'clock positions) notches or scarring were not observed in this group of normal children.[32] The horizontal hymenal diameter was variable, but ranged from 1 to 6.5 mm. The linea ves-

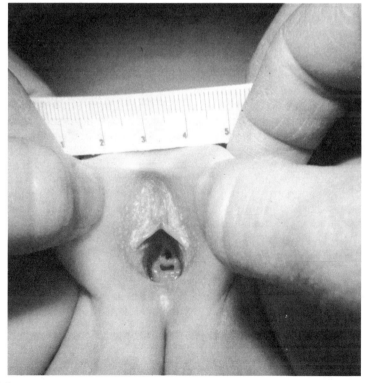

FIG 2.
Normal prepubertal introital anatomy.

tibularis, a white line or spot in the midline of the posterior vestibule, recently was identified as a normal neonatal introital landmark.[33] Examination should be performed with magnification, whether with optical loupes, the colposcope, or a cystoscope. McCann advocates the colposcopic photograph as a teaching, legal, and research tool.[29] Over time, introital injuries may resolve with little scar formation, although a skilled examiner usually can document those subtle changes that seem to persist.[34] Urethral prolapse can be confused with acute introital trauma (and vice versa). Prolapse, however, is a fairly distinct lesion with symmetrical circular eversion of urethral epithelium (we have no histologic justification to call this mucosa) and a central meatus. The lesion is asymptomatic and isolated, although it may occur after straining. Bloody spotting may be present.[35]

Boys

In boys, one specifically seeks evidence of penile or anal injury. This may be quite dramatic, or there may be no physical evidence at all of abuse. We have seen genital injuries from corporal punishment related to enuresis or encopresis. These have consisted of blunt trauma to the penis with corporal cavernosal rupture or cigarette burns to the glans penis (Fig 3). More overt sexual abuse may take the form of genital sucking and biting, and this may result in gross penoscrotal cellulitis (Fig 4). Acute forced anal penetration usually causes visible injury, but repetitive anal injury may be virtually undetectable. The two classic penile traumas of childhood are injuries from falling toilet seats or zipper entanglements, but these generally are easy to identify (Fig 5). Another penile trauma is a tourniquet injury. These usually are self-applied and consist of a hairband or string. It is rare that a complete confession will be obtained, although we have seen these applied to stop bed-wetting in several boys and in one boy who thought he could circumcise himself.

Sexual abuse of boys is more likely to occur in public places and is more likely to cause physical injury than is abuse of girls. Ellerstein's review was one of the important early studies of male sexual abuse.[36] Spencer and Dunklee evaluated 140 abused boys and found no physical evidence in 32%, perianal erythema and abrasion in 27%, perianal scars and skin tags in 11%, and rectal laceration or fissure in 11%. Bruising of the penis or perineum was observed in 7% and semen was found, by smear of fluorescence, in 5%.[37]

Genitourinary Clues to Sexual Abuse: A Clinical Review

In search of genitourinary clues, we surveyed the records of 150 children who had undergone evaluation by our child protection team for sexual abuse.[38] There were 30 boys (age range 1 to 14 years, mean 6.8 years) and 120 girls (age range 7 months to 17 years, mean 6.1 years). Because proof of sexual abuse is a legal matter, it was impossible to know if abuse

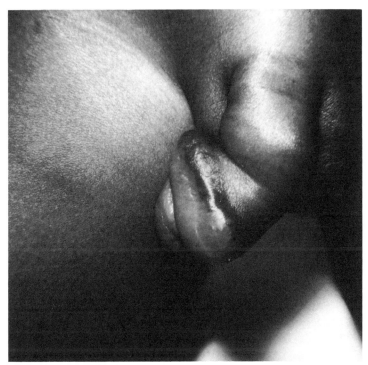

FIG 3.
Six-year-old boy with injury to corpora cavernosa secondary to beating with a stick by father for encopresis.

actually had occurred in all of these children. Legal action was initiated in 46% of the cases. Pertinent genitourinary historical findings are listed in Table 3. Significant genitourinary historical findings include enuresis, encopresis, urinary retention, voiding complaints, vaginal discharge, urinary tract infections, hematuria, sexually explicit play, and a prior history of abuse. Some of these are common complaints in pediatric urologic practice. Nonetheless, the incidences and patterns may be atypical enough in some children to raise a question of possible abuse. Klevan and DeJong ascertained that 20% of victims of sexual abuse had genitourinary complaints such as vaginal pain, urinary frequency, dysuria, and enuresis. Urinary tract infection, however, was uncommon and occurred in only 2 of 85 symptomatic victims.[39] Genital bleeding in girls may be evidence of penetrative injury or its residue, sexually transmitted pelvic inflammatory disease.[40-42] Among boys subjected to sexual abuse, our series of patients indicated a surprisingly high (23.3%) incidence of encopresis, compared to an incidence of only 1.6% in girls. Others also have made this association.[43]

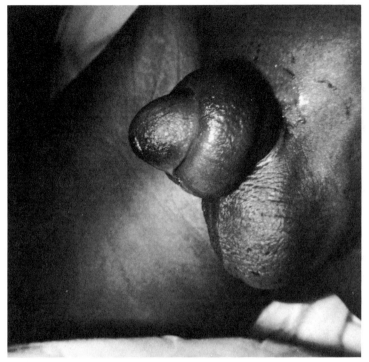

FIG 4.
Two-year-old boy with penile cellulitis secondary to genital bites from uncle.

Physical findings are listed in Table 4. Abnormal introital dimensions in prepubertal, sexually inactive females are unusual and dictate further evaluation (Fig 6). Other physical findings include contusions, lacerations, chronic inflammation, hymenal scars, perianal laxity, and vaginal discharge. Sperm in the urine or introital washing is obvious proof of sexual activity. Perhaps the most important thing to remember regarding physical findings of sexual abuse is that a large percentage of girls who are likely subjects of abuse (31%, in our experience) have absolutely no findings indicative of abuse, in spite of very skilled examination.

When To Suspect Sexual Abuse

Although sexual abuse of children extends through all socioeconomic strata, some families are at particular risk. Low income alone does not seem to increase risk, but families with social isolation, adolescent parents, parents who were abused or maltreated during their childhoods, parental violence, and parental mental illness increase the risk for sexual abuse of children. Additional factors such as sexual abuse of a sibling or other family

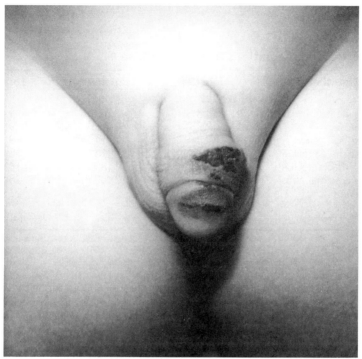

FIG 5.
Seven-year-old boy with penile ecchymosis from toilet seat injury.

member, overcrowding, and alcohol/drug misuse increase the chance for sexual abuse. Prematurity, neonatal hospitalization, colic, mental retardation, and congenital anomalies in a child also increase the risk of sexual abuse.[6] Suboptimal day care situations render many children vulnerable to abuse.

Many symptoms related to sexual abuse are common complaints in urologic practice and by themselves are not proof of abuse. In some children, a constellation of these symptoms, amidst other clues, suggests abuse. We are concerned with unusual patterns or a late onset of enuresis, particularly in a vulnerable child and family. Recurrent urinary infections or symptoms of infection without positive urine findings also occur in sexually abused children. Unusual patterns of voiding dysfunction may provide additional clues. Encopresis is more likely a concomitant of sexual abuse in boys than in girls. Goodwin taught that urinary retention in girls can be a manifestation of sexual abuse,[44] and we occasionally find such a situation. Be suspicious of an atypical pattern of symptoms in a vulnerable family and child.

Most instances of sexual abuse in children leave no physical signs. It is critical, therefore, to realize that *a normal physical examination does not rule out sexual abuse.* Genital injury, vaginal lacerations or contusions,

TABLE 3.
Historical Manifestations of Sexual Abuse

Manifestation	Male (%)	Female (%)	Total (%)
Wet—day	—	5 (4.2)	5 (3.3)
Wet—night	1 (3.3)	8 (6.6)	9 (6.0)
Encopresis	7 (23.3)	2 (1.6)	9 (6.0)
Voiding symptoms	1 (3.3)	17 (14.2)	18 (12)
Vaginal discharge	—	18 (15)	18 (12)
Urinary tract infection	—	10 (8.3)	18 (12)
Previous sexual abuse	2 (6.6)	13 (10.8)	15 (10)
Hematuria	—	2 (1.6)	2 (1.3)

vaginal discharge or bleeding, and rectal injury are evidence of acute injury. Spotty vaginal bleeding in the newborn usually is a transient and benign phenomenon. Vaginal bleeding in prepubertal children may be due to sexual abuse, although it also can be caused by trauma, foreign body, coagulopathy, malignancy, or precocius puberty. These same causes may be present after puberty. Dysfunctional uterine bleeding, that is, any deviation in the normal menstrual cycle, often can be due to an immature hypothalamic-pituitary-ovarian axis.[45, 46] "Urethral prolapse" actually may be a contused meatus. Torn, stained, or bloody underclothing should be noted and evidence of semen on clothes or patients can be found by means of a Wood's lamp. Examination of the urine is important and the presence of semen in the urine or introital washings of a young girl is evidence of abuse. Chronic changes are more subtle and may include widened transverse vaginal diameter and other hymenal alterations. Genital or perianal scars, skin tags, and hyperpigmentation raise the suspicion of abuse. Condyloma acuminatum and other sexually transmitted diseases in a young

TABLE 4.
Physical Manifestations of Sexual Abuse

Manifestation	Male (%)	Female (%)	Total (%)
Trauma	6 (20)	17 (14)	23 (15)
Widened horizontal diameter	—	53 (44)	—
Condyloma	1 (3.3)	6 (5)	7 (4.6)
Normal examination	11 (37)	35 (29)	46 (31)

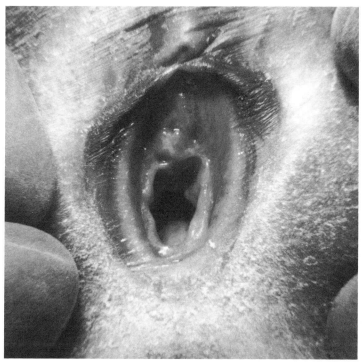

FIG 6.
Seven-year-old girl with recurrent sexual abuse by mother's boyfriend.

child also may be direct evidence of abuse, although we think condyloma in some instances can be transmitted innocently during daily care activities. Other signs of general abuse or neglect should increase suspicion.

Mistaken and False Accusations

Sexual abuse of children is a devastating charge and one that must be levied with care and deliberation. Some lesions, including accidental perineal trauma, allergic vulvar reactions, urethral prolapse, lichen sclerosus et atrophicus, varicella, congenital discolorations, bacterial skin infections, straddle injury, female epispadias, and other dermatologic conditions can masquerade as sexual abuse.[47-50] Persistent enuresis can produce chronic skin inflammation, hyperpigmentation, and genital ulceration. Chadwick suggested that 8% of allegations made by children are fictitious, but he believes these instances are discerned easily by careful interview.[51] Some false accusations are engendered by marital disharmony, divorce, and custody disputes. A notorious epidemic of false accusations occurred in Cleveland, England, based on the supposition that reflex anal dilation was proof of prior anal penetration. Subsequent review determined that the initial evaluations were flawed, although sexual abuse was not disproven amidst the public clamor.[52] Green found that false allegations comprise only 6% of overall reports of child sexual abuse, although the incidence is 55% among children evaluated for custody/visitation disputes. He identified specific characteristics by which to distinguish true abuse from incest hoax.[53]

Evaluation and Management of Sexual Abuse in Children

Once child abuse is suspected, evaluation should proceed in concert with a child protection team. State laws mandate that suspected abuse be reported. The child should be examined and interviewed carefully. Interview techniques vary with age and are performed best by a child abuse specialist. Anatomically correct dolls permit a child to describe what happened. Physical examination must be careful and sensitive to the patient's emotional state; if indicated, we do not hesitate to perform examinations under anesthesia, during which acute injuries can be treated. Specimens and cultures must be obtained before a patient is prepped. Chronic changes secondary to sexual abuse may be subtle. Careful documentation is an absolute requirement, because careless and inaccurate descriptions will jeopardize subsequent legal proceedings. The fundamental requirement in evaluation for sexual abuse is protection of the child. When suspicion of abuse is low and injury is not acute, we proceed with careful outpatient evaluation coordinated with the child protection team. If suspicion is strong and the likelihood of further abuse is great, we do not hesitate to hospitalize the child for further evaluation, even though third-party payors may balk at reimbursement. The American Academy of Pediatrics recommends hospitalization to rule out suspected abuse and states that compensation is indicated even when there is no physical diagnosis.[54] Sibling risk and victimization of mothers of abused children also must be assessed; childhood sexual abuse usually is a family disorder.[55]

The very nature of the specialty places urologists in a unique position either to recognize or to overlook a substantial number of children who are sexually abused. Urologists, and pediatric urologists in particular, must become knowledgeable in this area and take their place on the child protection team. In addition, the pediatric specialist should become an advocate for the recognition of child sexual abuse. The American Academy of Pediatrics provides an excellent brochure discussing child sexual abuse that can be distributed to families or made available in waiting rooms.[56] The most recent guidelines of the American Academy of Pediatrics should be mandatory reading for those who evaluate and treat children, regardless of their subspecialty.[57]

References

1. Forbes TR: Inquests into London and Middlesex homicides, 1673–1783. *Yale J Biol Med* 1977; 50:207–220.

2. Caffey J: Multiple fractures in the long bones of infants suffering from chronic subdural hematoma. *AJR Am J Roentgenol* 1946; 56:163–173.
3. Kempe CH, Silverman FN, Steele BF, et al: The battered child syndrome. *JAMA* 1962; 181:17–24.
4. Helfer RE: The developmental basis of child abuse and neglect: An epidemiological approach, in Helfer RE, Kempe RS (eds): *The Battered Child*, 4th ed. Chicago, University of Chicago Press, 1988, p 61.
5. Gavs SM: Reporting child abuse. *Mich Med* 1988; 87:191.
6. AMA Council on Scientific Affairs: AMA diagnostic and treatment guidelines concerning child abuse and neglect. *JAMA* 1985; 254:796–800.
7. Feldman W, Feldman E, Goodman JT, et al: Increased prevalence of sexual abuse due to increased reporting. *Pediatrics* 1991; 88:29–33.
8. Helfer RE: The epidemiology of child abuse and neglect. *Pediatr Ann* 1984; 13:745–751.
9. Hobbs CJ, Wynne JM: Buggery in childhood—a common syndrome of child abuse. *Lancet* 1986; 2:792–796.
10. Finkelhor D: The sexual abuse of children: Current research reviewed. *Psychiatr Ann* 1987; 17:233–241.
11. Marshall WN, Pul T, Davidson C: New child abuse spectrum in an era of increased awareness. *Am J Dis Child* 1988; 142:664–667.
12. DeJong AR, Rose M: Frequency and significance of physical evidence in legally proven cases of child sexual abuse. *Pediatrics* 1989; 84:1022–1026.
13. Ladson S, Johnson CF, Doty RE: Do physicians recognize sexual abuse? *Am J Dis Child* 1987; 141:412–415.
14. Britton HL: Do physicians recognize sexual abuse (editorial)? *Am J Dis Child* 1987; 141:402–403.
15. Bloom DA, Seeley WW, Ritchey ML, et al: Toilet habits and continence in children: An opportunity sampling in search of normal parameters. *J Urol* 1993, in press.
16. Goldberg CC, Yates A: The use of anatomically correct dolls in the evaluation of sexually abused children. *Am J Dis Child* 1990; 144:1334–1336.
17. Sterne GG, Chadwick DL, Krugman RD, et al: Oral and dental aspects of child abuse and neglect. *Pediatrics* 1986; 78:537–539.
18. Emans SJ: Evaluation of the sexually abused child and adolescent. *Adolesc Pediatr Gynecol* 1988; 1:157–163.
19. Schiff AF: Examination and treatment of the male rape victim. *South Med J* 1980; 73:1498–1502.
20. Koop CE: *The Surgeon General's Letter on Child Sexual Abuse.* Washington DC, U.S. Department of Health and Human Services, 1988, Publication No HRS-M-CH-88-13.
21. Bays J, Chadwick D: The serologic test for syphilis in sexually abused children and adolescents. *Adolesc Pediatr Gynecol* 1991; 4:148–151.
22. Gutman LT, St Claire KK, Weedy C, et al: Human immunodeficiency virus transmission by child sexual abuse. *Am J Dis Child* 1991; 145:137–141.
23. Ricci LR: Photographing the physically abused child. Principles and practice. *Am J Dis Child* 1991; 145:275–281.
24. Marshall WA, Tanner JM: Variations in the pattern of pubertal changes in boys. *Arch Dis Child* 1970; 45:13–23.
25. Marshall WA, Tanner JM: Variations in the pattern of pubertal changes in girls. *Arch Dis Child* 1969; 44:291–303.
26. McCann J, Voris J, Simon M, et al: Perianal findings in prepubertal children selected for nonabuse: A descriptive study. *Child Abuse Negl* 1989; 13:179–193.

27. Flaherty EG, Weiss H: Medical evaluation of abused and neglected children. *Am J Dis Child* 1990; 144:330–334.
28. Goff CW, Burke KR, Rickenback C, et al: Vaginal opening measurement in prepubertal girls. *Am J Dis Child* 1989; 143:1366–1368.
29. McCann J, Voris J, Simon M, et al: Comparison of genital examination techniques in prepubertal girls. *Pediatrics* 1990; 85:182–187.
30. Emans SJ, Woods ER, Flagg NT, et al: Genital findings in sexually abused, symptomatic and asymptomatic, girls. *Pediatrics* 1987; 79:778–785.
31. Berenson A, Heger A, Andrews S: Appearance of the hymen in newborns. *Pediatrics* 1991; 87:458–465.
32. Berenson AB, Heger AH, Hayes JM, et al: Appearance of the hymen in prepubertal girls. *Pediatrics* 1992; 89:387–394.
33. Kellogg ND, Parra JM: Linea vestibularis: A previously undescribed normal genital structure in female neonates. *Pediatrics* 1991; 87:926–929.
34. McCann J, Voris J, Simon M: Genital injuries resulting from sexual abuse: A longitudinal study. *Pediatrics* 1992; 89:307–317.
35. Johnson CF: Prolapse of the urethra: Confusion of clinical and anatomic characteristics with sexual abuse. *Pediatrics* 1991; 87:722–725.
36. Ellerstein NJ, Canavan W: Sexual abuse of boys. *Am J Dis Child* 1980; 134:255–257.
37. Spencer MJ, Dunklee P: Sexual abuse of boys. *Pediatrics* 1986; 78:133–138.
38. Bloom DA, Knectel J: Urological manifestations of sexual abuse. Presented at American Urological Association Annual Meeting, Boston, June 1988.
39. Klevan JL, DeJong AR: Urinary tract symptoms and urinary tract infection following sexual abuse. *Am J Dis Child* 1990; 144:242–244.
40. Cowan BD, Morrison JC: Management of abnormal genital bleeding in girls and women. *N Engl J Med* 1991; 324:1710–1715.
41. Cates W Jr, Peterson HB: Abnormal genital bleeding in girls and women. *N Engl J Med* 1991; 325:1655.
42. Frothingham TE, Herman-Giddens ME: Abnormal genital bleeding in girls and women. *N Engl J Med* 1991; 325:1665.
43. Brayden R, Altemeier WA: Encopresis and child sexual abuse. *JAMA* 1989; 262:2446.
44. Goodwin WE: Personal communication (residency aphorisms). UCLA Department of Urology, 1978.
45. Badawy SZA, Refaie A: Dysfunctional uterine bleeding in adolescent and teenage girls. *Adolesc Pediatr Gynecol* 1990; 3:65–69.
46. Jaffe SB, Jewelewicz R: Dysfunctional uterine bleeding in the pediatric and adolescent patient. *Adolesc Pediatr Gynecol* 1991; 4:62–69.
47. Anders KH, Smith JG Jr: Dermatologic conditions misdiagnosed as evidence of child abuse. *JAMA* 1989; 261:3547.
48. Koblenzer PJ: Dermatologic conditions misdiagnosed as evidence of child abuse. *JAMA* 1989; 261:3547–3548.
49. Herman-Giddens ME, Berson NL: Dermatologic conditions misdiagnosed as evidence of child abuse. *JAMA* 1989; 261:3548.
50. Bays J, Jenny C: Genital and anal conditions confused with child sexual abuse trauma. *Am J Dis Child* 1990; 144:1319–1322.
51. Chadwick DL: Book review: *Accusations of Child Sexual Abuse*, Wakefield and Underwager. *JAMA* 1989; 261:3035.
52. Fulginiti VA, Krugman RD: Cleveland, England: Child abuse in the public eye. *Am J Dis Child* 1989; 143:651–652.

53. Green AH: True and false allegations of sexual abuse in child custody disputes. *J Am Acad Child Adolesc Psychiatry* 1986; 25:449–456.
54. Evans HE, American Academy of Pediatrics Committee on Hospital Care: Medical necessity for the hospitalization of the abused and neglected child. *Pediatrics* 1987; 79:300.
55. McKibben L, De Vos E, Newberger EH: Victimization of abused children: A controlled study. *Pediatrics* 1989; 84:531–535.
56. *Child Sexual Abuse.* Elk Grove Village, Ill. American Academy of Pediatrics Department of Publications,
57. Krugman RD, Bays JA, Chadwick DL, et al: American Academy of Pediatrics Committee on Abuse and Neglect. Guidelines for the evaluation of sexual abuse of children. *Pediatrics* 1991; 87:254–260.

Neurotransmitters and the Rationale for Medical Treatment in Impotence

Andrew L. Freedman, M.D.

Resident, Department of Surgery/Urology, University of California, Los Angeles
School of Medicine, Los Angeles, California

Louis J. Ignarro, Ph.D.

Professor of Pharmacology, University of California, Los Angeles School of
Medicine, Los Angeles, California

Jacob Rajfer, M.D.

Professor of Surgery/Urology, University of California, Los Angeles School of
Medicine, Los Angeles, California; Chief, Division of Urology, Harbor-University
of California, Los Angeles Medical Center, Torrance, California

The preceding decade has seen an explosion in our understanding of and
ability to treat impotence. This has come on the heels of advances in research that have enabled us to understand the basic physiology of erection
and, in doing so, have allowed us to begin designing medical therapies that
address the symptoms and causes of impotence. As a result, the future
holds the promise of not only rational forms of therapy, but very possibly
the prophylactic prevention of the dysfunction itself.

History

Despite recent advances in neurophysiology, there still remain large gaps
in our understanding of how a normal erection occurs. Many of these gaps
and controversies are a continuation of the debates that began more than
100 years ago with the early investigations in erectile physiology. In 1863,
Eckhard was the first to show that galvanic stimulation of the pelvic nerves,
the so-called "nervi erigentes" or nerves of erection, could produce erections, thereby launching the search for the actual electrical events that induce an erection. Lue and his colleagues in the early 1980s described the
three physiologic phases of an erection and highlighted the importance of
smooth muscle relaxation in this phenomenon.[118-127] Very soon thereafter, Virag and associates[210-214] showed that papaverine, a smooth muscle
relaxant, could produce an erection when injected directly into the caver-

nosal smooth muscle. In 1981, Benson and coworkers,[23] and in the mid-1980s, Saenz de Tejada and colleagues[174-180] focused our attention on the nonadrenergic, noncholinergic nerves as the actual nerves that are involved in cavernosal smooth muscle relaxation. Most recently, nitric oxide has been shown to be the chemical mediator of cavernosal smooth muscle relaxation. Yet, these remarkable findings only accent the hundreds of careful observations and experiments that have laid the fertile foundation of what we now know and what remains to be discovered regarding this important physiologic event.

Anatomy

The physiology of a normal erection is a complex multisystem event involving the coordinated interaction of the endocrine, psychologic, neurologic, and vascular systems. Alteration in any one of these systems can have profound deleterious effects upon the whole reaction. The unique anatomic arrangement of the penis allows for its ability to expand temporarily in both girth and length when ready to perform its physiologic function.

Neuroanatomy

The neurologic regulation of penile erection remains an elusive topic of research due to its extreme complexity, species variation, and, until recently, lack of appropriate animal models. Despite these limitations, significant progress in understanding the intricate neurologic pathways has been made. The basic organization in vertebrates consists of spinal copulatory reflexes that are inhibited tonically by central pathways.[20, 39, 79, 173] Release of these inhibitory conditions, elicited by appropriate stimuli, results in erection. To describe these pathways best, it is necessary to divide the system into those processes originating in the supraspinal central nervous system and those initiated in the spinal cord.

Central Neural Processes

In a general sense, erotic stimuli can be received through somatosensory, olfactory, auditory, or visual receptors, or they can be generated internally via psychologic processes. These sensations then are carried by specific pathways to the hypothalamus, where they are integrated. Projections from the hypothalamus travel through spinal tracts to autonomic nuclei in the cord, where they regulate the spinal copulatory reflexes. In turn, afferent information is carried from the periphery through the intermediolateral cell column of the sacral cord back to the caudal thalamus (lamina V and VII). Specifically, the integrating function is thought to occur in the medial preoptic-anterior hypothalamic area.[83, 130] Stimulation of this area results in penile erection. Projections from the medial preoptic-anterior hypothalamic area travel via the medial forebrain bundle to the midbrain tegmental area and then through the ventrolateral pons and medulla to the lumbosacral autonomic centers through the dorsolateral funiculus.[194] Central inputs into the hypothalamus include somatosensory and visual stimuli from thalamic nuclei II and olfactory information from the rhinencephalon, and the limbic system provides memory and emotional elements.

Descending central inhibition of the spinal reflexes is thought to be mediated by the paragigantocellular reticular nucleus in the ventral medulla.[131]

The role of specific neurotransmitters in the central system is complex and uncertain. Important centrally acting inhibitors include serotonin,[24, 57] norepinephrine, and gamma-aminobutyrate.[25] Neurotransmitters that act centrally to stimulate erections include dopamine, acetylcholine, and oxytocin.[15,134] Dopamine appears to act most importantly at the paraventricular nucleus of the hypothalamus, causing the release of oxytocin, which has effects both in the hypothalamus and distally. Other central neurotransmitters include adrenocorticotropic hormone, corticotropin-releasing factor, and opioids.

Once stimulated, the major effect of the central system is to release and stimulate the spinal reflexes that produce the erection and other copulatory behavior.

Spinal Cord

Within the spinal cord, there are two main areas that mediate the erectile reflex: the thoracolumbar sympathetics and the sacral parasympathetics. The sympathetic nucleus is located at the T10 to L2 level in the nucleus intermediolateralis thoracolumbalis pars principalis and the nucleus intercalatus spinalis.[126, 127] The sympathetic outflow is carried by the hypogastric nerve and branches from the sacral sympathetic chain and autonomic inferior mesenteric plexus.[217] The sympathetic fibers join the parasympathetic nerves that arise from the nucleus intermediolateralis sacralis pars principalis at the level of S2 to S4. The parasympathetic fibers are carried by the pelvic splanchnic nerves that emerge from the S2 to S4 foramina to join the hypogastric nerve and form the pelvic plexus. The pelvic plexus forms a broad rectangular plate that is located lateral to the rectum. In addition to the nerves for erection, the pelvic plexus contains the autonomic fibers for the pelvic organs and vessels, including the bladder, prostate, urethra, seminal vesicles, and rectum. Somatic fibers for the pelvic musculature also are carried within the pelvic plexus. The fibers that eventually innervate the corpora cavernosa form a bundle from the most caudal fibers of the pelvic plexus.

Distal Nerves

The distal innervation of the penis arrives from two discrete sources. The cavernosal nerves formed from the most caudal pelvic plexus fibers travel as a bundle within the endopelvic fascia and course posterolateral to the prostate within the groove between the prostate and rectum at the 5- and 7-o'clock position.[112] Throughout its course, fibers are given off that innervate the prostate proper. At the level of the membranous urethra, the bundle moves anteriorly and travels through the urogenital diaphragm at the 3- and 9-o'clock position. The nerve passes external to the striated sphincter in close apposition to the membranous urethra. Once through the sphincter, the nerves travel further anterior, lying over the proximal bulbous urethra at the 1- and 11-o'clock position. At the hilum of the penis, some branches are distributed to the corpus spongiosum, but the bulk of the nerves enter the corpora cavernosa along with the deep cavernosal arteries. Once inside the corpora, the nerves divide into terminal branches that innervate the helicine arteries and the corporal smooth muscle.

The second system begins as the pudendal nerve that is formed by the anterior divisions of S2 to S4 and is part of the lumbosacral plexus, but distinct from the pelvic plexus formed from the hypogastric nerve and the other sacral autonomic fibers. The pudendal nerve exits the pelvis through the greater sciatic foramina and reenters through the lesser sciatic foramina. Passing through Alcock's canal, the pudendal nerve divides into three branches: the inferior hemorrhoidal, the perineal, and the dorsal nerve of the penis. The dorsal nerve, the first branch, then travels forward, penetrating the transversus perinei muscle to reach the dorsum of the penis. It continues along the dorsolateral surface of the penis, giving off sensory branches to the skin before finally terminating in the glans.[93] Although the dorsal nerve primarily serves to carry penile sensation, interconnections between it and the cavernous nerves often can be found, though the function of these connections is unknown.[33]

Vascular Anatomy

Arterial

The importance of arterial blood flow to the penis in erection long has been appreciated and the anatomy of the extrapenile arterial system well-described. In brief, the main source of arterial flow originates from the internal pudendal artery. This artery typically arises from the last division of the internal iliac artery. The internal pudendal artery then travels through Alcock's canal adjacent to the pudendal nerve, where it gives off the perineal artery and continues as the common penile artery until reaching the urethral bulb, where it divides into its three terminal branches. The branches include the bulbourethral artery, the dorsal artery, and the deep or cavernosal artery. The bulbar portion of the bulbourethral artery quickly enters the bulb of the penis, where it is responsible for blood supply to the proximal urethra and Cowper's gland, whereas the urethral portion, also called the spongiosal artery, runs within the corpus spongiosum lateral to the urethra, where it is responsible for the arterial supply to the urethra, corpus spongiosum, and glans. The dorsal artery runs the length of the penis, lying between the medially placed deep dorsal vein and the lateral dorsal nerve. Distally, the artery travels laterally along with the branches of the dorsal nerve to enter the glans at the dorsal lateral aspect. Along its path, the dorsal artery gives off circumflex branches that travel laterally. The primary function of the dorsal artery is to supply blood to the glans, though the circumflex branches may supply some flow to the cavernous bodies. The dorsal arteries and the spongiosal (urethral) arteries anastomose within the glans. There are no extracavernous connections between the dorsal penile and the cavernosal artery systems. The cavernosal artery enters the penis in the hilum at a point adjacent to the joining of the two cavernous bodies and then travels distally within the center of the cavernous body. Throughout its course, it gives off multiple terminal branches better known as the helicine arteries. The helicine arteries empty into the sinusoidal spaces and are responsible for the blood supply to the cavernosal bodies and for the majority of the arterial contribution to penile erection. Anatomic variations of this arterial tree are relatively common, the most common being the presence of an accessory internal pudendal artery. This accessory artery may be present in addition to the paired internal pudendal arteries, or it may replace one of these. It may provide additional blood supply or it may serve as the origin for one or more of the ipsilateral terminal cavernosal arteries. The accessory artery most commonly arises from the ipsilateral obturator artery, though it also may arise from the superior or inferior vesical artery. In a detailed anatomic review, an accessory pudendal artery was seen in seven of ten cadavers, occurring unilaterally in six and bilaterally in one.[33] Other anomalies include aberrant origins of the bulbar or urethral artery and extracavernosal branches of the cavernosal artery entering the contralateral corpora cavernosa.

Venous

The anatomy of the venous system has become increasingly important in understanding the physiology of erection as well as in the treatment of venogenic impotence. The venous system can be divided into three distinct systems, though intercommunications certainly do occur. The superficial system consists of multiple small veins lying primarily along the dorsum of the penis between Colles' and Buck's fascia. The superficial veins are responsible for the venous drainage of the skin, subcutaneous tissue, and prepuce. The veins coalesce at the root of the penis to form a single superficial dorsal vein, which subsequently drains into one of the saphenous veins. Occasionally, the veins form two superficial dorsal veins, each of which drains into its ipsilateral saphenous vein. The intermediate system consists of the deep dorsal vein and the circumflex veins. The deep dorsal vein is formed from the union of numerous small veins that drain the glans and merge to form a retrocoronal plexus that drains into the deep dorsal vein. The deep dorsal vein then runs within a groove between the two corpora cavernosa between Buck's fascia and the tunica albuginea. It typically runs as a single vein, though there often can be paired veins or an additional vein arising from the proximal penis. The deep dorsal vein enters the pelvis between the suspensory ligament to drain into the periprostatic plexus. The plexus subsequently drains into the lateral perivesical plexus, which terminates into the internal iliac vein. The circumflex veins arise from the corpus spongiosum and travel laterally around the corpus cavernosum perpendicular to the long axis of the penis. They communicate with longitudinally running veins, the lateral veins of the penis, and their partners, both ipsilateral and contralateral, to form common channels that empty into the deep dorsal vein at an oblique angle. Prior to their drainage in the deep dorsal vein, the circumflex veins receive flow from emissary veins that arise as venules from the sinusoidal space and travel to form a subalbugineous plexus.[62] They then traverse the tunica in an oblique manner as emissary veins to enter the circumflex veins. The subalbugineous plexus is crucial to producing venous outflow resistance during erection, as will be discussed later. The circumflex veins are present only at the distal two thirds of the penis, with the emissary veins of the proximal one third draining into the deep system. The deep dorsal vein also is noted to have valves, as do the pelvic veins.[58] These valves often are found to be incompetent in patients with impotence, though their role in erection remains unknown.[4, 5, 59, 60] The deep venous system beings with the emissary veins of the proximal penis, which coalesce to form 2 to 5 cavernous veins arising from the hilum of the penis. These veins further merge to form one or two large, medially placed cavernous veins, which then run laterally to drain into the internal pudendal vein. Additionally, several small veins arise from the dorsolateral aspect of the crura and merge to form the crural veins, which drain into the internal pudendal vein. The internal pudendal vein in turn empties into the internal iliac vein.

Sinusoidal System

The sinusoids consist of spaces that are formed by trabeculae made up of bundles of smooth muscle and connective tissue. The connective tissues form a fibrous skeleton with connection to the undersurface of the tunica albuginea, and the perivascular and perineural sheaths.[72] The smooth muscle bundles insert into the fibrous skeleton in at least two places.[73] The sinusoidal spaces are lined by a layer of endothelium similar to that seen in the peripheral vasculature. Each space is in communication with multiple other spaces, effectively creating a single continuous channel.[62] The spaces are fed by the helicine arteries and drain into small venules that drain into the subalbugineous plexus. The sinusoidal dilatation during erection is limited by only the inelastic tunica albuginea.

Physiology of Normal Erection

Normal erection in its simplest terms requires three events: (1) increased arterial inflow, (2) decreased venous outflow, and (3) corporal smooth muscle relaxation. The relative importance of each event long has been debated, though it is a somewhat moot point, as all three are necessary to achieve an adequate erection and defects in any one can prevent the development of a normal erection. Nonetheless, recent evidence is developing to support the concept that active relaxation of the corporal smooth muscle may be the critical event in developing a normal erection. How this mechanism is impaired in various forms of impotence remains to be explained.

Hemodynamics

The hemodynamic mechanisms of normal erection have been controversial. In the 19th century, it was felt that primary venous occlusion was responsible.[29, 216] Later investigators credited increased arterial inflow[46, 50, 148] for maintaining erections. Some believed that these hemodynamic effects were mediated by intravascular ridges or polsters either in the arteries,[215] veins,[46] or both[40] that regulated blood flow through a form of arteriovenous shunting that controlled erection. Since then, the existence of polsters has been questioned seriously, as the typical histologic findings have been shown more likely to represent either vessel branch points, intimal cushions, atherosclerotic changes, or response to stress.[23, 150] Further understanding of smooth muscle physiology has made the concept of polsters virtually obsolete.

The pioneering work of Lue in the monkey,[125] dog,[126, 127, 209] and human[126a] has revolutionized our understanding of the hemodynamics of normal erection. The rate of arterial inflow is regulated by the degree of constriction of the penile arterial tree and the sinusoidal smooth muscle. In the flaccid state, the sinusoidal spaces are contracted by the smooth muscle trabecula, creating high resistance to the arterial flow. Additionally, the arterial tree is in a normally constricted state. The venous channels are open, as the contracted sinusoids are not compressing the subalbugineous plexus against the tunica albuginea. At the initiation of erection, the sinusoidal smooth muscle relaxes by an active process. This serves three purposes: (1) by reducing resistance of the artery, it greatly increases arterial inflow; (2) by expanding the sinusoidal capacity to store blood, it allows penile engorgement[180]; and (3) by expanding, it shuts off venous outflow by compressing the venous plexuses against the inelastic tunica albuginea.[62, 94, 118, 123] In essence, it initiates the three mechanisms deemed necessary to develop an erection. During detumescence, the reverse occurs, with a contraction of the sinusoidal smooth muscle causing increased arterial resistance and decreased venous plexus pressure allowing egress of the trapped sinusoidal blood.

Neurophysiology

Of all the aspects of the physiology of erection, its neurologic regulation remains the most controversial and difficult to elucidate. In particular, the emerging importance of active smooth muscle relaxation is challenging the traditional models of neural regulation. Increasingly, there is awareness that there exists a third system beyond the traditional cholinergic (parasympathetic) and adrenergic (sympathetic) autonomic systems. The neurotransmitters involved in this nonadrenergic, noncholinergic system are not well-known and are thought to be primarily peptides. Additionally, the role of secondary messengers arising from the nerves, vessels, or smooth muscle is coming to the fore, and these may play significant, yet unknown roles. Research has extended beyond in vivo observation, using various animal models,* organ baths,[177] cell culture,[65, 107] and even the latest techniques of molecular biology in an effort to elucidate the final pathways of erection.

In a broad sense, the various neural control systems work together to produce the hemodynamic changes, increased arterial inflow, and venous constriction through smooth muscle relaxation, as described above. The sympathetic nervous system, through norepinephrine, serves to maintain smooth muscle tone during flaccidity; the parasympathetic system, through acetylcholine, augments arterial dilation and inhibits the sympathetic system; and the nonadrenergic noncholinergic system initiates smooth muscle relaxation. What mediates nonadrenergic, noncholinergic neural transmission remains controversial, though recent evidence has pointed to an endothelial-independent mechanism using nitric oxide. Many other substances have been investigated, including vasoactive intestinal polypeptide, though none to date has met all the requirements to be considered the neurotransmitter of erection.

Adrenergic Control

The sympathetic nervous system consists of a prejunctional and postjunctional neuron. The prejunctional fiber arises from the thoracolumbar cord and travels to its assigned ganglion, which usually is at some distance from its target organ. Within the ganglion, the prejunctional nerve synapses with the postjunctional fiber. All prejunctional fibers use acetylcholine as their neurotransmitter and, thus, are cholinergic. In the sympathetic system, the postjunctional fibers use norepinephrine as their neurotransmitter to the target organ and, thus, are adrenergic. The effect of adrenergic transmission is dependent on the subtype of receptor present on the target organ. The primary receptor types are α and β. α Receptors can be divided further into a postsynaptic α_1 and a presynaptic α_2 subtype. The α_1 receptors mediate the excitatory response from adrenergic stimulation, whereas the α_2 receptors serve to inhibit neurotransmitter release when stimulated. β Receptors can be divided into β_1, which are predominantly at cardiac sites, and β_2, which are located elsewhere. In general, α_1 receptors cause smooth muscle and vascular constriction, and β receptors cause smooth muscle and vascular relaxation. Norepinephrine, which is formed and stored in the neuron from hydroxylation of dopamine by the enzyme dopamine β-hydroxylase, can stimulate both α and β receptors, though it is primarily a potent agonist of α receptors, with minimal β_2 effect.[219]

In the penis, the primary function of the adrenergic fibers is to initiate detumescence and maintain flaccidity.[96] Experimentally, it has been shown that adrenergic nerves and α receptors are abundant,[22] norepinephrine

*References 50, 125–127, 162, 207, 208.

levels increase during detumescence,[48] and norepinephrine in vitro causes dose-dependent contraction of corpora cavernosal smooth muscle.[6] The effect of norepinephrine is blocked by α_1 antagonists,[86] which can cause[34] or potentiate[47, 49] erections when injected intravenously or intracavernosally. α_2 Agonists attenuate norepinephrine release and its effects.[176, 179] The β effect of norepinephrine is minimal and, given the great predominance of α to β receptors,[113] it is assumed that β-adrenergic stimulation plays little, if any, role in erection.[174, 175, 178]

Therefore, it is believed that the primary role of the sympathetic input is to produce contraction of the penile arterial tree and trabecular smooth muscle, thus decreasing arterial inflow and allowing venous runoff, resulting in detumesence. Suppression of the sympathetic influence also is thought to be necessary for the initiation of erection.[9]

Cholinergic Control

Although acetylcholine is the neurotransmitter in somatic nerves and prejunctional sympathetic nerves, the term cholinergic nerves is used to describe the autonomic parasympathetic nerves that use acetylcholine as their postjunctional neurotransmitter. Acetylcholine is formed by the acetylation of choline with acetyl coenzyme A and is stored in synaptic vesicles. Upon release, the neurotransmitter exerts its effects by binding to specific acetylcholine receptors. These receptors can be subdivided into muscarinic and nicotinic receptors. Nicotinic receptors are present in autonomic ganglia and on somatic muscle end plates, whereas parasympathetic autonomic end organs contain muscarinic receptors.[220] In autonomic ganglia, acetylcholine can have both excitatory and inhibitory effects. In peripheral vascular and corpora cavernosal smooth muscle, the effect of acetylcholine is to cause relaxation. This relaxation has been shown to be endothelium-dependent[68] and is attributed to the effect of an endothelium-derived relaxing factor.[67] This endothelium-derived relaxing factor is thought to be nitric oxide[89, 91, 155] and will be discussed at greater length later.

The role of cholinergic nerves in erection has experienced many revisions since Eckhard first showed in 1863 that galvanic stimulation of parasympathetic nerves could produce erection in dogs. One cause of the controversy has been conflicting experimental reports on the effects of acetylcholine and acetylcholine receptor blockers in vivo and in vitro. It is well-accepted that cholinergic nerves exist within the corpora cavernosa,[22, 190] as well as muscarinic and nicotinic receptors.[7] Muscarinic receptors have been shown to be present on the trabecular smooth muscle as well as the lacunar endothelium.[204] Cholinergic fibers in the penis also have been shown to synthesize and release acetylcholine.[26] What has been controversial is the physiologic effect of released acetylcholine. In vivo animal studies have shown either no effect,[82] a partial effect,[13] or a full erection[199] with exogenous acetylcholine, whereas atropine, a muscarinic receptor blocker, also has been shown to have either no effect,[35, 50] a partial effect,[14] or full blockade[207, 208] on the erection. Other data show that the effect of acetylcholine in the corpora is mediated by both muscarinic and nicotinic receptors.[195] In vitro studies with acetylcholine and atropine likewise have had conflicting results.[7, 22, 81, 105, 132] However, with the knowledge that the effects of acetylcholine are endothelium-dependent, more recent investigations[104, 174, 175, 178] with intact endothelium have begun to reveal a consistent pattern. In smooth muscle strips from the corpus cavernosum placed in organ baths and precontracted with norepinephrine, acetylcholine causes concentration-dependent relaxation that is blocked completely by atropine and enhanced by physostigmine, an acetylcholinesterase inhibitor. Smooth muscle supposedly denuded of endothelium appears not to relax in response to acetylcholine, confirming a purported endothelial dependence. Electrical field stimulation, however, causes a dose-dependent biphasic reaction, with an initial contraction and subsequent relaxation. The contractile phase is blocked by bretylium and prazosin, an inhibitor of norepinephrine release and a specific α_1 blocker, respectively, suggesting that contraction is mediated by an adrenergic mechanism. The relaxation is blocked completely by tetrodotoxin, a nonspecific nerve blocker, but only partially by atropine. Additional β blockade with propranolol has no effect. This would suggest the presence of a noncholinergic, nonadrenergic mechanism that is primarily responsible for relaxation of the corporal smooth muscle.

Synthesis of the available experimental data has led to the suggestion of a more limited role of the cholinergic system.[174, 175, 178] It appears that acetylcholine may (1) act prejunctionally to inhibit adrenergic activity, (2) act prejunctionally to enhance nonadrenergic, noncholinergic activity, and (3) act directly to produce endothelium-dependent relaxation.

Nonadrenergic, Noncholinergic Control

As elicited by the in vitro work described previously, it is apparent that there exists a powerful third system of neurotransmitters that is primarily responsible for the active smooth muscle relaxation that produces normal erection. Nonadrenergic, noncholinergic effects are not limited to erection and are a major source of neural control both in the central nervous system and in the periphery. Many of the nonadrenergic, noncholinergic transmitters, especially in the central nervous system, are well-known and include peptides, amino acids, opioids, histamine, and serotonin. Nonadrenergic, noncholinergic systems also are described in the regulation of intestinal function, typically involving peptides such as glucagon, secretin, and vasoactive intestinal polypeptide.

In cavernosal smooth muscle relaxation, the identity of the mediators of nonadrenergic, noncholinergic transmission has not been proven and many candidates have been suggested, including nitric oxide, vasoactive intestinal polypeptide, calcitonin gene-related peptide, bradykinin, neuropeptide Y, substance P, and serotonin.

Nitric Oxide

Nitric oxide recently has drawn considerable attention, since it has been shown to be the endothelium-derived relaxing factor[89, 91] and to mediate nonadrenergic, noncholinergic relaxation in human corpora cavernosa smooth muscle.[90, 104, 163] Nitric oxide is formed by cell-mediated oxidation of endogenous L-arginine by nitric oxide synthetase and has an effective half-life of .1 to 5 seconds.[85] The nitric oxide synthase system has been found in vascular endothelium[154] and smooth muscle,[224] and can be inhibited by N-substituted analogues of L-arginine such as N-amino-L-arginine.[66] Smooth muscle relaxation due to nitric oxide has been shown to be mediated by cyclic guanosine monophosphate.[77, 90] Nitric oxide is believed to be an important mediator of nonadrenergic, noncholinergic smooth muscle relaxation in such organs as the gastric fundus,[30, 114] lower esophageal sphincter,[44,203] trachea,[115] anococcygeus,[70] and ileocolonic junction.[30, 31]

In corpus cavernosum muscle strips, electrical field stimulation produces relaxation despite adrenergic and cholinergic blockade. This relaxation is associated with an increase in nitric oxide and cyclic guanosine monophosphate formation.[90] This effect can be blocked by inhibitors of nitric oxide formation such as L-N-nitro arginine[87, 90] and can be restored by nitric oxide or its precursor L-arginine.[163] Although the endothelial-dependent relaxation was mediated by nitric oxide, the nitric oxide–induced relaxation was not endothelium-dependent.[90, 104] Suggestions have been made that nitric oxide may be the neurotransmitter of nonadrenergic, noncholinergic neurons, but its short half-life makes it unlikely to serve as a preformed neurotransmitter. Thus, there still exists the possibility of an intermediary neurotransmitter that acts by stimulating nitric oxide formation and release. One such possible intermediary transmitter may be vasoactive intestinal polypeptide.

Vasoactive Intestinal Polypeptide

Vasoactive intestinal polypeptide is a 28–amino acid polypeptide with vasodilating activity that originally was isolated from the small intestine.[181] Since then, it has been found throughout the body,[183] though it is most highly concentrated in the gastrointestinal and genitourinary systems,[10, 55, 111] where it acts as a mediator of smooth muscle relaxation and vasodilation.[165] There has been great interest in a possible role for vasoactive intestinal polypeptide as a neurotransmitter in penile erection, as it has been found to cause atropine-resistant vasodilation due to parasympathetic stimulation in other organ systems.[28, 128] Vasoactive intestinal polypeptide–containing nerves have been shown to be abundant in the penis, principally surrounding the pudendal artery and the erectile cavernosal smooth muscle.[159] Levels of the polypeptide, though, have been found to be decreased in men with organic impotence unrelated to the specific cause of erectile dysfunction.[78, 189] Vasoactive intestinal polypeptide also has been observed to be released during erection in men[152, 210, 212] and in animals,[13, 14, 76] though other authors have refuted these findings.[101, 103] In vivo experiments have had mixed results, with intracavernous injections of the polypeptide producing good erections in dogs,[14, 92] but a generally poor response in humans. Ottesen, using potent volunteers, found increased tumescence in all research subjects, but full erection in only one of five with intracavernous vasoactive intestinal polypeptide injection.[152] Similar results of mild tumescence without erection following vasoactive intestinal polypeptide injection have been reported by others,[8, 102, 170] though Kiely reported that it did enhance tumescence due to papaverine or papaverine/phentolamine injection.[102] Of interest was the finding of Juenemann that the primary effect of exogenous vasoactive intestinal polypeptide was decreased venous outflow, presumably due to cavernosal smooth muscle relaxation, with minimal change in arterial inflow.[92] In addition, vasoactive intestinal polypeptide antibody blocked the increase in venous resistance due to pelvic nerve stimulation.[92]

In vitro results using isolated strips of corpus cavernosum smooth muscle consistently have shown vasoactive intestinal polypeptide to be a potent mediator of relaxation.[8, 222] Exogenous vasoactive intestinal polypeptide appears to affect the smooth muscle directly, most likely through a specific receptor, as it is not inhibited by atropine, adrenoreceptor blockers, or tetrodotoxin.[56] Although antiserum to vasoactive intestinal polypeptide was able to block its exogenous effects, it was unable to inhibit the relaxing effect of electrical field stimulation.[8] In gastric fundus smooth muscle strips, vasoactive intestinal polypeptide relaxation was enhanced by L-arginine and partially inhibited by N-monomethyl-L-arginine, whereas antivasoactive intestinal polypeptide antibodies only partially inhibited nonadrenergic, noncholinergic relaxation, which then was blocked fully by the addition of N-monomethyl-L-arginine.[14] This suggests that both nitric oxide and vasoactive intestinal polypeptide are involved in nonadrenergic, noncholinergic relaxation and, although it cannot be excluded that vasoactive intestinal polypeptide stimulates the release of nitric oxide, it is more likely that they work independently. Therefore, although vasoactive intestinal polypeptide has many features suggesting that it is an important neurotransmitter of erection, its specific role awaits further investigation.

Miscellaneous Neurotransmitters

Many other substances have been suggested as important mediators of erection, including calcitonin gene-related peptide,[197, 200] prostaglandin I$_2$,[138] prostaglandin E$_1$,[169] and substance P.[14] Further study is necessary to elucidate a role for any of these substances.

Physiology of Impotence

Impotence has been divided in many different schema. Originally, the etiology of impotence was divided into organic or psychogenic, with 90% of cases being attributed to psychogenic causes. As our understanding of and ability to treat impotence has grown, appreciation for the organic causes has increased to the point at which it now is believed that 90% of cases of impotence are nonpsychogenic.[95] Likewise, our classification has expanded to consider separately hormonal, neurologic, vascular, and psychologic causes. Among patients with organic causes, a vascular etiology is believed to be present in up to 85%, though this may be more a reflection of our current diagnostic techniques rather than a physiologic phenomenon. In fact, our improved understanding of the cellular physiology involved in erection has necessitated a new classification for neurovascular impotence. This classification is based upon the normal physiology as described previously and can be labeled as either (1) failure to fill, (2) failure to relax, or (3) failure to store. The advantage of a physiologically based system is the ability to understand the role of multifactorial risk factors such as diabetes mellitus and radiation, while also suggesting a site of action for previously poorly understood causes such as diabetes mellitus, hypertension, and smoking. Primary hormonal and psychogenic impotence will be discussed separately.

Neurovascular Impotence

Failure to fill implies an inability of the arterial system to provide an adequate increase in blood flow to sustain an erection. This is associated most commonly with diffuse atherosclerotic peripheral vascular disease. Risk factors for arterial insufficiency–related impotence include hypertension, hyperlipidemia, diabetes mellitus, cigarette smoking, trauma, and pelvic irradiation.[75, 172, 188, 211] Therapy has been directed at restoring adequate perfusion, though results have been generally disappointing, possibly due to associated small vessel and smooth muscle disease.[108]

Failure to relax refers to any impairment of the active smooth muscle relaxation within the corpora cavernosa that is so central to normal erection. Included also are defects of the intracavernosal vasculature, which fails to increase in luminal size due to intrinsic damage and persistently elevated vessel wall resistance. Impairment can occur from functional or anatomic alterations anywhere along the pathway, such as in neurologic input, as occurs in spinal cord injury, peripheral neuropathy, diabetes, multiple sclerosis, pelvic surgery, and antihypertensive medications, or in the endothelial-smooth muscle interactions, as is postulated to occur in dysfunction related to diabetes, hypertension, cigarettes use,[186] renal failure, alcohol abuse, hypercholesterolemia,[16] and, possibly, aging.[168] In fact, the effects of chronic arterial insufficiency may be mediated by intrapenile endothelial and smooth muscle deterioration, as seen on electron microscopy,[156] and may explain why technically adequate revascularization often fails to correct impotence.[45] Similarly, a wide range of ultrastructural deterioration can be seen with the other risk factors listed above.[41, 137] Therapy to date has been directed at ameliorating the associated underlying risk factors if present, restoring erections with a prosthesis or vacuum erection device, or attempting to induce smooth muscle relaxation pharmacologically with intracavernosal injections of direct smooth muscle relaxers such as papaverine, phentolamine, or prostaglandin E_1. This form of medical therapy will be discussed in detail later. It is hoped that, with better understanding of the basic physiology of impotence, a more specific therapy aimed at the true deficit will be devised. It still remains to be discovered whether impairment of cavernosal smooth muscle relaxation is primarily a smooth muscle, endothelial, or neurotransmitter defect.

Failure to store refers to the ability to maintain veno-occlusion once it has been initiated by smooth muscle relaxation. Defects most commonly consist of venous leakage or, less frequently, cavernosal-spongiosal fistulas or shunts. Despite its frequent occurrence in impotent men (25% to 86%),[123, 164] the actual mechanism of this incompetence is unknown. Therapy has been directed at surgical ligation of leaking veins identified by cavernosography, but long-term results have been disappointing.[167, 205]

Endocrinopathic Impotence

Impotence can result from a number of discrete endocrinopathies. The most common results from low serum testosterone levels from either hypogonadotropic or hypogonadal hypogonadism, castration, or as a side effect of hormonal deprivation for prostate cancer. Testosterone is believed to influence libido through a central action upon the hypothalamus and limbic system.[166, 182] Peripherally, its effects upon erection are unknown and, although patients with low testosterone levels can achieve erections,[19] they typically show decreased erections on nocturnal tumescence testing.[109] Erections often can be restored with exogenous hormone replacement in patients with low serum testosterone levels.[43]

Hyperprolactinemia also often can result in impotence. Elevated prolactin appears to work through two mechanisms: (1) by lowering gonadotropin-releasing hormone, luteinizing hormone, and testosterone levels, and (2) by having a direct antitestosterone effect such that testosterone replacement in the face of elevated prolactin is ineffective. Common causes of increased prolactin include pituitary adenoma, chronic renal failure, medications, and idiopathic hyperprolactinemia.[64] Therapy is directed at removing the inciting cause, such as an adenoma, or medically reducing prolactin levels with bromocriptine.

Irregularities of the thyroid, either hyperthyroidism or hypothyroidism, can result in impotence. Hypothyroidism can act to decrease testosterone,[158] whereas the mechanism by which hyperthyroidism affects sexual function is less well-understood, though it may function through increased testosterone-binding globulin due to increased thyroxine, resulting in decreased free serum testosterone. Treatment is aimed at correcting the underlying thyroid abnormality.

Psychogenic Impotence

The physiology of psychogenic impotence remains poorly understood. One theory is that the heightened anxiety often associated with psychogenic dysfunction, such as in performance anxiety, results in increased sympathetic tone interfering with smooth muscle relaxation, which requires a withdrawal of alpha-adrenergic stimulation.[49] Therapy has been directed, with generally good results, toward behavioral therapy, particularly a program of sensate focusing aimed at reducing the anxiety associated with maintaining an erection. Medical therapies have included the use of yohimbine, an α_2 receptor blocker that has been shown to have mild[202] to no effectiveness[141] in treating organic impotence, but to be effective in treating psychogenic impotence.[142]

Diabetes Mellitus

Diabetes is one of the most common causes of impotence, with one in two diabetic men experiencing this complication during the course of their disease and 75% of diabetic men over 60 years of age afflicted.[171] The mechanism of impairment has been a source of great speculation, with small-vessel disease or peripheral neuropathy the most common suspects. Hormonal alterations are not thought to play a significant role[174, 175, 178] and, although psychogenic impotence may occur in these patients, it does not do so at a significantly increased rate.[129] Evidence suggesting a vascular impairment has been the finding of cavernosal artery insufficiency recorded by Doppler study and angiography,[2, 84] along with changes in vascular morphology.[172] Support for a neuropathic cause has come from the finding of an increased incidence of other peripheral neuropathies, such as neurogenic bladder, which occurs in up to 82% of impotent diabetic men,[52, 54] as compared to potent diabetic men.[133] The bulbocavernosal reflex also has been found to be abnormal in 70%[12] of diabetics, though other investigators have discounted the significance of that reflex.[151] Morphologic changes in the penile nerves of impotent diabetic men,[53] including decreased norepinephrine,[135, 136] decreased acetylcholinesterase-positive nerve fibers,[116] and decreased vasoactive intestinal polypeptide and vasoactive intestinal polypeptide fibers,[78, 84, 116] also support a neurologic etiology for diabetes-associated impotence.

Recently, however, in vitro studies with corporal tissue from impotent diabetic men have shown impaired autonomic relaxation with impairment of endothelial-dependent relaxation[176] and impaired uptake, synthesis, and release of acetylcholine.[27] The smooth muscle itself, on the other hand, responded normally to direct smooth muscle relaxers such as papaverine and nitroprusside.[179] This suggests that the significant defect is within the endothelial-dependent mechanism prior to the smooth muscle, such as the neuron, neurotransmitter, or endothelial cell.

Treatment traditionally has been aimed at improving glucose control, which, on occasion, can reverse transient impotence associated with hyperglycemia, though in general, impotence is not related to the degree of severity of the diabetes or to its treatment.[106, 171] Successful therapies for these patients include penile prostheses, vacuum devices, and pharmacologic injection therapy.

Hypertensive Impotence

The effects of hypertension appear to be mediated by two mechanisms: a high association with arteriosclerosis and the adverse side effects of antihypertensive medications. In terms of arteriosclerosis, 85% of hypertensive impotent men were shown to have an impaired arterial response to papaverine when evaluated by duplex ultrasonography.[143] The addition of diabetes or smoking was associated with a worse arterial response. This is despite an earlier finding that 91% of hypertensive patients had a normal pelvic arteriogram.[211]

Patients on antihypertensive medications, especially thiazides, had an even more impaired arterial response thought to be due to a direct effect of the medications on the erectile tissue.[42] Patients on β-blockers and vasodilating medications had the best arterial response, though none developed erections, suggesting interference with the veno-occlusive mechanism.[143] Treatment is directed at maintaining blood pressure control using medications with the fewest erectile side effects, such as calcium channel blockers[63] or atenolol.[218]

Impotence and Aging

There clearly is an increased incidence of impotency associated with aging, with 41% of men 60 to 70 years old having erectile dysfunction.[97] The causes are not specific to any factor of aging and encompass all the same causes of impotence as in younger men. Combined neurovascular impairment is most common, accounting for 30% of all impotence in older men; vascular insufficiency alone accounts for 21%, diabetes accounts for 17%, neuropathy accounts for 10%, psychogenic causes account for 3%, and hormonal causes contribute 2.6%.[146] Aging also is associated with decreased gonadal steroids and reduced nerve conduction velocity.[145] Of clinical importance is that libido is generally preserved.[97] Therapeutic options for the geriatric patient should not be limited by the patient's age alone and treatment always should begin with an effort to correct the frequently present reversible causes such as medications or hormonal imbalances.

Postoperative Impotence

The majority of postoperative impotence is due to nerve damage sustained during pelvic surgeries, such as radical prostatectomy, cystoprostatectomy, urethral reconstruction, or abdominal perineal resection. Arterial insufficiency can follow vascular procedures such as aortobifemoral bypass or any injury to the pudendal vessels. Treatment is aimed at prevention by improved understanding of the neural anatomy and improved surgical technique.[121] In cases in which nerve injury is unavoidable, if the vascular supply is intact, patients may respond well to pharmacotherapy; otherwise, prosthesis placement or vacuum erection devices often are quite satisfactory.[119, 120]

Medical Therapy

The therapeutic options available for the successful treatment of erectile impotence have expanded greatly over the past decade. Successful surgical approaches include penile revascularization,[74] venous ligation,[221] and penile prostheses.[157, 184] Medical therapy encompasses the use of any nonsurgical technique to restore erectile function. Options include the use of oral medications such as yohimbine,[193] transcutaneous agents such as nitroglycerine,[38, 153] noninvasive vacuum constriction devices,[223] or intracavernosal injection of vasoactive agents.[225] Effective intracavernosal agents have included papaverine, phentolamine, prostaglandin E_1, or a combination of all three (Table 1). Less effective agents have included vasoactive intestinal polypeptide, calcitonin gene-related peptide, and α blockers alone. For the purpose of this chapter, discussion of medical treatment will be limited to intracavernosal injection therapy.

Recalling that the crucial step in developing a normal erection is active cavernosal smooth muscle relaxation, and that the neural element-endothelium-smooth muscle axis is the most likely site of impairment in the most common forms of impotence, it is clear that the production of smooth muscle relaxation should be the major goal of any medical therapy. Successful pharmacotherapy not only should produce smooth muscle relaxation, but it should do so in a way that causes a minimum of immediate side effects and no long-term damage to the tissues. Additionally, the effects should be transient to avoid ischemic injury. As the specific defect of smooth muscle relaxation in most forms of impotence remains unknown, the agent's effects have been aimed at the smooth muscle directly in order to bypass the endothelium-dependent mechanisms. In order to understand their effects, it is necessary to recall the basic pharmacology of these agents.

Pharmacology

Papaverine is the salt of a benzylisoquinoline alkaloid that can be obtained from opium or synthesized directly. It acts as a nonspecific smooth muscle relaxer and vasodilator through its inhibition of the cyclic nucleotide phosphodiesterase, guanylcyclase, which in turn increases intracellular cyclic

TABLE 1.
Mechanisms of Action of
Clinically Used Vasoactive Agents

Drug	Action
Papaverine	Phosphodiesterase inhibition
Phentolamine	α_1 Receptor blockade
Prostaglandin E_1	Direct smooth muscle relaxation and α receptor blockade

guanosine monophosphate, leading to increased dephosphorylation of the myosin light chain[147] and interference with calcium flux.[191]

Phentolamine is a blocker of α_1 receptors on the smooth muscle. Alone it has only a minimal effect on erection due to poor veno-occlusion, though it serves well to potentiate the effect of papaverine when given in combination.

Prostaglandin E_1, an autocoid produced through arachidonic acid metabolism, has numerous and diverse effects throughout the body. Of particular interest, it has been shown to be a potent vasodilator and direct smooth muscle relaxant. The effects of prostaglandins are mediated through regulation of cyclic adenosine monophosphate synthesis through its effects on adenylate cyclase. In addition, there is growing evidence of specific smooth muscle membrane receptors for prostaglandins that may play an as yet unknown role.[140]

Clinical Uses

Diagnostic

In addition to their therapeutic functions, intracavernosal injections of vasoactive agents have proved to be a powerful diagnostic tool. The chief diagnostic uses are (1) single injection to evaluate arterial competence, (2) adjunct to angiography to evaluate arterial occlusion, (3) adjunct to Doppler ultrasound evaluation of arterial dilation, and (4) adjunct to cavernosography and cavernosometry to evaluate the veno-occlusive mechanism.

Single-Injection Penodynamics.—Both papaverine and prostaglandin E_1 have been used alone in an attempt to distinguish vasculogenic impotence quickly and easily from neurogenic or psychogenic impotence. With this technique, a single injection of a vasoactive substance[1, 36, 88] is administered intracavernosally and, if a full erection occurs within 10 to 20 minutes and lasts for greater than 30 minutes, a vascular defect is ruled out. Patients with suspected neurologic disease have a tendency to be supersensitive to these agents; thus, lower test doses are recommended in these patients. If a full erection fails to develop or fails to maintain following this vasoactive injection, then further vascular evaluation is necessary.

Duplex Doppler Ultrasound..—A less invasive means by which to evaluate arterial competence is the combination of real-time ultrasound and color Doppler ultrasound. The gray-scale ultrasound is used to locate the cavernosal arteries, which then can be evaluated for diameter and, with the addition of Doppler, for peak flow. The adequacy of response to intracavernosal injection of vasoactive substances through these vessels is used to assess arterial competence. The criterion for a response to be considered normal or adequate has been suggested to be a peak velocity of greater than 25 cm/sec.[37, 124, 161] Changes in arterial diameter were found to be less predictive.[21] Initial good arterial response with subsequent early loss of turgidity was associated with venous leakage.[185] Ultrasound findings have been shown to correlate favorably with angiography[144] and nocturnal penile tumescence monitoring.[187]

Cavernosography/Cavernosometry.—For the patient with vasculogenic impotence due to venous incompetence, further evaluation can be performed with pharmacocavernosometry and cavernosography. Cavernosometry is the dynamic measurement of intracorporeal pressure during saline infusion.[149, 160, 214] Pressure should rise rapidly and be able to be maintained with a minimal flow in a patient with normal veno-occlusion. The addition of vasoactive substances intracorporally prior to testing has increased greatly the accuracy and usefulness of this study in identifying those patients with significant venous leakage.[196, 198] By having the vasoactive substances directly relax the corporal smooth muscle, the venous-dependent portion of the veno-occlusive mechanism can be assessed in a physiologically more accurate manner.[118, 123] Likewise, the addition of papaverine or prostaglandin E_1 injection prior to cavernosography, in which contrast material is injected into the corporal space in order to identify radiographically anatomically the site of venous leakage, has greatly increased accuracy,[196] to the point at which cavernosography without pharmacologic smooth muscle relaxation is not recommended.[201]

Angiography.—Patients suspected of having an arterial occlusive etiology of their impotence who may benefit from a penile revascularization procedure must undergo a selective pudendal angiography. Such patients may include those with a history of pelvic trauma, primary impotence, significant peripheral vascular disease, or an isolated arteriogenic dysfunction as determined on Doppler ultrasound testing.[17] The addition of pharmacologically induced partial tumescence greatly improves the image quality and accuracy of these examinations.[32] A full erection can be detrimental to intrepreting the arteriogram as there may be a decrease in cavernosal flow during full erection.[122]

Therapeutic

Since the early observations of Virag and Brindley,[34, 210] intracavernous pharmacotherapy has been shown to be a safe, effective, and widely accepted treatment for erectile dysfunction. Successful management requires proper patient selection, careful dose titration, and thorough patient education. Complications can occur, and this treatment should remain in the hands of a urologist who can recognize best and treat any complications that may occur.

Patient Selection.—Virtually all impotent patients potentially are candidates for pharmacotherapy. Patients with neurogenic impotence tend to have the best erectile response and usually respond to lower doses. Trials in the spinal cord–injured population, which tends to include younger men, have shown the treatment to be generally well-accepted and without increased risks or complications.[117, 192] Patients with vasculogenic impotence can be evaluated as described above with a single injection of papaverine or prostaglandin E_1. Those with adequate erection are excellent candidates for therapy, whereas those with poor response often can achieve adequate erections with the addition of manual stimulation or the application of a vacuum erection device.[120] Patients with therapeutic androgen deprivation, such as may be caused by treatment for prostate cancer, can achieve erections with injection therapy, though libido remains reduced.[71] Injection therapy also has been used in patients with psychogenic impotence, in whom, although there is good erectile response and acceptance with improved self-esteem, sexual satisfaction, and decreased anxiety, the treatment has not been shown to have much effect upon the underlying psychologic dysfunction and may not be recommended as first-line therapy.[11, 18, 206] In the geriatric population, treatment response and complication rates have been shown to be comparable to those in younger men, though higher drug doses are required and patients tend to use the injections less frequently.[100]

Contraindications to therapy include sickle cell anemia, bleeding diathesis, Peyronie's disease, a history of transient ischemic attacks, and unstable cardiovascular disease.[139]

Dose Titration.—Many drugs and drug combinations can be used in pharmacotherapy of impotence. The most common are papaverine alone, papaverine with phentolamine, prostaglandin E_1 alone, or a combination of prostaglandin E_1 and papaverine. All protocols require careful dose titration to produce an erection that is adequate for intromission, yet spontaneously undergoes detumescence within 1 to 2 hours, although, in our clinic, we do not become concerned until the erection has lasted 6 hours. Reported initial doses of papaverine range from 18 to 60 mg. Reported combination papaverine/phentolamine doses range widely, with 30 mg of papaverine and 0.5 mg of phentolamine noted most commonly. Prostaglandin E_1 has been used at doses of 5 to 30 µg, though most physicians begin with 10 µg in vasculogenic impotence and with 5 µg in suspected neurogenic impotence. Papaverine and prostaglandin E_1 also can be used in combination. If the initial dose produces a prolonged erection, the dose is cut in half. If the response is inadequate, the dose can be increased in increments until a satisfactory dose is reached. Once careful dose titration is achieved, the patient is ready to try self-injections at home.

Patient Education.—Comprehensive patient education is necessary to minimize complications of pharmacotherapy for impotence. Of critical importance is that the patient understand the dangers of priapism and seek attention for any prolonged erections within 4 to 6 hours. Patients also should be instructed that further dose modification may be necessary if the injection does not produce an adequate erection, but that a second injection should not be given, as this can lead to severe priapism and has led to one reported death.[80] Other important tips are to hold the needle perpendicular to the shaft, avoid obvious veins, maintain sterile technique, and hold pressure over the injection site for 2 to 3 minutes to reduce hematoma formation. Anticoagulation or stable heart disease are not contraindications to this form of treatment.

Clinical Results.—As stated previously, pharmacotherapy has enjoyed a high degree of success and acceptance. Papaverine, when used alone, has demonstrated significant effectiveness, with 27% of patients achieving full erections and 65% achieving partial erections.[99] The addition of phentolamine greatly improves its effectiveness, with 48% to 70% of patients achieving full erections that are not due to a placebo effect.[99, 103] Prostaglandin E_1 also has shown significant effectiveness, even in patients who are unresponsive to papaverine. In comparison studies, prostaglandin E_1 was shown to produce better erections in 46% to 55.8% of men, whereas papaverine was equally or more effective in 14% to 17.8% of men.[51, 98] Additionally, in patients who demonstrated a preference, 55% preferred prostaglandin E_1, whereas only 27% preferred papaverine. The combination of prostaglandin E_1 and papaverine has shown even greater efficacy, with 77.5% of patients achieving full erections without increased complications and with less penile pain than with prostaglandin E_1 injections alone due to a decreased prostaglandin E_1 dose.[61]

Complications from therapy most commonly consist of priapism, fibrosis, hematoma, elevation of liver function tests, penile pain, hypotension, and vasovagal reaction. Chronic use of papaverine is associated more commonly with fibrosis (31% ± 8.6% at 1 year), elevated liver enzymes (9.8%), and hematomas (20.9%)[110] than is chronic use of prostaglandin E_1, which is associated more commonly with penile pain (17% severe, 22% mild to moderate).[69] Priapism should be infrequent after dose stabilization, though incidence reports range from 3% to 10%.[120] Experimentally, chronic papaverine use has been shown to produce smooth muscle atrophy and collagen replacement, whereas prostaglandin E_1 did not produce any histologic changes.[3] Although drop-out rates of 50%[69, 110] have been reported, the majority of patients either failed to follow up after dose titration or discontinued therapy while still achieving erection; only 26% to 28% quit due to complications or inadequate erections. Overall satisfaction in those who continue therapy is high. In the largest and longest series reported to date, 84.8% of patients report satisfaction, with only 2.8% developing fibrosis and a rate of prolonged erections of 3 per 1,000 injections.[213] Improvement in spontaneous erections was reported to have occurred in 65% of patients, with 15% no longer requiring therapy.[213]

Conclusion

Improved understanding of the physiology of erection, and particularly the pivotal role of active smooth muscle relaxation, has allowed the development of safe and effective medical therapy for impotence due to a wide variety of causes. It is hoped that, in the future, greater understanding of the specific neurotransmitters involved in erection will allow specific targeting of medical therapy, providing greater efficacy with fewer side effects and simpler administration. Ideally, one day medical therapy can be targeted to the causes of dysfunction in order to prevent clinical impotence before it happens.

References

1. Abber JC, Lue TF, Orvis BR, et al: Diagnostic tests for impotence: A comparison of papaverine injection with the penile-brachial index and nocturnal penile tumescence monitoring. *J Urol* 1986; 135:923–925.
2. Abelson D: Diagnostic value of the penile pulse and blood pressure: A Doppler study of impotence in diabetics. *J Urol* 1975; 113:636.
3. Aboseif SR, Breza J, Bosch RJLH, et al: Local and systemic effects of chronic intracavernous injection of papaverine, prostaglandin E1, and saline in primates. *J Urol* 1989; 142:403–408.
4. Aboseif SR, Lue TF: Fundamentals and hemodynamics of penile erection. *Cardiovasc Intervent Radiol* 1988; 11:185.
5. Aboseif SR, Lue TF: Hemodynamics of penile erection. *Urol Clin North Am* 1988; 15:1.
6. Adaikan PG, Karim SMM: Adrenoreceptors in the human penis. *J Auton Pharmacol* 1981; 1:199.
7. Adaikan PG, Karim SMM, Kottegoda SR, et al: Cholinoreceptors in the corpus cavernosum muscle of the human penis. *J Auton Pharmacol* 1983; 3:107.
8. Adaikan PG, Kottegoda SR, Ratnam SS: Is vasoactive intestinal polypeptide the principal transmitter involved in human penile erection? *J Urol* 1986; 135:638–640.
9. Adaikan PG, Ratnam SS: Pharmacology of penile erection in humans. *Cardiovasc Intervent Radiol* 1988; 11:191–194.
10. Alm P, Alumets J, Hakanson R, et al: Peptidergic (vasoactive intestinal polypeptide) nerves in the genitourinary tract. *Neuroscience* 1977; 2:751.
11. Althof SE, Turner LA, Levine SB, et al: Sexual, psychological, and marital impact of self-injection of papaverine and phentolamine: A long-term prospective study. *J Sex Marital Ther* 1991; 17:101–112.
12. Andersen JT, Bradley WE: Early detection of diabetic visceral neuropathy: An electro physiologic study of bladder and urethral innervation. *Diabetes* 1976; 25:1100.
13. Andersson PO, Bjornberg J, Bloom SR, et al: Vasoactive intestinal polypeptide in relation to penile erection in the cat evoked by pelvic and hypogastric nerve stimulation. *J Urol* 1987; 138:419.
14. Andersson PO, Bloom SR, Mellander S: Hemodynamics of pelvic nerve induced penile erection in the dog: Possible mediation by vasoactive intestinal polypeptide. *J Physiol (Lond)* 1984; 350:209–224.
15. Argiolas A, Melis MR, Gessa GL: Yawning and penile erection: Central dopamine-oxytocin-adrenocorticotropin connection. *Ann N Y Acad Sci* 1988; 525:330–337.
16. Azadzoi KM, Saenz de Tejada I: Hypercholesterolemia impairs endothelium-dependent relaxation of rabbit corpus cavernosum smooth muscle. *J Urol* 1991, 146:238–240.
17. Bahren W, Gall H, Scherb W, et al: Arterial anatomy and arteriographic diagnosis of arteriogenic impotence. *Cardiovasc Intervent Radiol* 1988; 11:195–210.
18. Bahren W, Scherb W, Gall H, et al: Effects of intracavernous pharmacotherapy on self-esteem, performance anxiety and partnership in patients with chronic erectile dysfunction. *Eur Urol* 1989; 16:175–180.

19. Bancroft J, Wu FC: Changes in erectile responsiveness during androgen replacement therapy. *Arch Sex Behav* 1983; 211:59–66.
20. Beach FA: Cerebral and hormonal control of reflexive mechanisms involved in copulatory behavior. *Physiol Rev* 1967; 47:289–316.
21. Benson CB, Vickers MA: Sexual impotence caused by vascular disease: Diagnosis with duplex sonography. *AJR Am J Roentgenol* 1989; 153: 1149–1153.
22. Benson GS, McConnell J, Lipshultz LI, et al: Neuromorphology and neuropharmacology of the human penis. *J Clin Invest* 1980; 65:506–513.
23. Benson GS, McConnell JA, Schmidt WA: Penile polsters: Functional structures or atherosclerotic changes. J Urol 1981; 125:800.
24. Berendsen HHG, Jenck F, Broekkamp CLE: Involvement of 5-HT1c-receptors on drug-induced penile erections in rats. *Psychopharmacology* 1990; 101:57–61.
25. Bitran D, Hull EM: Pharmacological analysis of male rat sexual behavior. *Neurosci Biobehav Rev* 1987; 11:365–389.
26. Blanco R, Saenz de Tejada I, Goldstein I, et al: Cholinergic neurotransmission in human corpus cavernosum. II. Acetylcholine synthesis. *Am J Physiol* 1988; 254:H468–H472.
27. Blanco R, Saenz de Tejada I, Goldstein I, et al: Dysfunctional penile cholinergic nerves in diabetic impotent men. *J Urol* 1990; 144:278–280.
28. Bloom SR, Edwards AV: Vasoactive intestinal peptide in relation to atropine resistant vasodilation in the submaxillary gland of the cat. *J Physiol (Lond)* 1980; 300:41–53.
29. Bochdalek V: Ergebnesse uber einem bis getzt uberschenen Teil des Erektion sapparates des Penis und der Clitoris. *Vierteljahrschr Prakt Heilunde* 1845; 43:115.
30. Boeckxstaens GE, Pelckmans PA, Bodgers JJ, et al: Release of nitric oxide upon stimulation of nonadrenergic noncholinergic nerves in the rat gastric fundus. *J Pharmacol Exp Ther* 1991; 256:441–447.
31. Boeckxstaens GE, Pelckmans PA, Ruytjens IF, et al: Bioassay of nitric oxide released upon stimulation of nonadrenergic noncholinergic nerves in the canine ileocolonic junction. *Br J Pharmacol* 1991; 103:1085–1091.
32. Bookstein JJ, Valji K, Parsons L, et al: Pharmacoarteriography in the evaluation of impotence. *J Urol* 1987; 137:333–337.
33. Breza J, Aboseif SR, Orvis BR, et al: Detailed anatomy of penile neurovascular structures: Surgical singificance. *J Urol* 1989; 141:437.
34. Brindley GS: Cavernosal alpha-blockade: A new technique for investigating and treating erectile impotence. *Br J Psychol* 1983; 143:332–337.
35. Brindley GS: Pilot experiments on the action of drugs injected into the human corpus cavernosum penis. *Br J Pharmacol* 1986; 87:495.
36. Buvat J, Buvat-Herbaut M, Dehaene JL, et al: Is intracavernous injection of papaverine a reliable screening test for vascular impotence? *J Urol* 1986; 135:476–478.
37. Chiang PH, Chiang CP, Wu CC, et al: Colour duplex sonography in the assessment of impotence. *Br J Urol* 1991; 68:181–186.
38. Claes H, Baert L: Transcutaneous nitroglycerin therapy in the treatment of impotence. *Urol Int* 1989; 44:309–312.
39. Clark TK, Caggiula AR, McConnell RA, et al: Sexual inhibition is reduced by rostral midbrain lesions in the male rat. *Science* 1975; 190:169–171.

40. Conti G: L'erection du penis humain et ses bases morphologico-vasculaires. *Acta Anat (Basel)* 1952; 14:217.
41. Conti G, Virag R: Human penile erection and organic impotence: Normal histology and histopathology. *Urol Int* 1989; 44:303–308.
42. Creed KE, Carati CJ, Adamson GM, et al: Responses of erectile tissue from impotent men to pharmacological agents. *Br J Urol* 1989; 63:428–431.
43. Davidson JM, Camargo CA, Smith ER: Effects of androgen on sexual behavior in hypogonadal men. *J Clin Endocrinol Metab* 1979; 48:955–958.
44. De Man JG, Pelckmans PA, Boeckxstaens GE, et al: The role of nitric oxide in inhibitory nonadrenergic noncholinergic neurotransmission in the canine lower oesophageal sphincter. *Br J Pharmacol* 1991; 103:1092–1096.
45. Dewar ML, Blundell PE, Lidstone D, et al: Effects of abdominal aneurysmectomy, aortoiliac bypass grafting and angioplasty on male sexual potency: A prospective study. *Can J Surg* 1985; 28:154–156.
46. Deysach LJ: Comparative morphology of erectile tissue of penis with especial emphasis on probable mechanism of erection. *Am J Anat* 1939; 64:111.
47. Diederichs W, Lue TF: Reduction of sympathetic influences on penile erection by phentolamine. *Urol Int* 1991; 46:64–66.
48. Diederichs W, Stief CG, Lue TF, et al: Norepinephrine involvement in penile detumescence. *J Urol* 1990; 143:1264–1266.
49. Diederichs W, Stief CG, Lue TF, et al: Sympathetic inhibition of papaverine induced erection. *J Urol* 1991; 146:195–198.
50. Dorr L, Brody M: Hemodynamic mechanisms of erection in the canine penis. *Am J Physiol* 1967; 213:1526.
51. Earle CM, Keogh EJ, Wisniewski ZS, et al: Prostaglandin E1 therapy for impotence, comparison with papaverine. *J Urol* 1990; 143:57–59.
52. Ellenberg M: Impotence in diabetes: The neurologic factor. *Ann Intern Med* 1971; 75:213.
53. Faerman I, Glocer L, Fox D, et al: Impotence and diabetes: Histological studies of the autonomic nervous fibers of the corpora cavernosa in impotent diabetic males. *Diabetes* 1974; 23:971.
54. Faerman I, Vilar O, Rivarola MA, et al: Impotence and diabetes: Studies of androgenic function in diabetic impotent males. *Diabetes* 1972; 21:23.
55. Fahrenkrug J: Vasoactive intestinal polypeptide: Measurement, distribution and putative neurotransmitter function. *Digestion* 1979; 19:149.
56. Fahrenkrug J, Ottesen B, Palle C: Vasoactive intestinal polypeptide and the reproductive system. *Ann N Y Acad Sci* 1988; 525:393–404.
57. Finberg JPM, Vardi Y: Inhibitory effect of the 5-hydroxytryptamine on penile erectile function in the rat. *Br J Pharmacol* 1990; 101:698–702.
58. Fitzpatrick TJ: Venography of the deep dorsal venous and valvular systems. *J Urol* 1974; 111:518.
59. Fitzpatrick TJ: A cavernosogram study on the valvular competence of the human deep dorsal vein. *J Urol* 1975; 113:497.
60. Fitzpatrick TJ: The corpus cavernosum intercommunicating venous drainage system. *J Urol* 1975; 113:494.
61. Floth A, Schramek P: Intracavernous injection of prostaglandin E1 in combination with papaverine: Enhanced effectiveness in comparison with papaverine plus phentolamine and prostaglandin E1 alone. *J Urol* 1991; 145:56–59.
62. Fournier GR Jr, Juenemann K-P, Lue TF, et al: Mechanisms of venous occlusion during canine penile erection: An anatomic demonstration. *J Urol* 1987; 137:163.

63. Fovaeous M, Andersson KE, Hedlund H: Effects of some calcium channel blockers on isolated human penile erectile tissues. *J Urol* 1987; 138:1267.
64. Franks S, Jacobs HS, Martin N, et al: Hyperprolactinemia and impotence. *Clin Endocrinol (Oxf)* 1978; 8:277–287.
65. Freedman AL, Sikka SC, Rajfer J: Development of rat cavernosal smooth muscle cell culture and its response to papaverine. *Surg Forum* 1988; 39:658–659.
66. Fukuto JM, Wood KS, Byrns RE, et al: N-amino-L-arginine: A new potent antagonist of L-arginine-mediated endothelium-dependent relaxation. *Biochem Biophys Res Commun* 1990; 168:458–465.
67. Furchgott RF: Role of endothelium in responses of vascular smooth muscle. *Circ Res* 1983; 53:557–573.
68. Furchgott RF, Zawadski JV: The obligatory role of endothelial cells in the relaxation of arterial smooth muscle by acetylcholine. *Nature* 1980; 288:373–376.
69. Gerber GS, Levine LA: Pharmacological erection program using prostaglandin E1. *J Urol* 1991; 146:786–789.
70. Gibson A, Mirzazadeh S: N-methylhydroxylamine inhibits and M&B 22948 potentiates relaxation of the mouse anococcygeus to nonadrenergic noncholinergic field stimulation and to nitrovasodilator drugs. *Br J Pharmacol* 1989; 96:637–644.
71. Gilbert W, Gillatt DA, Desai KM, et al: Intracorporeal papaverine injection in androgen deprived men. *J R Soc Med* 1990; 83:161.
72. Goldstein AMB, Meehan JP, Zakhary R, et al: New observations on microarchitecture of corpora cavernosa in man and possible relationship to mechanism of erection. *Urology* 1982; 20:259–266.
73. Goldstein AMB, Padma-Nathan H: The microarchitecture of the intracavernosal smooth muscle and the cavernosal fibrous skeleton. *J Urol* 1990; 144:1144–1146.
74. Goldstein I: Penile revascularization. *Urol Clin North Am* 1987; 14: 805–813.
75. Goldstein I, Feldman MI, Deckers PJ, et al: Radiation associated impotence: A clinical study of its mechanism. *JAMA* 1984; 251:903–910.
76. Goldstein I, Saenz de Tajada I, Krane RJ, et al: Changes in corporal vasoactive intestinal polypeptide (VIP) concentration following pelvic nerve stimulation. *J Urol* 1985; 133:218A.
77. Gruetter CA, Barry BK, McNamara DB, et al: Relaxation of bovine coronary artery and activation of coronary arterial guanylate cyclase by nitric oxide, nitroprusside and a carcinogenic nitrosoamine. *J Cyclic Nucleotide Res* 1974; 5:211–224.
78. Gu J, Lazarides M, Pryor JP, et al: Decrease of vasoactive intestinal polypeptide (VIP) in the penises from impotent men. *Lancet* 1984; 2:315–317.
79. Hart BL, Kitchell RL: Penile erection and contraction of penile muscles in the spinal and intact dog. *Am J Physiol* 1966; 210:257–262.
80. Hashmat AI, Abrahams J, Fani K, et al: A lethal complication of papaverine-induced priapism. *J Urol* 1991; 145:146–147.
81. Hedlund H, Andersson KE: Comparison of the responses to drugs acting on adrenoreceptors and muscarinic receptors in human isolated corpus cavernosum and cavernous artery. *J Auton Pharmacol* 1985; 5:81–88.
82. Henderson VE, Repke MH: On the mechanism of erection. *Am J Physiol* 1933; 106:441.
83. Herbert J: The role of the dorsal nerves of the penis in the sexual behavior of the male rhesus monkey. *Physiol Behav* 1973; 10:292–300.

84. Herman A, Adar R, Rubinstein Z: Vascular lesions associated with impotence in diabetic and nondiabetic arterial occlusive disease. *Diabetes* 1978; 27:975.
85. Hoffmann MR, Menon NK, Bing RJ: Nitric oxide as an endothelium-derived relaxing factor: Theoretical and experimental considerations. *J Appl Cardiol* 1990; 5:455–460.
86. Holmquist F, Hedlund H, Andersson KE: Effects of the alpha 1-adrenoceptor antagonist R-(-)-YM12617 on isolated human penile erectile tissue and vas deferens. *Eur J Pharmacol* 1990; 186:87–93.
87. Holmquist F, Hedlund H, Andersson KE: L-N-nitro arginine inhibits nonadrenergic noncholinergic relaxation of human isolated corpus cavernosum. *Acta Physiol Scand* 1991; 141:441–442.
88. Hwang TI, Yang C, Wang S, et al: Impotence evaluated by the use of prostaglandin E1. *J Urol* 1989; 141:1357–1359.
89. Ignarro LJ, Buga GM, Wood KS, et al: Endothelium-derived relaxing factor produced and released from artery and vein is nitric oxide. *Proc Natl Acad Sci U S A* 1987; 84:9265–9269.
90. Ignarro LJ, Bush PA, Buga GM, et al: Nitric oxide and cyclic GMP formation upon electrical field stimulation cause relaxation of corpus cavernosum smooth muscle. *Biochem Biophys Res Commun* 1990; 170:843–850.
91. Ignarro LJ, Byrns RE, Buga GM, et al: Endothelium-derived relaxing factor from pulmonary artery and vein possesses pharmacological and chemical properties identical to those of nitric oxide radical. *Circ Res* 1987; 61: 866–879.
92. Juenemann KP, Lue TF, Luo JA, et al: The role of vasoactive intestinal polypeptide as a neurotransmitter in canine penile erection: A combined in vivo and immunohistochemical study. *J Urol* 1987; 138:871–877.
93. Juenemann KP, Lue TF, Schmidt RA, et al: Clinical significance of sacral and pudendal nerve anatomy. *J Urol* 1988; 139:74.
94. Juenemann KP, Luo JA, Lue TF, et al: Further evidence of venous outflow restriction during erection. *Br J Urol* 1986; 58:320–324.
95. Juenemann KP, Persson-Juenemann C, Alken P: Pathophysiology of erectile dysfunction. *Semin Urol* 1990; 8:89–93.
96. Juenemann KP, Persson-Juenemann C, Lue TF, et al: Neurophysiological aspects of penile erection: The role of the sympathetic nervous system. *Br J Urol* 1989; 64:84–92.
97. Kaiser FE, Viosca SP, Morley JE, et al: Impotence and aging: Clinical and hormonal factors. *J Am Geriatr Soc* 1988; 36:511–519.
98. Kattan S, Collins JP, Mohr D: Double-blind, cross-over study comparing prostaglandin E1 and papaverine in patients with vasculogenic impotence. *Urology* 1991; 37:516–518.
99. Keogh EJ, Watters GR, Earle CM, et al: Treatment of impotence by intrapenile injections. A comparison of papaverine versus papaverine and phentolamine: A double-blind, crossover trial. *J Urol* 1989; 142:726–728.
100. Kerfoot WW, Carson CC: Pharmacologically induced erections among geriatric men. *J Urol* 1991; 146:1022–1024.
101. Kiely EA, Blank MA, Bloom SR, et al: Studies of intracavernosal VIP levels during pharmacologically induced penile erections. *Br J Urol* 1987; 59:334–339.
102. Kiely EA, Bloom SR, Williams G: Penile response to intracavernosal vasoactive intestinal polypeptide alone and in combination with other vasoactive agents. *Br J Urol* 1989; 64:191–194.

103. Kiely EA, Ignotus P, Williams G: Penile function following intracavernosal injection of vasoactive agents or saline. *Br J Urol* 1987; 59:473–476.
104. Kim N, Azadzoi KM, Goldstein I, et al: A nitric oxide-like factor mediates nonadrenergic-noncholinergic neurogen relaxation of penile corpus cavernosum smooth muscle. *J Clin Invest* 1991; 88:112–118.
105. Klinge E, Sjostrand NO: Comparative study of some isolated mammalian smooth muscle effectors of penile erection. *Acta Physiol Scand* 1977; 100:354–367.
106. Kolodny RC, Kahn CB, Goldstein HH, et al: Sexual dysfunction in diabetic men. *Diabetes* 1974; 23:306.
107. Krall JF, Fittingoff M, Rajfer J: Characterization of cyclic nucleotide and inositol 1,4,5-triphosphate-sensitive calcium-exchange activity of smooth muscle cells from the human corpora cavernosa. *J Biol Reprod* 1988; 39: 413–422.
108. Krane RJ, Goldstein I, Saenz de Tejada I: Impotence. *N Engl J Med* 1989; 321:1648–1659.
109. Kwan M, Greenleaf WJ, Mann J, et al: The nature of androgen action in male sexuality: A combined laboratory-self-report study on hypogonadal men. *J Clin Endocrinol Metab* 1983; 57:557–562.
110. Lakin MM, Montague DK, Medendorp SV, et al: Intracavernous injection therapy: Analysis of results and complications. *J Urol* 1990; 143:1138–1141.
111. Larsson LI, Fahrenkrug J, Schaffalitzky de Muckadell OB: Occurrence of nerves containing vasoactive intestinal polypeptide immunoreactivity in the male genital tract. *Life Sci* 1977; 21:503.
112. Lepor H, Gregeman M, Crosby R, et al: Precise localization of the autonomic nerves from the pelvic plexus to the corpora cavernosa: A detailed anatomic study of the adult male pelvis. *J Urol* 1985; 133:207.
113. Levine RM, Wein A: Adrenergic alpha receptors outnumber beta receptors in human penile corpus cavernosum. *Invest Urol* 1980; 18:225.
114. Li CG, Rand MJ: Nitric oxide and vasoactive intestinal polypeptide mediate nonadrenergic noncholinergic inhibitory transmission to smooth muscle of the rat gastric fundus. *Eur J Pharmacol* 1990; 191:303–309.
115. Li CG, Rand MJ: Evidence that part of the NANC relaxant response of guinea pig trachea to electrical field stimulation is mediated by nitric oxide. *Br J Pharmacol* 1991; 102:91–94.
116. Lincoln J, Crowe R, Blackway PE, et al: Changes in the vipergic, cholinergic and adrenergic innervation of human penile tissue in diabetic and non-diabetic impotent males. *J Urol* 1987; 137:1053.
117. Lloyd LK, Richards JS: Intracavernous pharmacotherapy for management of erectile dysfunction in spinal cord injury. *Paraplegia* 1989; 27:457–464.
118. Lue TF: The mechanism of penile erection in the monkey. *Semin Urol* 1986; 4:217–224.
119. Lue TF: Impotence after prostatectomy. *Urol Clin North Am* 1990; 17:613–620.
120. Lue TF: Intracavernous drug administration: Its role in diagnosis and treatment of impotence. *Semin Urol* 1990; 8:100–106.
121. Lue TF: Impotence after radical pelvic surgery: Physiology and management. *Urol Int* 1991; 46:259–265.
122. Lue TF, Hricak K, Marich KW, et al: Vasculogenic impotence evaluated by high-resolution ultrasonography and pulsed Doppler spectrum analysis. *Radiology* 1985; 155:777–781.

123. Lue TF, Hricak K, Schmidt RA, et al: Functional evaluation of penile veins by cavernosography in papaverine-induced erection. *J Urol* 1986; 135:479–482.
124. Lue TF, Mueller SC, Jow YR, et al: Functional evaluation of penile arteries with duplex ultrasound in vasodilator-induced erection. *Urol Clin North Am* 1989; 16:799–807.
125. Lue TF, Takamura T, Schmidt RA, et al: Hemodynamics of erection in the monkey. *J Urol* 1983; 130:1237.
126. Lue TF, Takamura T, Umraiya M, et al: Hemodynamics of canine corpora cavernosa during erection. *Urology* 1984; 24:347.
126a. Lue TF, Tanagho EA: Physiology of erection and pharmacological management of impotence. *J Urol* 1987; 137:829–836.
127. Lue TF, Zeineh SJ, Schmidt RA, et al: Neuroanatomy of penile erection: Its relevance to iatrogenic impotence. *J Urol* 1984; 131:273.
128. Lunderg JM, Ahggard A, Fahrenkrug J, et al: Vasoactive intestinal polypeptide in cholinergic neurons of exocrine glands: Functional significance of co-existing transmitters for vasodilation and secretion. *Proc Natl Acad Sci U S A* 1980; 77:1651–1655.
129. Maatman TJ, Mintague DK, Martin LM: Erectile dysfunction in men with diabetes mellitus. *Urology* 1987; 29:589–592.
130. Maclean PD, Denniston RH, Dua S: Further studies on cerebral representation of penile erection: Caudal thalamus, midbrain, and pons. *J Neurophysiol* 1963; 26:274–293.
131. Marson L, McKenna KE: The identification of a brainstem site controlling spinal sexual reflexes in male rats. *Brain Res* 1990; 515:303.
132. McConnell J, Benson GS, Wood J: Autonomic innervation of the mammalian penis: A histochemical and physiological study. *J Neural Transm* 1979; 45:227.
133. McCullock DK, Young RJ, Prescott RS: The natural history of impotence in diabetic men. *Diabetologia* 1984; 26:437.
134. Meada N, Matsouka N, Yamaguchi I: Septohippocampal cholinergic pathway and penile erections induced by dopaminergic and cholinergic stimulants. *Brain Res* 1990; 537:163.
135. Melman A, Henry DP, Felten DL, et al: Alteration of the penile corpora in patients with erectile impotence. *Invest Urol* 1980; 17:474.
136. Melman A, Henry DP, Felten DL, et al: Effect of diabetes upon penile sympathetic nerves in impotent patients. *South Med J* 1980; 73:307.
137. Mersdorf A, Goldsmith PC, Diederichs W, et al: Ultrastructural changes in impotent penile tissue: A comparison of 65 patients. *J Urol* 1991; 145:749–758.
138. Mikhailidis DP, Jeremy JY, Shoukry K, et al: Eicosanoids, impotence and pharmacologically induced erection. *Prostaglandins Leukot Essent Fatty Acids* 1990; 40:239–242.
139. Miller-Catchpole R: Vasoactive intracavernous pharmacotherapy for impotence: Papaverine and phentolamine. *JAMA* 1990, 264.752–754.
140. Moncada S, Flower RJ, Vane JR: Prostaglandins, prostacyclin, thromboxane A2 and leukotrienes, in Gilman AG, Goodman LS, Rall TW, et al (eds): *The Pharmacological Basis of Therapeutics,* 7th ed. New York, Macmillan, 1985, pp 660–673.
141. Morales A, Condra M, Owen JA, et al: Is yohimbine effective in the treatment of organic impotence? Results of a controlled trial. *J Urol* 1987; 137:1168–1172.

142. Morales A, Condra M, Owen JA, et al: Oral and transcutaneous pharmacological agents in the treatment of impotence. *Urol Clin North Am* 1988; 15:87–93.
143. Mueller SC, El-Damanhoury H, Ruth J, et al: Hypertension and impotence. *Eur Urol* 1991; 19:29–34.
144. Mueller SC, van Wallenberg-Pachaly H, Voges GE, et al: Comparison of selective internal iliac pharmacoangiography, penile brachial index and duplex sonography with pulsed doppler analysis for the evaluation of vasculogenic (arteriogenic) impotence. *J Urol* 1990; 143:928–932.
145. Mulligan T, Katz PG: Erectile failure in the aged: Evaluation and treatment. *J Am Geriatr Soc* 1988; 36:54–62.
146. Mulligan T, Katz PG: Why aged men become impotent. *Arch Intern Med* 1989; 149:1365–1366.
147. Needleman P, Corr PB, Johnson Jr EM: Drugs used for the treatment of angina: Organic nitrates, calcium channel blockers, and beta adrenergic antagonists, in Gilman AG, Goodman LS, Rall TW, et al (eds): *The Pharmacological Basis of Therapeutics*, 7th ed. New York, Macmillan, 1985, pp 806–826.
148. Newman HF, Northup JD, Devlin J: Mechanism of human penile erection. *Invest Urol* 1964; 1:350.
149. Newman HF, Reiss H: Artificial perfusion in impotence. *Urology* 1984; 24:469–471.
150. Newman HF, Tchertkoff V: Penile vascular cushion and erection. *Invest Urol* 1980; 18:43–45.
151. Nogueira MC, Herbaut AG, Wespes E: Neurophysiological investigations of two hundred men with erectile dysfunction. *Eur Urol* 1990; 18:37–41.
152. Ottesen B, Wagner G, Virag R, et al: Penile erection: Possible role for vasoactive intestinal polypeptide as a neurotransmitter. *BMJ* 1984; 288:9–11.
153. Owen JA, Saunders C, Harris J, et al: Topical nitroglycerin: A potential treatment for impotence. *J Urol* 1989; 141:546–548.
154. Palmer RMJ, Ashton DS, Moncada S: Vascular endothelial cells synthesize nitric oxide from L-arginine. *Nature* 1988; 333:664–666.
155. Palmer RMJ, Ferrege AG, Moncada S: Nitric oxide release accounts for the biological activity of endothelium-derived relaxing factor. *Nature* 1987; 327:524–526.
156. Persson C, Diederichs W, Lue TF, et al: Correlation of altered penile ultrastructure with clinical arterial evaluation. *J Urol* 1989; 142:1462–1468.
157. Petrou SP, Barrett DM: The use of penile prostheses in erectile dysfunction. *Semin Urol* 1990; 8:138–152.
158. Pogach LM, Vaitukaitis JL: Endocrine disorders associated with erectile dysfunction, in Krane RJ, Siroky MB, Goldstein I (eds): *Male Sexual Dysfunction*. Boston, Little, Brown, 1983, pp 63–76.
159. Polak JM, Mina S, Gu J, et al: VIPergic nerves in the penis. *Lancet* 1981; 2:217–219.
160. Puech-Leao P, Chao S, Glina S, et al: Gravity cavernosometry—a simple diagnostic test for cavernosal incompetence. *Br J Urol* 1990; 65:391–394.
161. Quam JP, King BF, James EM, et al: Duplex and color doppler sonographic evaluation of vascular impotence. *AJR Am J Roentgenol* 2989; 153:1141–1147.
162. Quinlan DM, Nelson RJ, Partin AW, et al: The rat as a model for the study of penile erection. *J Urol* 1989; 141:656–661.

163. Rajfer J, Aronson WJ, Bush PA, et al: Nitric oxide as a mediator of relaxation of the corpus cavernosum in response to nonadrenergic noncholinergic neurotransmission. *N Engl J Med* 1992; 326:90–94.
164. Rajfer J, Rosciszewski A, Mehringer M: Prevalence of corporal venous leakage in impotent men. *J Urol* 1988; 140:69–71.
165. Rattan S, Said SI, Goyal RK: Effect of vasoactive intestinal polypeptide (VIP) on the lower esophageal sphincter pressure (LESP). *Proc Soc Exp Biol Med* 1977; 155:40.
166. Rees HD, Michael RP: Brain cells of the male rhesus monkey accumulate 3H-testosterone or its metabolites. *J Comp Neurol* 1982; 206:273–277.
167. Rossman B, Mieza M, Melman A: Penile vein ligation for corporeal incompetence: An evaluation of short-term and long-term results. *J Urol* 1990; 144:679–682.
168. Rousseau P: Impotence in elderly men. *Postgrad Med* 1988; 83:212–219.
169. Roy AC, Adaikan PG, Sen DK, et al: Prostaglandin 15-hydroxydehydrogenase activity in human penile corpora cavernosa and its significance in prostaglandin-mediated penile erection. *Br J Urol* 1989; 64:180–182.
170. Roy JB, Petrone RL, Said SI: A clinical trial of intracavernosal vasoactive intestinal peptide to induce penile erection. *J Urol* 1990; 143:302–304.
171. Rubin A, Babbott O: Impotence and diabetes mellitus. *JAMA* 1958; 168:498.
172. Ruzbarsky V, Michal V: Morphologic changes in the arterial bed of the penis with aging: Relationship to the pathogenesis of impotence. *Invest Urol* 1977; 15:194.
173. Sachs BD, Garinello LD: Spinal pacemaker controlling sexual reflexes in male rats. *Brain Res* 1979; 171:152–156.
174. Saenz de Tejada I, Blanco R, Goldstein I, et al: Cholinergic neurotransmission in human corpus cavernosum. I. Response of isolated tissue. *Am J Physiol* 1988; 254:H459–H467.
175. Saenz de Tejada I, Goldstein I: Diabetic penile neuropathy. *Urol Clin North Am* 1988; 15:17–22.
176. Saenz de Tejada I, Goldstein I, Azadzoi K, et al: Impaired neurogenic and endothelium-mediated relaxation of penile smooth muscle from diabetic men with impotence. *N Engl J Med* 1989; 320:1025–1030.
177. Saenz de Tejada I, Goldstein I, Blanco R, et al: Smooth muscle of the corpora cavernosae: Role in penile erection. *Surg Forum* 1985; 36:623–624.
178. Saenz de Tejada I, Goldstein I, Krane RJ: Local control of penile erection. *Urol Clin North Am* 1988; 15:9–15.
179. Saenz de Tejada I, Kim N, Lagan I, et al: Regulation of adrenergic activity in penile corpus cavernosum. *J Urol* 1989; 142:1117–1121.
180. Saenz de Tejada I, Moroukian P, Tessier J, et al: Trabecular smooth muscle modulates the capacitor function of the penis. Studies on a rabbit model. *Am J Physiol* 1991; 260:H1590–H1595.
181. Said SI, Mutt V: Polypeptide with broad biological activity: Isolation from small intestine. *Science* 1970, 169.1217.
182. Sar M, Stumpf WE: Distribution of androgen target cells in rat forebrain and pituitary after (3H)-dihydrotestosterone administration. *J Steroid Biochem* 1977; 8:1131–1135.
183. Schultzberg M: The peripheral nervous system, in Emson PC (ed): *Chemical Neuroanatomy*. New York, Raven Press, 1983.
184. Scott FB, Bradley WE, Timm GW: Management of erectile impotence: Use of implantable inflatable prothesis. *Urology* 1973; 2:80.

185. Shabsigh R, Fishman IJ, Quesada ET, et al: Evaluation of vasculogenic erectile impotence using penile duplex ultrasonography. *J Urol* 1989; 142:1469–1474.
186. Shabsigh R, Fishman IJ, Schum C, et al: Cigarette smoking and other vascular risk factors in vasculogenic impotence. *Urology* 1991; 38:227–231.
187. Shabsigh R, Fishman IJ, Shotland Y, et al: Comparison of penile duplex ultrasonography with nocturnal penile tumescence monitoring for the evaluation of erectile impotence. *J Urol* 1990; 143:924–927.
188. Sharplip ID: Penile arteriography in impotence after pelvic trauma. *J Urol* 1981; 126:477–481.
189. Shirai M, Maki A, Takanami M, et al: Content and distribution of vasoactive intestinal polypeptide (VIP) in cavernous tissue of human penis. *Urology* 1990; 35:360–363.
190. Shirai M, Sasaki K, Rikimaru A: Histochemical investigation on the distribution of adrenergic and cholinergic nerves in human penis. *Tohoku J Exp Med* 1972; 107:403–404.
191. Sidi AA: Vasoactive intracavernous pharmacotherapy. *Urol Clin North Am* 1988; 15:95–100.
192. Sidi AA, Cameron JS, Dykstra DD, et al: Vasoactive intracavernous pharmacotherapy for the treatment of erectile impotence in men with spinal cord injury. *J Urol* 1987; 138:539–542.
193. Sonda LP, Mazo R, Chancellor MB: The role of yohimbine for the treatment of erectile impotence. *J Sex Marital Ther* 1990; 16:15–21.
194. Steers WD: Neural control of penile erection. *Semin Urol* 1990; 8:66–79.
195. Stief C, Benard F, Bosch R, et al: Acetylcholine as a possible neurotransmitter in penile erection. *J Urol* 1989; 141:1444–1448.
196. Stief C, Benard F, Diederichs W, et al: The rationale for pharmacologic cavernosography. *J Urol* 1988; 140:1564–1566.
197. Stief C, Benard F, Ruud JLH, et al: A possible role for calcitonin-gene-related peptide in the regulation of the smooth muscle tone of the bladder and penis. *J Urol* 1990; 143:392–397.
198. Stief C, Diederichs W, Benard F, et al: The diagnosis of venogenic impotence: Dynamic or pharmacologic cavernosometry? *J Urol* 1988; 140:1561–1563.
199. Stief C, Diederichs W, Benard F, et al: Possible role for acetylcholine as a neurotransmitter in canine penile erection. *Urol Int* 1989; 44:357–363.
200. Stief C, Wetterauer U, Schaebsdau FH, et al: Calcitonin-gene-related peptide: A possible role in human penile erection and its therapeutic application in impotent patients. *J Urol* 1991; 146:1010–1014.
201. Stief C, Wetterauer U, Sommerkamp H: Intra-individual comparative study of dynamic and pharmacocavernography. *Br J Urol* 1989; 64:93–97.
202. Susset JG, Tessier CD, Wincze J, et al: Effect of yohimbine hydrochloride on erectile impotence: A double-blind study. *J Urol* 1989; 141:1360–1363.
203. Tottrup A, Svane D, Forman A: Nitric oxide mediating NANC inhibition in opossum lower esophageal sphincter. *Am J Physiol* 1991; 260:G385–G389.
204. Traish AM, Carson MP, Kim N, et al: Characterization of muscarinic acetylcholine receptors in human penile corpus cavernosum: Studies on whole tissue and cultured endothelium. *J Urol* 1990; 144:1036–1040.
205. Treiber U, Gilbert P: Venous surgery in erectile dysfunction: A critical report on 116 patients. *Urology* 1989; 34:22–27.
206. Turner LA, Althof SE, Levine SB, et al: Self-injection of papaverine and

phentolamine in the treatment of psychogenic impotence. *J Sex Marital Ther* 1989; 15:163–176.

207. Vardi Y, Belur R, Siroky MB: Pelvic nerve induced relaxation of canine corporal smooth muscle is blocked by atropine. *Fed Proc* 1987; 46:338.

208. Vardi Y, Siroky MB: A canine model for hemodynamic study of isolated corpus cavernosum. *J Urol* 1987; 138:663.

209. Vardi Y, Siroky MB: Hemodynamics of pelvic nerve induced erection in a canine model. 1. Pressure and flow. *J Urol* 1990; 144:794–797.

210. Virag R: Intracavernous injection of papaverine for erectile failure. *Lancet* 1982; 2:938.

211. Virag R, Bouilly P, Frydman D: Is impotence an arterial disorder? *Lancet* 1985; 1:181–184.

212. Virag R, Ottesen B, Fahrenkrug J, et al: Vasoactive intestinal polypeptide release during penile erection in man. *Lancet* 1982; 2:1166.

213. Virag R, Shoukry K, Floresco J, et al: Intracavernous self-injection of vasoactive drugs in the treatment of impotence: 8-Year experience with 615 cases. *J Urol* 1991; 145:287–293.

214. Virag R, Spencer P, Friedman D: Artificial erection in diagnosis and treatment of impotence. *Urology* 1984; 24:157–161.

215. Von Ebner V: Uber Klappenartige Vorrichtungen in den Arterien der Schwellkorger. *Anat Anz* 1900; 18:79.

216. Waldeyer W: Topographisch-anatomisch mit besonderes Berucksichtigung der Chirurgie un gynakologie Dargestellt, in Das Becken, 1899, p 354.

217. Walsh PC, Donker PJ: Impotence following radical prostatectomy: Insight into etiology and prevention. *J Urol* 1982; 128:492.

218. Wassertheil-Smoller S, Blaufox MD, Oberman A, et al: Effect of antihypertensives on sexual function and quality of life: The TAIM study. *Ann Intern Med* 1991; 114:613–620.

219. Weiner N: Norepinephrine, epinephrine and the sympathomimetic amines, in Gilman AG, Goodman LS, Rall TW, et al (eds): *The Pharmacological Basis of Therapeutics*, 7th ed. New York, Macmillan, 1985, pp 145–180.

220. Weiner N, Taylor P: Neurohumoral transmission: The autonomic and somatic motor nervous systems, in Gilman AG, Goodman LS, Rall TW, et al (eds): *The Pharmacological Basis of Therapeutics*, 7th ed. New York, Macmillan, 1985, pp 66–99.

221. Wespes E, Schulman CC: Venous leakage: Surgical treatment of a curable cause of impotence. *J Urol* 1985; 133:796.

222. Willis E, Ottesen B, Wagner G, et al: Vasoactive intestinal polypeptide (VIP) as a possible neurotransmitter involved in penile erection. *Acta Physiol Scand* 1981; 113:545–547.

223. Witherington R: Vacuum constriction device for management of erectile impotence. *J Urol* 1989; 141:320.

224. Wood KS, Buga GM, Byrns RE, et al: Vascular smooth muscle-derived relaxing factor (MDRF) and its close similarity to nitric oxide. *Biochem Biophys Res Commun* 1990, 170:80–88.

225. Zorgniotti AW, Lefleur RS: Auto-injection of corpus cavernosum with a vasoactive drug combination for vasculogenic impotence. *J Urol* 1985; 133:39–41.

The Long-Term Outcome in Vasovasostomy and Vasoepididymostomy

John W. Konnak, M.D.

Professor, Surgery-Urology, The University of Michigan Medical Center, Ann Arbor, Michigan

Bilateral vasectomy for sterilization has been practiced in America for over 75 years, but its popularity as a method of birth control increased dramatically after 1970. For the past 20 years, approximately 500,000 to 1 million vasectomies per year have been performed on American men. It is estimated that 0.5% of these men will seek reversal of vasectomy for a variety of reasons, including, most commonly, divorce and remarriage. Successful vasovasostomy first was reported in 1919, but since that time, techniques and understanding of vasectomy reversal have been refined to the point at which technical success with return of sperm to the ejaculate approaches 90%, with pregnancy rates between 50% and 80%. This chapter will discuss factors that affect these results, including surgical techniques, length of time obstructed, histologic changes in the vasectomized testis, intraoperative findings, antisperm antibodies, and other considerations. In addition, the indications and results of vasoepididymostomy will be discussed.

Surgical Technique

Surgical techniques of vasovasostomy may be classified according to the method of optical technique used and the actual method of anastomosis. Optical techniques include unmagnified, loupe magnification, and microsurgical. Direct comparison of the optical techniques is difficult because earlier series of operations tended to use no magnification, whereas later reports generally described the use of loupes or the operating microscope. Comparison also is made difficult because the authors interpret their data in different ways. Whether the pregnancy rate is based on the entire series or just on patients with sperm in the ejaculate, and how patients who are lost to follow-up are counted can make significant differences in study results. Selected series are shown in Table 1. The series of unmagnified vasovasostomy procedures report return of sperm to the ejaculate in 38% to 90% of patients, with pregnancy rates in partners of 19% to 55%.[1-5, 7, 8]

TABLE 1.
Selected Series of Vasovasostomy

Author	Year	Number of Patients	Optical Aid	Patency Rate, %	Pregnancy Rate, %
Silber[12]*	1989	282	Microscope	91	81
Fallon[10]	1981	36	Loupe	63	57
Phadke and Phadke[1]	1967	46	None	83	55
Lee and McLaughlin[5]	1980	26	Microscope	96	54
Amelar and Dubin[3]	1979	26	Loupe	88	53
Uruhart-Hay[9]	1981	50	Loupe	84	52
Belker et al.[13]	1991	1,247	Microscope	86	52
Lee, H.Y.[7]	1986	324	Microscope	90	51
Lee and McLaughlin[5]	1980	41	None	90	46
Fenster et al.[4]	1981	41	None	90	46
Requeda et al.[6]	1983	47	Microscope	80	46
Cos et al.[14]	1983	87	Microscope	75	46
Middleton et al.[8]	1987	73	None	81	45
Kessler and Freiha[11]	1981	96	Loupe	92	45
Martin[15]	1981	40	Microscope	90	43
Lee, H.Y.[7]	1986	300	Loupe or none	84	35
Amelar and Dubin[3]	1979	93	None	84	33
Derrick et al.[2]	1973	1,630	None	38	19

*Patients with no sperm in vas fluid excluded.

The results of studies employing loupe magnification include patency rates of 63% to 92%, with pregnancy rates of 45% to 57%.[3, 7, 9–11] Using the operating microscope, patency rates of 75% to 96% are reported, with pregnancy rates of 43% to 81%.[5–7, 12–15] The 1980 series of Lee and McLaughlin[5] includes patients operated upon in the same time frame by the same surgeons using both macroscopic and microscopic techniques. Using macroscopic techniques, the patency rate was 90%, with a pregnancy rate of 46%; using the microsurgical method, respective rates were 96% and 54%. H.Y. Lee, in a much larger series, reports macrosurgical (unmagnified or loupe) success rates of 84% for patency and 35% for pregnancy, and microsurgical success rates of 90% for patency and 51% for pregnancy.[7] Although there is considerable overlap, the results tend to favor the microsurgical techniques. This may be due to the fact that micro-surgical techniques allow for the use of finer suture material and permit a more precise mucosa-to-mucosa approximation. Another advantage of the routine use of the operating microscope is that it keeps microsurgical skills current so that they can be employed for other procedures that require microsurgical technique, such as tuble-to-tubule vasoepididymostomy. The main disadvantages of microsurgical techniques are that they require expensive equipment, generally are more time-consuming, and require training and practice to master.

The anastomosis may be done in one or two layers. The two-layer approach usually requires microsurgical technique. The single-layer approach is performed more accurately under the microscope, but may be accomplished macroscopically or with loupes as well. In the single-layer anastomosis (Fig 1), four interrupted 7–0 to 9–0 sutures are placed through the entire wall of the vas. Interrupted 8–0 to 9–0 sutures may be placed in the muscular layer between the primary four sutures to obtain a watertight anastomosis. Sealing the vas with a CO_2 laser after placing the initial sutures has been reported[16] and may be somewhat less time-consuming, but offers no other advantage and requires special equipment. In the two-layer method (Fig 2), a mucosa-to-mucosa anastomosis of the lumen is per-

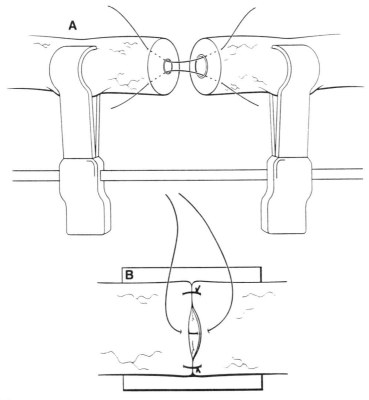

FIG 1.
In the single-layer anastomosis, four interrupted 7–0 to 9–0 nylon sutures are placed at 90 degrees through the full thickness of the vas. Suture size depends on whether magnification is used or not. **A,** placement of the first two sutures. **B,** interrupted 7–0 to 9–0 sutures then may be placed in the muscular layer between the primary sutures to obtain a watertight anastomosis.

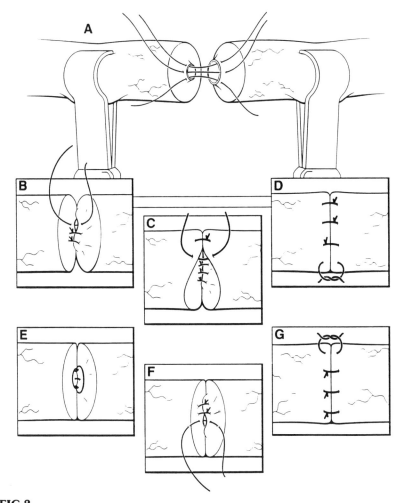

FIG 2.
In the two-layer anastomosis, three interrupted 10–0 nylon sutures are placed through the mucosa (**A**) anteriorly and tied (**B**). The muscular layer is closed over this with 9–0 nylon sutures (**C** and **D**). The vas then is turned over (**E**) and two or three more mucosal sutures are placed (**F**). The muscular layer closure then is completed (**G**). If desired, all the mucosal sutures may be placed before the muscular closure is performed.

formed using five or six interrupted 10–0 sutures. A second layer of interrupted 9–0 sutures is placed in the muscular layer. The patency and pregnancy rates with single- and double-layer anastomoses appear to be similar.[13, 17] The two-layer anastomosis may have an advantage in creating a more precise anastomosis when there is a large size discrepancy between the ends of the vas, or when the anastomosis must be made in the convoluted portion. For surgeons who perform vasovasostomy only occasionally, the single-layer approach probably is preferable. For those who perform frequent procedures and vasoepididymostomies, the two-layer anastomosis has advantages. Indwelling stents are not used routinely. They have no clear-cut advantage[18] and, in one experimental study, had a detrimental effect on patency.[19]

Interval of Obstruction and Histologic Changes in the Vasectomized Testis

The interval of obstruction between the time of vasectomy and vasovasostomy is the single most important factor in predicting technical success and long-term outcome with pregnancy following vasovasostomy.[20] This is illustrated in Figure 3 from the Vasovasostomy Study Group.[13] The reason for the deleterious effect of time is not known. Silber has demonstrated that absence of sperm in the vas fluid at operation is associated with histologic epididymal changes.[20] He believes that these changes are due to extravasation of sperm-containing fluid in the epididymis and that this causes obstruction of the epididymis, which accounts for the absence of sperm. Sharlip believes that the likelihood of this scenario with a concomitant decrease in return of sperm to the ejaculate increases with time, especially if the interval is greater than 12 years.[12] As shown in Figure 3, the Vasovasostomy Study Group has confirmed this decreased incidence of return of sperm to the ejaculate. However, both Sharlip's study and that of the Study Group demonstrate return of sperm to the semen in a significant number of men, and the Study Group found that pregnancy occurred in 30% of the wives of patients with bilateral absence of sperm from the vas fluid.

The histology of the vasectomized testis has been described[22-24] and, in a study by Jarow et al.,[25] biopsies from vasectomized men's testes were compared with those from normal fertile control subjects. Histologic differences were noted in this study, including an increase of thickness of seminiferous tubular walls, an increase in the mean cross-sectional area of the tubules, a reduction in the number of Sertoli's cells and spermatids, and focal fibrosis. Only focal fibrosis correlated with a decrease in the technical success rate and fertility in this study, and this did not seem to increase with time or age of the patient.

Despite these observations, pregnancy has been reported in 30% of partners of patients whose interval of obstruction was 15 years,[13] so a prolonged interval is not a definite contraindication to vasovasostomy.

Intraoperative Findings

Attempts have been made to predict the success of vasovasostomy based on a number of intraoperative observations. These include the presence or absence of a sperm granuloma, and the appearance and quality of the vas

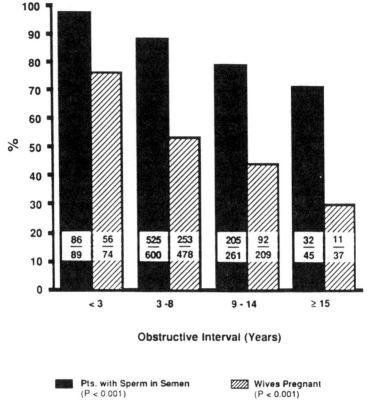

Obstructive Interval (Years)

■ Pts. with Sperm in Semen   ▨ Wives Pregnant
(P < 0.001)   (P < 0.001)

FIG 3.
Pregnancy and patency rates of patients (pts) undergoing vasovasostomy at increasing intervals since vasectomy. Numerator equals number of patients achieving patency or pregnancy; denominator equals total number of patients in each group. (From Belker AM, Thomas AJ, Fuchs EF, et al: *J Urol* 1991; 145:505–511. Used by permission.)

fluid obtained at operation from the proximal cut end of the vas deferens.

A sperm granuloma is believed to form at the vasectomy site due to the extravasation of sperm there. This finding is documented histologically in about 25% of patients undergoing vasovasostomy, and intraoperative vasal fluid quality generally is better if a granuloma is present.[26] The proposed mechanism is a pressure-reducing effect of sperm leaking into the tissue.[20] Despite this, the Vasovasostomy Study Group could demonstrate no beneficial effect on return of sperm to the ejaculate or fertility associated with histologically documented sperm granuloma.[13]

The appearance of the vas fluid ranges from watery to opalescent to creamy, or fluid may be absent. Attempts have been made to correlate the appearance of the fluid with results.[21, 27] There does not seem to be any association between the appearance of the fluid and the interval of obstruction or sperm granuloma.[13, 28] Bilaterally creamy fluid is associated with somewhat poorer quality and lower return of sperm and pregnancy rates (70% and 45%, respectively).[13]

Sperm in the vas fluid range in quality from normal motile sperm, to nonmotile sperm, to mostly sperm heads, all sperm heads, and no sperm. The Vasovasostomy Study Group has used a grading system for vas fluid quality devised by Silber[20] and has shown a decrease in patency and pregnancy rates when quality deteriorates (Fig 4).[13] As discussed previously, patency and pregnancy rates are considerably poorer when sperm is absent bilaterally (60% and 30%, respectively), or when only heads are present. Vasoepididymostomy has been advocated in patients with no sperm in the vas fluid bilaterally,[29 30] but the results with primary vasovasostomy reported by the study group are almost as good as those of most series of

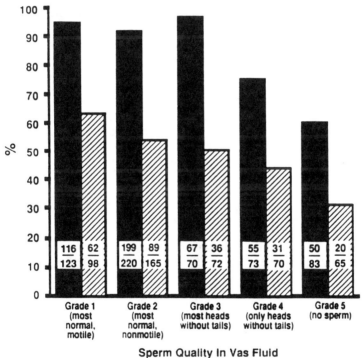

Sperm Quality In Vas Fluid

■ Pts. with Sperm in Semen   ▨ Wives Pregnant

FIG 4.
Patency and pregnancy rates according to quality of sperm in intraoperative vas fluid when sperm quality is identical bilaterally. Numerator equals number of patients (pts) achieving patency or pregnancy; denominator equals total number of patients in each group. (From Belker AM, Thomas AJ, Fuchs EF, et al: *J Urol* 1991; 145:505–511. Used by permission.)

bilateral vasoepididymostomy, and this has led them to advocate primary vasovasostomy in these patients.[13] Possible exceptions are patients with creamy vas fluid and a long interval of obstruction. Silber reports somewhat better results with primary vasoepididymostomy,[30] but his series includes patients operated for reasons other than vasectomy reversal and his results are not confirmed by most other researchers (Table 2.).

Antisperm Antibodies

The production of antibodies to sperm following vasectomy in humans and animals has been well documented for many years.[41] Although antibodies can arise spontaneously, they usually are associated with an injury to the genital tract, such as obstruction, infection, torsion, vasectomy, and other causes.[42] In vasectomy reversal, the original vasectomy, obstruction of the genital tract, sperm granuloma, and the subsequent reversal surgery all may be conducive to the production of antibodies. Ansbacher[43] and others[41, 44, 45] demonstrated circulating serum antibodies in approximately 50% of vasectomized men. Others have demonstrated their presence in seminal plasma in a much lower percentage of patients (~7%).[46–48] Serum antibody titers peak at 6 to 12 months after vasectomy and then decline, persisting in about 30% of patients.[42] Following vasovasostomy, the percentage of patients with detectable serum antibodies remains the same, whereas the percentage of those with seminal plasma antibodies increases to about 30%.[49] Sperm antibodies have been detected and quantified by

TABLE 2.
Selected Series of Vasoepididymostomy

Author	Year	Number of Patients	Optical Aid*	Patency Rate, %	Pregnancy Rate, %
Silber[31]	1989	190	Micro	76	49
Hagner[32]	1936	33	Macro	64	49
Thomas[33]	1986	50	Micro	66	42
Fogdestam[34]	1986	50	Micro	85	37
Schoysman[35]	1986	565	Macro	56	18
Kar and Phadke[36]	1975	281	Macro	49	14
Lee[37]	1978	82	Macro	30	13
Dubin and Amelar[38]	1984	46	Micro	39	13
Hondry[39]	1983	83	Macro	35	11
Dubin and Amelar[38]	1984	69	Macro	20	10
Hanley[40]	1955	71	Macro	16	7

*Micro = microsurgical technique; macro = macrosurgical technique.

sperm agglutination, sperm immobilization, indirect immunofluorescence, enzyme-linked immunosorbent assay, and the immunobead antisperm antibody test. The sperm agglutination and immobilization tests measure serum antibodies that may not be present on the sperm cell surface; for this reason, these tests have been criticized for lack of specificity and sensitivity.[42] The indirect immunofluorescence and enzyme-linked immunosorbent assays use solubilized sperm antigens and probably bear little relationship to infertility and the clinical status of the patient.[42] The immunobead test can be used to detect antisperm antibodies bound to sperm in semen (direct test) or to detect antibodies indirectly in serum, semen, or other fluids. In a recent study, Broderick and McClure[50] used the indirect immunobead test to demonstrate significant (20% binding or more) serum antibodies in 35% of 55 vasectomized men who were undergoing vasovasostomy, and used the direct test to demonstrate significant sperm surface antibodies in 38% of 31 men who had undergone successful vasovasostomy. In addition, they found that preoperative serum assays correctly classified the antibody status of 69% of their patients undergoing vasovasostomy, for a specificity of 79%, the same percentage reported by Helstrom.[51] They also demonstrated an inverse relationship between quantities of sperm surface antigen and percentage of sperm motility, but did not show a correlation with interval of obstruction or patient age. Although agglutinating and immobilizing antisperm antibody tests may lack specificity, Fuchs and Alexander and others[6, 46, 52, 53] demonstrated that fertility rates were lower in patients who had undergone successful vasovasostomy and had low or high antibody titers in serum or seminal plasma. This association has not been supported universally, however, and other studies show no effect on pregnancy of serum antisperm antibodies[12, 54] or sperm-bound antibodies measured by the direct immunobead test.[55]

The effect on fertility of these antibodies is not entirely clear. Surface antibodies should not lyse sperm cells and would not affect sperm count. Gross agglutination or immobilization of sperm, however, very likely would decrease fertility. Immune complexes in the testis might affect fertility, but although these can be demonstrated in the testes of vasectomized guinea pigs[56] and rabbits,[57] they have not been demonstrated in men.[58] Other possible areas of effect include impaired cervical mucus and ova penetration. Bronson demonstrated that sperm rarely were seen in cervical mucus in postcoital testing when all sperm were antibody-bound, compared with normal results when less than 50% of sperm were antibody-bound.[59] Abnormal hamster egg penetration also has been described in association with immune globulin–associated sperm.[60] In vitro fertilization has been shown to be affected adversely when high percentages of sperm are antibody-coated.[61] The clinical implications of these observations are unclear. Future treatments of men who remain infertile following successful vasovasostomy and who have antibody-coated sperm might be directed at reducing the percentage of antibody-coated sperm and then employing assisted reproductive techniques such as in vitro fertilization.

Other Considerations

Other considerations include postoperative semen analysis and female fertility factors.

Following vasovasostomy, initial evaluation of the semen within the first 2 months often reveals low sperm counts with poor motility. The counts and motility improve with time and reach a plateau approximately 1 year following the procedure. This could account for the observation that it took 24 months for the majority of pregnancies to occur in the Vasovasostomy Study Group's series.[13] Patients with sperm counts of 10 million or less have a poorer prognosis for inducing pregnancy than do patients with counts greater than 10 million (31% vs. 55% to 70%). Once the initial counts are greater than 10 million, pregnancy rates are not significantly different regardless of whether the sperm count is 11 to 20 million or more than 60 million (Fig 5).[12, 13] Silber reports similar findings when pregnancy

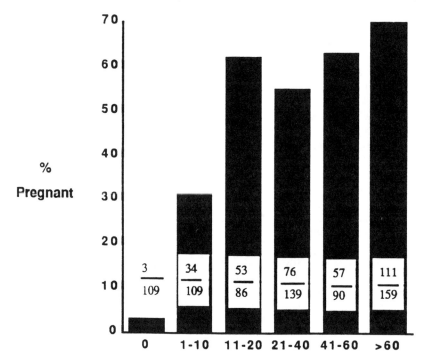

Sperm Count (million/cc)

FIG 5.
Correlation of postoperative sperm count with occurrence of pregnancy after vasectomy reversal. Numerator equals the number of patients achieving pregnancy; denominator equals the total number in the group. (Adapted from Belker AM, Thomas AJ, Fuchs EF, et al: *J Urol* 1991; 145:505–511. Used by permission.)

rates are correlated with sperm motility.[12] The pregnancy rate is reduced only when motility falls below 20%. These observations are based on isolated semen analyses, and may not reflect the semen quality at the time of conception.

Patients with azoospermia or very low sperm counts may be candidates for repeat vasovasostomy, although the results are not as good as with the initial procedure.[13] If these patients have no sperm in the vas fluid, consideration should be given to vasoepididymostomy.

Female factors undoubtedly play a role in the fertility rate following vasovasostomy. There is little information documenting this in the literature. The Vasovasostomy Study Group showed that wives who had been pregnant previously had somewhat better pregnancy rates than did those who had not, but the difference was not statistically significant.[13]

Epididymal Obstruction

The epididymal tubule originates at the coalescence of the efferent ducts from the testis. The tubule itself is convoluted and is contained in the epididymis. The total length of the tubule if it were straightened out would be approximately 4 m. The more proximal portion is contained within the head or caput of the epididymis, whereas the more distal portion is within the body or corpus and the tail or cauda. Epididymal obstruction may develop following vasectomy, as discussed earlier in this chapter. Other causes include inflammation, congenital obstruction, Young's syndrome, and trauma. Inflammatory causes include epididymitis and specific infections such as gonorrhea and tuberculosis. Infections such as tuberculosis, which cause obstruction throughout the length of the tubule, are less amenable to surgical treatment than are infections such as gonorrhea, which usually affect the distal portion. Prompt treatment of these infections has reduced the likelihood of obstruction due to these causes. Congenital obstruction ranges from complete absence of the body and tail of the epididymis to areas of atresia at the distal epididymis or segmentally within the epididymis.[33, 62] Obstruction also may occur proximally at the rete testis, or distally with nonunion of the vas and epididymis or absence of the vas deferens. To be surgically correctable, an appropriate portion of the vas must be present, together with an acceptable portion of the epididymis that connects to the testis. Young's syndrome is a cause of obstruction that often is found in association with bronchitis or bronchiectasis.[63, 64] In this condition, sperm, some partially phagocytized, are found in the caput but not in the distal epididymis. Traumatic causes are rare and must affect both sites to be significant. Most common are iatrogenic injuries that occur during surgery in the scrotum.

Incomplete epididymal obstruction has been implicated as a cause of oligospermia in up to 20% of oligospermic men.[33] In addition, it may be a cause of oligospermia following vasovasostomy for vasectomy reversal. Incomplete obstruction may be suspected based on a history of a certain cause of epididymal obstruction, or in severely oligospermic men who have testes of normal size and normal gonadotropin levels. Testicular biopsy can be considered in selected patients.

The diagnosis of epididymal obstruction usually is based on normal testicular biopsy results together with azoospermia and a normal semen volume. Presence of the vas deferens is determined by palpation and a positive fructose test. In the absence of a history of vasectomy, epididymal obstruction is confirmed by surgical exploration. Intraoperative vasograms need not be done routinely unless vasal obstruction is suspected. The epididymis is explored and samples of epididymal fluid are obtained from the distal portion and examined microscopically. If sperm are not present, samples are obtained more proximally until sperm is encountered. A microsurgical anastomosis between the vas deferens and the epididymal tubule is made at this level.

Technique of Vasoepididymostomy

Early methods of vasoepididymostomy were based on the technique of Martin first reported in 1903.[65] In this method, a fistula is created between the side of the vas deferens and the side of the epididymis. An end-to-side fistula also has been employed (Fig 6). The results of selected larger series

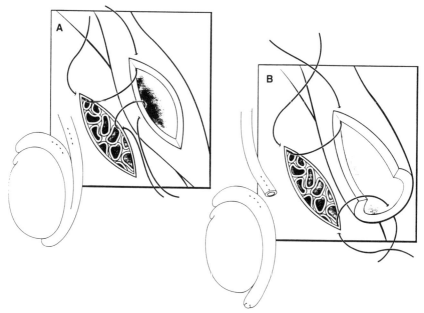

FIG 6.
A, side-to-side method of creating a fistula between the epididymis and vas deferens. A single layer of interrupted 7−0 to 9−0 nylon or polypropylene suture may be employed, depending on whether magnification is used or not. **B,** end-to-side method.

are shown in Table 2.[32, 35–40] Patency rates range from 16% to 64%, with pregnancy rates of 7% to 49%. More recently, microsurgical anastomosis of the vas deferens to the epididymal tubule has been employed. The "specific tubule" technique described by Silber[29] involves serial transection of the epididymis until sperm is encountered. The "specific tubule" from which sperm-laden fluid is demonstrated by microscopic smear is selected for a microsurgical end-to-end anastomosis with the lumen of the vas using 10–0 suture (Fig 7). The muscular layer of the vas is sutured to the investing layer of the epididymis. Others, including this author, have used an end-to-side technique wherein the epididymis is opened at an appropriate level and a portion of the tubule is mobilized and opened longitudinally[33] (see Fig 7). If sperm is demonstrated, the lumen of the vas is anastomosed to the side epididymal tubule using 10–0 suture and the muscular layer is

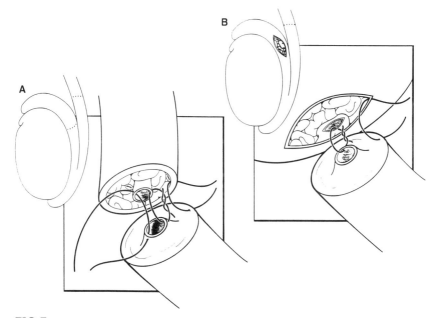

FIG 7.
A, the "specific tubule" method of Silber for creating a vasoepididymostomy. The epididymis is divided and the patent tubule is identified and confirmed by microscopic demonstration of sperm cells. Then the vas is divided and the mucosa of the vas lumen is anastomosed to the patent tubule using interrupted 10–0 nylon sutures. The muscular and adventitial layer is sutured to the epididymal tunic using interrupted 9–0 nylon sutures. **B,** the end-to-side method. The epididymal tunic is incised carefully so as to expose the epididymal tubule without injuring it. A knuckle of tubule is selected, mobilized slightly, and incised under the operating microscope. The fluid from the tubule is examined for sperm. If sperm is present, an anastomosis is made between the tubule and the mucosa of the vas using interrupted 10–0 nylon sutures. The epididymal tunic then is sutured to the muscular and adventitial layer of the vas using interrupted 9–0 nylon sutures.

sutured to the investing layer of the epididymis with 9–0 suture. Selected larger series using these microsurgical techniques are shown in Table 2.[31, 33, 34, 38] Patency rates range from 39% to 85%, with pregnancy rates of 13% to 49%. As in the case of vasovasostomy series, direct comparison of these results is difficult, because the authors interpret their data differently.

The advantage of the side-to-side or end-to-side fistula is simplicity and technical ease of performance. The results are somewhat better with the microsurgical technique, but microsurgical equipment is necessary and the anastomosis is technically difficult and requires microsurgical training and experience to accomplish successfully.

Factors Affecting Results of Vasoepididymostomy

Some of the factors affecting the results of vasovasostomy also may affect the results of vasoepididymostomy. These include histologic changes in the testis, antisperm antibody formation, and sperm count. Reports of the incidence of antisperm antibodies in men with congenital absence of the vas are conflicting, with a rate of 11% in one series[66] and 71% in another.[67] In men with epididymal obstruction who have surgical correction, a postoperative rise in the incidence of sperm antibodies might be expected.[49] As discussed previously, the effect of sperm antibodies on fertility is controversial.

Sperm count apparently affects the pregnancy rate only when the count is very low. Silber reports a decrease in fertility after vasoepididymostomy only when sperm was absent from the ejaculate.[30]

The level of obstruction and anastomosis should have an effect on surgical results. It has been demonstrated that sperm maturation and motility progress as the cells pass through the epididymis. If passage through the epididymis is necessary for fertility, the results of anastomosis to the more proximal caput should be worse than the results of more distal anastomosis. This has been shown to be true to some extent in several studies.[29, 35] In a recent series, Silber reported patency and pregnancy rates of 73% and 31%, respectively, for anastomosis at the caput and 78% and 56%, respectively, for anastomosis at the corpus.[29] These studies demonstrate that transit through the full length of the epididymis is not necessary for fertility, and that even sperm that have not undergone transit through the entire caput may be fertile.

Future Trends

Future trends will deal with improving fertility in patients with successful vasovasostomy and vasoepididymostomy and with using epididymal sperm for achieving pregnancy in the partners of men with absence of the vas deferens. Assisted reproductive techniques such as intrauterine insemination[68] and in vitro fertilization[69] already have shown some success in male factor infertility and are being applied in patients who have undergone vasovasostomy and vasoepididymostomy. Epididymal sperm has been employed successfully in achieving in vitro fertilization and successful pregnancies.[70] Using these techniques, fertility rates approaching normal may be possible in these patients.

References

1. Phadke GM, Phadke AG: Experience in the reanastomosis of the vas deferens. *J Urol* 1967, 97:888–890.
2. Derrick FC, Yarbrough W, D'Agostine J: Vasovasostomy: Results of questionnaire of members of the American Urological Association. *J Urol* 1973; 110:556–557.
3. Amelar RD, Dubin L: Vasectomy reversal. *J Urol* 1979; 121:547–550.
4. Fenster H, McLoughlin MG: Vasovasostomy—is the microscope necessary? *Urology* 1981; 18:60–64.
5. Lee L, McLaughlin MG: Vasovasostomy: A comparison of macroscopic and microscopic techniques at one institution. *Fertil Steril* 1980; 33:54–55.
6. Requeda E, Charron J, Roberts K: Fertilizing capacity and sperm antibodies in vasovasostomized men. *Fertil Steril* 1983; 39:197–203.
7. Lee HY: A 20-year experience with vasovasostomy. *J Urol* 1986; 136: 413–415.
8. Middleton RG, Smith JA, Moore MH, et al: A 15-year followup of a nonmicrosurgical technique for vasovasostomy. *J Urol* 1987; 137:886–887.
9. Uruhart-Hay D: A low power magnification technique of reanastomosis of the vas. *Br J Urol* 1981; 53:466–469.
10. Fallon B, Miller RK, Gerber W: Nonmicroscopic vasovasostomy. *J Urol* 1981; 126:361–362.
11. Kessler R, Freiha F: Macroscopic vasovasostomy. *Fertil Steril* 1981; 36:531–532.
12. Silber SJ: Pregnancy after vasovasostomy for vasectomy reversal: A study of factors affecting long-term return of fertility in 282 patients followed for 10 years. *Hum Reprod* 1989; 4:318–322.
13. Belker AM, Thomas AJ, Fuchs EF, et al: Results of 1469 microsurgical vasectomy reversals by the vasovasostomy study group. *J Urol* 1991; 145: 505–511.
14. Cos LR, Valvo JR, Davis RS: Vasovasostomy: Current state of the art. *Urology* 1983; 22:567–575.
15. Martin DC: Microsurgical reversal of vasectomy. *Am J Surg* 1981; 142:48–50.
16. Rosemberg SK: Clinical use of carbon dioxide (CO2) laser in microsurgical vasovasostomy. *Urology* 1987; 29:372–374.
17. Sharlip ID: Vasovasostomy: Comparison of two microsurgical techniques. *Urology* 1981; 17:347–352.
18. Roland SI: Splinted and non-splinted vasovasostomy. *Fertil Steril* 1961; 12:191–195.
19. Fernandes M, Shaw KN, Draper JW: Vasovasostomy: Improved microsurgical technique. *J Urol* 1968; 100:763–766.
20. Silber SJ: Microscopic vasectomy reversal. *Fertil Steril* 1977; 28:1191–1201.
21. Sharlip ID: The significance of intravasal azoospermia during vasovasostomy: Answer to a surgical dilemma. *Fertil Steril* 1982; 38:496–498.

22. Gupta AS, Kothare LK, Dhruva A, et al: Surgical sterilization and its effect on the structure and function of the testis in man. *Br J Surg* 1975; 62:59–63.
23. Jenkins IL, Muir VY, Blacklock NJ, et al: Consequences of vasectomy: An immunological and histological study related to subsequent fertility. *B J Urol* 1979; 51:406–410.
24. Mehrotra R, Nath P, Tandon P, et al: Ultrastructural appearances of interstitial tissue of testis in vasectomized individuals. *Indian J Med Res* 1983; 77: 347–352.
25. Jarow JP, Budin RE, Dym M, et al: Quantitative pathologic changes in the human testis after vasectomy. *N Engl J Med* 1985; 313:1252–1285.
26. Belker AM, Konnak JW, Sharlip ID, et al: Intraoperative observations during vasovasostomy in 334 patients. *J Urol* 1983; 129:524–527.
27. Silber SJ: Epididymal extravasation following vasectomy as a cause for failure of vasectomy reversal. *Fertil Steril* 1979; 31:309–315.
28. Sharlip ID, Belker AM, Konnak JW, et al: Relationship of gross appearance of the vas fluid during vasovasostomy to sperm quality, obstructive interval, and sperm granuloma. *J Urol* 1984; 131:681–683.
29. Silber SJ: Microscopic vasoepididymostomy: Specific microanastomosis to the epididymal tubule. *Fertil Steril* 1978; 30:565–576.
30. Silber SJ: Results of microsurgical vasoepididymostomy: Role of epididymis in sperm maturation. *Hum Reprod* 1989; 4:298–303.
31. Silber SJ: Results of microsurgical vasoepididymostomy: Role of epididymis in sperm maturation. *Hum Reprod* 1989; 4:298–303.
32. Hagner FR: The operative treatment of sterility in the male. *JAMA* 1936; 107:1851.
33. Thomas AJ: Vasoepididymostomy. *Urol Clin North Am* 1987; 14:527–538.
34. Fogdestam I, Fall M, Nilsson S: Microsurgical epididymovasostomy in the treatment of occlusive azoospermia. *Fertil Steril* 1986; 46:925–929.
35. Schoysman RJ, Bedford JM: The role of the human epididymis in sperm maturation and sperm storage as reflected in the consequences of epididymovasostomy. *Fertil Steril* 1986; 46:293–299.
36. Kar JK, Phadke AM: Vasoepididymal anastomosis. *Fertil Stenl* 1975; 26:743–756.
37. Lee HY: Corrective surgery of obstructive azoospermia. *Arch Androl* 1978; 1:115–121.
38. Dubin L, Amelar RD: Magnified surgery for epididymovasostomy. *Urology* 1984; 23:525–528.
39. Hendry WF, Parslow JM, Stedronska J: Exploratory scrototomy in 168 azoospermic males. *Br J Urol* 1983; 55:785–791.
40. Hanley HG: The surgery of male infertility. *Ann R Coll Surg Engl* 1955; 17:159.
41. Alexander NJ, Anderson DJ: Vasectomy: Consequences of autoimmunity to sperm antigens. *Fertil Steril* 1979; 32:253–260.
42. Haas GG: Antibody-mediated causes of male infertility. *Urol Clin North Am* 1987; 14:539–550.
43. Ansbacher R, Hodge P, Williams A, et al: Vas ligation: Humoral sperm antibodies. *Int J Fertil* 1976; 21:258–260.
44. Shulman S, Zappi E, Amed U, et al: Immunologic consequences of vasectomy. *Contraception* 1972; 5:269–278.
45. Tung KSK: Human sperm antigens and antibodies. 1. Studies on vasectomy patients. *Exp Immunol* 1975; 20:93–104.

46. Royle MG, Parslow JM, Kingscott MMB, et al: Reversal of vasectomy: The effect of sperm antibodies on subsequent fertility. *Br J Urol* 1981; 53:654–659.
47. Linnet L, Hort T: Sperm agglutinins in seminal plasma and serum after vasectomy. Correlation between immunological and clinical findings. *Clin Exp Immunol* 1977; 30:413–420.
48. Hellema HWJ, Samuel T, Rumke P: Sperm autoantibodies as a consequence of vasectomy. *Clin Exp Immunol* 1979; 38:31–36.
49. Linnet L, Hjort T, Fogh-Andersen P: Association between failure to impregnate after vasovasostomy and sperm agglutinins in semen. *Lancet* 1981; 1:117–119.
50. Broderick GA, Tom R, McClure RD: Immunological status of patients before and after vasovasostomy as determined by the immunobead antisperm antibody test. *J Urol* 1989; 142:752–755.
51. Helstrom JG, Overstreet JW, Samules SJ, et al: The relationship of circulating antisperm antibodies to sperm surface antibodies in infertile men. *J Urol* 1988; 140:1039–1044.
52. Fuchs EF, Alexander NJ: Immunologic considerations of vasovasostomy. *Fertil Steril* 1983; 40:497–499.
53. Sullivan MJ, Howe GE: Correlation of circulating antisperm antibodies to functional success in vasovasostomy. *J Urol* 1977; 117:189–191.
54. Thomas AJ, Pontes JE, Rose NR, et al: Microsurgical vasovasostomy: Immunologic consequences and subsequent fertility. *Fertil Steril* 1981; 35:447–451.
55. Newton RA: IgG antisperm antibodies attached to sperm do not correlate with infertility following vasovasostomy. *Microsurgery* 1988; 9:278–280.
56. Muir VY, Turk JL, Hanley HG: Comparison of allergic aspermatogenesis with that induced by vasectomy. 1. In vivo studies in the guinea pig. *Clin Exp Immunol* 1976; 24:72–80.
57. Bigazzi PE, Kosuda LL, Hsu KC, et al: Immune complex orchitis in vasectomized rabbits. *J Exp Med* 1976; 143:382–404.
58. Bagshaw HA, Masters JRW, Prior JP: Factors influencing the outcome of vasectomy reversal. *Br J Urol* 1980; 542:57–60.
59. Bronson RA, Cooper GW, Rosenfeld DL: Autoimmunity of spermatozoa: Effect on sperm penetration of cervical mucus as reflected by postcoital testing. *Fertil Steril* 1984; 41:609–614.
60. Haas GG: The inhibitory effect of sperm-associated immunoglobulins on cervical mucus penetration. *Fertil Steril* 1986; 46:334–337.
61. Clark GN, Lopata A, McBain JC, et al: Effect of sperm antibodies in males on human in vitro fertilization (IVF). *Am J Reprod Immunol* 1985; 8:62–66.
62. Michelson L: Congenital anomalies of the ductus deferens and epididymis. *J Urol* 1949; 61:384.
63. Young D: Surgical treatment of male infertility. *J Reprod Fertil* 1970; 23:541–542.
64. Hughes TM, Skolnick JL, Belker AM: Young's syndrome: An often unrecognized correctable cause of obstructive azoospermia. *J Urol* 1987; 137:1238–1240.
65. Martin E, Carnett JB, Levi NV: The surgical treatment of sterility due to obstruction at the epididymis. Together with a study of the morphology of human spermatozoa. *Univ Pennsylvania Med Bull* 1903; 15:2.
66. Patrizio P, Moretti-Rojas I, Ord T, et al: Low incidence of sperm antibodies in men with congenital absence of the vas deferens. *Fertil Steril* 1989; 52:1018–1021.

67. Girgis SM, Ekladios EM, Iskander R, et al: Sperm antibodies in serum and semen in men with bilateral congenital absence of the vas deferens. *Arch Androl* 1982; 8:301–305.
68. Belker AM, Cook CL: Sperm processing and intrauterine insemination for oligospermia. *Urol Clin North Am* 1987; 14:597–607.
69. Gibbons W: In vitro fertilization of male-factor infertility. *Urol Clin North Am* 1987; 14:563–567.
70. Ord T, Marillo E, Patrizio P, et al: The role of the laboratory in the handling of epididymal sperm for assisted reproductive technologies. *Fertil Steril* 1992; 57:1103–1106.

Microscopic Epididymal Sperm Aspiration and the Use of New Sperm Processing Techniques for Male Factor Infertility

Mark Sigman, M.D.

Assistant Professor of Urology, Division of Urology, Brown University;
Department of Urology, Rhode Island Hospital, Providence, Rhode Island

Vasal abnormalities are uncommon, but not rare, findings. Both unilateral and bilateral absence of the vas deferens occur. Only bilateral absence of the vas deferens will result in infertility unless a unilaterally absent vas is associated with a contralateral abnormality. Bilateral congenital absence of the vas (BCAV) is identified in about 1% of men who undergo infertility evaluation.[1-4] About 10% of infertile males have azoospermia. In most cases, this total sterility is due to defective spermatogenesis and not to obstruction. About 5% to 10% of patients with obstructive azoospermia, however, have BCAV.[4, 5] Since about 15% of couples are unable to conceive and, in about 30%, the cause is a pure male factor, this yields an incidence of BCAV in the general population of about 0.05%.

Embryology

The development of the genital ductal and urinary systems are intimately linked. During the fourth week of gestation, somites from condensed mesoderm form the pronephric duct. Although this structure presumably does not function in human embryos, its caudal portion forms the mesonephric (wolffian) duct. Soon after the mesonephric duct appears, mesonephric tubules begin to be seen. These tubules are induced by the advancing ampulla of the mesonephric duct. By the end of the fourth week, the mesonephric duct contacts the urogenital sinus. It is at this point that the metanephric duct (ureteral bud) appears. Whereas the mesonephros functions in the embryo, the caudal mesonephric nephrons degenerate as the cranial nephrons persist and contribute to the formation of the genital ductal system. The genital ducts are identical in the male and female embryo until the tenth week of development. Beginning during the fourth week of gestation, the gonadal ridges form. This is followed by the migration of germ cells from the endoderm of the yolk sac into the genital ridges. This process is complete by the end of the fifth week of human development. Male differentiation begins in the seventh week of gestation, when spermatogenic cords begin to form in the fetal testis. These cords differentiate into seminiferous tubules and the rete testis. After 12 weeks of gestation, the rete testis connects to the remnants of the mesonephric tubules, now known as the epigenitalis, to form the efferent ductules. The mesonephric duct develops proximally into the epididymis. The medial portion develops into the vas deferens, whereas the distal portion dilates to become the ampulla of the vas. The seminal vesicle develops as an outpouching of the distal portion of the mesonephric duct. The seminal vesicle and ampulla of the vas join to form the ejaculatory duct. At about 9 weeks of gestation, the rete cords join the remaining 5 to 12 cranial mesonephric tubules and become the efferent ductules. These tubules penetrate the tunica albuginea, elongate, convolute, and finally connect with the mesonephric duct.[6] Thus, the efferent ductules, when mature, consist of a combination of rete testes and mesonephric tubules. Since the rete testes are derived from the genital ridge, one may expect that, with isolated mesonephric duct abnormalities, the efferent ductules that make up the caput epididymis may not be affected.[7]

Anatomy

Although most cases of BCAV involve the entire vas deferens, there is considerable variation in the findings at its proximal and distal aspects. As can be predicted from an understanding of genital embryology, a defect occurring before 4 weeks of gestation may result in the absence of the genital ducts, as well as of the ureter and kidney. Embryologic abnormalities occurring after this period of time would be expected to be associated only with genital ductal abnormalities. Finally, one would expect the caput epididymis to be present in most cases, since it is an embryologic derivative of the mesonephric tubules and rete testes, and not of the mesonephric duct. The caput epididymis is present almost invariably, being reported in 88% to 100% of cases.[7, 8] Three patterns of epididymal anatomy are found in these patients. The presence of only the caput epididymis bilaterally is reported in about 61% of patients, whereas the presence of complete epididymides bilaterally is reported in about 32%; only 7% of patients demonstrate a complete epididymis on one side and a partial epididymis on the other.[4, 8, 9] The vas deferens may be completely absent or, in some cases, a thin fibrous cord may be present. Since the seminal vesicles are derivatives of the mesonephric duct, one would expect them also to be absent in these patients. With the use of computed tomographic scanning and, subsequently, of transrectal ultrasound, it has been found that, in the majority of patients, unilateral or bilateral seminal vesicles are present. Using computed tomographic scanning, Goldstein and Schlossberg[5] identified seminal vesicles bilaterally in 46% of patients with BCAV. A unilateral seminal vesicle was identified in 31% of patients, and complete bilateral absence or hypoplasia of the seminal vesicles was present in only 23%. It has been hypothesized that the low-volume ejaculates and fructose-negative semen often found in many of these patients may be due to an absence of the ejaculatory ducts in patients in whom the seminal vesicles are present. This hypothesis is difficult to prove, since nondilated ejaculatory ducts often are not visualized by present imaging techniques. Testicular biopsies generally reveal normal spermatogenesis.[4, 9] Electron microscopy of testicular biopsies of patients with BCAV has demonstrated mild acrosome abnormalities similar to the findings in patients who have undergone vasectomy, indicating that these changes are secondary to obstruction and not to an inherent defect in spermatogenesis.[10] Unilateral renal agenesis has been found in about 10% of patients, most commonly on the left side.[9]

Clinical Evaluation

Since BCAV generally is associated only with urogenital abnormalities, patients with this disorder present with primary infertility. Unilateral absence of the vas, if associated with a normal contralateral genital ductal system, is identified most often during evaluation for a vasectomy, not for infertility. Since the only common urinary tract abnormality is unilateral renal agenesis, this is diagnosed most often following the finding of BCAV. Although low seminal volume is associated with this condition, at the time of presentation, most patients do not realize that their ejaculate volume is low.

The key to diagnosis is the physical examination. Careful examination of the spermatic cords will reveal absence of the vas deferens. Although, in some cases, a thin, fibrous cord may be palpated, a careful examination of the cords generally will show clearly that the vas deferens is absent. It should be stressed that during evaluation , the vas deferens must be identified specifically because, in our experience, referring physicians have not always noted its absence. Palpation of the epididymides generally reveals whether they are complete or only partially present. In some patients, a small proximal portion of convoluted vas can be palpated in the region of the tail of the epididymis. Since occasional patients present with segmental vasal agenesis, the entire scrotal cord should be palpated for the presence of the vas deferens. Testicular volume and consistency usually are normal.[3] Semen analysis always reveals azoospermia. Although the average seminal volume is low (less than 1 cc), some patients will have normal seminal volumes.[3, 4, 8] Semen volume does not necessarily correlate with the presence or absence of the seminal vesicles, but may correlate with the presence or absence of ejaculatory ducts. Since the seminal vesicles contribute the seminal components responsible for coagulation, semen in these patients remains liquefied. Seminal vesicle fluid is alkaline, whereas prostatic secretions are acidic; therefore, the seminal pH may be on the acidic side compared with a normal seminal pH of 7.4 or greater. It must be emphasized, however, that this is not a universal finding, and some studies have reported alkaline pH levels ranging from 7.4 to 8.4 in these patients.[8] Seminal fructose often is absent, but may be present in low concentrations. Thus, qualitative tests for fructose may be positive in 25% of patients. Urinary gonadotropins and serum testosterone levels generally are normal. Acquired genital ductal obstruction such as that from vasectomy is associated with the development of antisperm antibodies in about two thirds of patients. Similar findings have been reported when patients with BCAV have been examined for the presence of serum agglutinating antisperm antibodies.[11, 12] In contrast, a recent study found no agglutinating or immobilizing antibodies in the sera of 20 patients with BCAV, and only 11% of these patients demonstrated serum antisperm antibodies as determined by the indirect immunobead assay.[13] Sperm agglutinins were identified in 29% of semen samples,[11] but none were found to have seminal antisperm antibodies when the indirect immunobead assay was used.

Diagnosis

Azoospermic patients with testes of normal size and nonpalpable vas deferens have congenital absence of the vas. Generally, low seminal volumes and normal serum follicle-stimulating hormone levels also are present. These findings are sufficient for the diagnosis of BCAV, and a scrotal exploration is neither indicated nor necessary. Any exploration will make subsequent epididymal aspiration procedures more difficult. A renal ultrasound generally should be performed once the diagnosis is made, since the patient should be informed if he has a unilateral kidney. Transrectal ultrasound, although of academic interest, will not change the diagnosis or treatment in these patients and, therefore, is not necessary.

Etiology

The etiology of BCAV has remained a mystery for many years. Although most cases appear to be isolated, reports of familial occurrence have appeared in the literature. Inheritance patterns have been described as autosomal recessive, X-linked recessive, autosomal dominant, or polygenic.[14, 15] Karyotypic studies of patients with BCAV generally have revealed normal karyotypes.[4] Occasional karyotypic abnormalities such as pericentric inversions,[16] mosaicism,[17] and Klinefelter's syndrome[18] have been reported.

Patients with cystic fibrosis (CF) almost invariably have absent vas deferens. In addition, epididymal and seminal vesicle abnormalities are similar to those in patients with BCAV. In contrast, patients with CF typically have pulmonary abnormalities, with a history of recurrent pulmonary infections due to inspissated secretions. Diabetes and gastrointestinal abnormalities resulting from malabsorption are common as well. A key finding in patients with CF is an inability to reabsorb sodium and chloride that results in perspiration containing higher than normal levels of sodium. The sweat test has been used for the diagnosis of CF for many years. Recently the CF gene has been mapped to chromosome 7.[19-21] Subsequent cloning of the gene has allowed genetic screening for CF.[22] The CF gene product is a transmembrane conductance regulator 1,480 amino acid residues long. There are about 11 known mutations found on the CF gene in patients with CF. The most common mutation is delta F508. Although a possible association between BCAV and CF has been hypothesized for many years,[23] screening was not possible until the cloning of the CF gene. Rigot and colleagues studied 19 patients with BCAV for the presence of the delta F508 mutation. Eight of the patients were found to be heterozygous for this mutation. Two patients were found to have abnormal sweat tests.[24] Anguiano and associates[25] performed genetic screening on 25 patients with BCAV and identified at least one CF mutation in 16 of them (64%). Three patients were found to be compound heterozygotes (containing two different mutations, one in the paternal and one in the maternal copy of the CF gene). In addition, they reported the identification of a new mutation not previously found in patients with CF. Three patients had abnormal sweat tests as well. Thus, it appears likely that BCAV is a variant of CF and that, as additional CF mutations are identified, the majority of patients with BCAV will be found to have mutations in this gene. This implies that dysfunction of the CF transmembrane conductance regulator protein may be responsible for the abnormal embryologic development of the wolffian duct structures. About 1 of every 25 people in the general population is a carrier of the CF trait (a mutation in one of the two copies of the CF gene). Thus, couples being evaluated for entrance into a microsurgical epididymal sperm aspiration program should undergo counseling and screening for CF. Both the patient and his spouse should be screened for CF mutations. In addition, the patient's siblings should be evaluated and counseled about the risk of having a child with CF and the subsequent pulmonary and gastrointestinal dysfunctions.

Treatment

Attempts have been made for many years to inseminate women using sperm obtained from patients with BCAV. In 1956, Hanley reported a successful pregnancy and delivery following insemination of sperm obtained from a spermatocele in a patient with BCAV.[26] Schoysman popularized the use of saphenous vein grafted onto the epididymis in an attempt to form a spermatocele; four pregnancies were achieved in 17 attempts.[27] Other investigators found that saphenous vein grafts degenerated and became fibrotic. Still other investigators have used different tissue, such as tunica vaginalis, but no successful pregnancies have been reported.[9, 28] Multiple variations of artificial spermatoceles have been devised. These have been based on the theory that an alloplastic spermatocele could be attached to the epididymis and sperm subsequently could be aspirated from the spermatocele and used for artificial insemination. Turner, in reviewing the literature, reported the use of 72 alloplastic spermatoceles in 52 patients with only 3 resulting term pregnancies.[29] Another review of 130 alloplastic spermatocele implantations reported a 7.7% pregnancy rate and a 4.4% live birth rate in 91 couples.[30] These authors found that pregnancies only occurred when intraoperative epididymal fluid demonstrated sperm with greater than 20% motility at the time of alloplastic spermatocele implantation. Frequent aspirations did not improve sperm motility. Materials such as polytetrafluoroethylene, silicone, and knitted polypropylene have been used to design spermatoceles. Poor sperm numbers and quality have been a consistent problem with the use of these devices. Research into the proper microenvironment, which will allow increased sperm viability as well as different methods of anastomosis to maintain a patent anastomosis, need to be investigated. These devices no longer are used on a routine clinical basis. Until alloplastic spermatoceles are improved such that multiple viable sperm with adequate fertilizing capacity can be obtained, these devices should not be implanted.

Although epididymal aspiration with subsequent insemination has been used sporadically for many years,[9] it was not until Pryor's report in 1984 that ductal aspiration was combined with modern assisted reproductive techniques.[31] In the first couple treated, azoospermia was secondary to acquired obstruction that was not surgically correctable. A pregnancy was initiated, but a miscarriage occurred. Temple-Smith reported an ongoing pregnancy that was achieved using microsurgical epididymal aspiration combined with in vitro fertilization in a male with secondary obstructed azoospermia.[32] The first successful pregnancies using microsurgical epididymal sperm aspiration (MESA) were reported in 1987.[33] MESA now is the treatment of choice for BCAV. Other potential candidates for MESA include anejaculatory patients who are unresponsive to electroejaculation and patients with obstructive azoospermia that is not surgically correctable, whether it is due to a failed vasectomy reversal, nonreconstructable vasal anomalies, or failed transurethral resection of the ejaculatory ducts.[34] More experience is needed to determine which patients will be optimal candidates for this procedure.

Technique

MESA involves close coordination between the urologist and the gynecologist. The female partner is given hormonal stimulation to induce super ovulation (the induction of multiple follicles per ovulatory cycle). Both oocyte aspiration and MESA occur on the same day. Since the time of oocyte retrieval is determined only 24 to 48 hours before the procedure, scheduling of operating room time usually is difficult. In some centers, the oocytes are retrieved first and MESA proceeds only if adequate eggs are retrieved. This approach ensures that the man will undergo surgery only when adequate eggs are guaranteed. On the other hand, eggs may be retrieved unnecessarily in those cases in which adequate numbers of sperm are not aspirated from the man. Other centers proceed with MESA first and perform egg retrieval only when adequate numbers of sperm are obtained. Often, the relative timing of oocyte and sperm aspiration is determined by the availability of the operating room. Although it is easy to perform multiple cycles of egg retrieval, each subsequent MESA procedure becomes increasingly more difficult because of tunical and epididymal scarring. Thus, we generally prefer that oocyte retrieval be performed first, and then we proceed with MESA once adequate oocytes have been retrieved.

MESA can be performed under local anesthesia but it requires the use of an operating room and operating microscope. Bilateral spermatic cord blocks at the level of the external inguinal ring are performed by the instillation of 0.5% bupivacaine (Marcaine) into each cord. A mixture of bupivacaine and lidocaine (Xylocaine) then may be used to infiltrate the scrotal skin, and a vertical hemiscrotal incision is made over the testes. We generally explore one side first and only proceed to the other side if adequate numbers of sperm are not obtained from the first side. The testis is delivered through the wound and the tunica vaginalis is opened. The epididymis then is examined to determine its anatomy. From this point on, the procedure is performed with the use of the operating microscope at 20 to 40× magnification. In early series, the epididymis was opened in its most distal aspect. It appears that in the majority of patients, however, motile sperm are found more proximally, toward the caput, and we usually do not open the tail of the epididymis, but begin epididymal exploration at the junction of the corpus and caput, and then proceed proximally if necessary. The tunica of the epididymis is grasped with microforceps and incised. Using blunt dissection, an individual epididymal tubule is freed from the surrounding connective tissue. The length of the incision is 2 to 5 mm, creating a trough into which epididymal fluid will collect and can be aspirated. Meticulous hemostasis with bipolar microforceps is essential. The wall of one individual epididymal tubule then is opened. This may be performed using a pointed microsurgical blade or microscissors. Others recommend against incising the tubule, and instead suggest using a micropipette to pierce the wall of the epididymal tubule and then aspiration of the fluid.[35] Once the tubule is incised, epididymal fluid will flow into the trough created by the incision of the tunica of the epididymis. A 24-gauge angiocath attached to a 3-cc syringe is used to aspirate a small volume of fluid, which is dropped into a sterile microscopic slide. This is examined under 400× magnification for the presence of motile sperm. If no motile sperm are identified, an epididymotomy is made in a more proximal portion of the epididymis. If motile sperm are obtained, they are aspirated into a syringe containing 0.3 to 0.5 cc of human tubule fluid with N-(2-hydroxyethyl) piperazine N'-(2-ethane sulfonic acid) (HEPES) buffer. Intermittently, the fluid in the syringe is expelled into a warmed tube containing additional human tubule fluid. Aspiration proceeds for 30 to 60 minutes. In general, if the epididymal fluid is thick and pasty, sperm will not be present; however, clarity of the fluid does not guarantee the presence of motile sperm. The flow of fluid from the epididymal tubule may be intermittent and occasionally is assisted by milking the epididymis. Following aspiration, the epididymotomy is closed with a single 10-0 double-armed nylon suture and the tunica of the epididymis is closed with several 9-0 nylon sutures. The testis should be placed back into the tunica vaginalis, which is closed with a running 4-0 chromic suture. The testis is placed back in the scrotum and the scrotum is closed in a standard fashion. The sperm then are transferred to the andrology laboratory for processing. The number of sperm retrieved varies considerably between patients. In an initial series, Silber reported obtaining progressively motile sperm in 62% of 32 patients. Numbers of sperm retrieved varied from 0 to 119 million, with motilities ranging from 0% to 30% and forward progressions being 0 to 3. In the majority of cases, motilities were 20% or less. Pregnancies were more likely when sperm demonstrated greater than 10% motility.[36] Using computer-assisted semen analysis, Davis and colleagues found that fertilization was more likely to occur in those patients with a higher proportion of motile cells and in whom the sperm were capable of undergoing capacitation.[37] Thus it is clear that the quality of sperm obtained appears to be quite poor.

Semen Processing

Following the collection of epididymal fluid, the sperm must be processed prior to insemination of the eggs. Although there are various semen processing techniques, they all involve the removal of epididymal fluid and subsequent concentration of the remaining sperm into a small volume (Table 1). More sophisticated processing techniques also select only the motile sperm, removing nonmotile sperm, cellular debris, and white blood cells.

TABLE 1.
Semen Processing Techniques

Sperm wash
Swim-up
Sedimentation
Percoll gradient centrifugation
Glass wool filtration
Nycodenze gradient centrifugation
Ficoll swim-up
Swim-down
Hyaluronic acid swim-up
Sephadex column filtration

For fertilization to occur, sperm must undergo capacitation and the acrosome reaction. Capacitation is a complete series of events involving changes in cell surface carbohydrates, proteins, and lipids.[38, 39] Other changes that take place during capacitation include an increase of adenylate cyclase activity, an influx of calcium ions, and the formation of acrosin from proacrosin.[40, 41] Following capacitation, sperm may undergo the acrosome reaction when exposed to appropriate inducers. The acrosome reaction consists of a fusion of the sperm plasma membrane and the acrosomal membrane, producing vesicles and the eventual release of the acrosomal contents. The zona pellucida, which is a glycoprotein layer surrounding human eggs, is an inducer of the acrosome reaction.[42] Acrosome-reacted sperm then burrow through the zona pellucida, reaching the para-vitelline space, where they then may penetrate the oolemma. Although capacitation normally occurs within the female reproductive tract, the appropriate use of semen-processing media makes it possible for capacitation to occur in vitro. The acrosome reaction generally is not induced in the absence of human ova, but is allowed to occur when the sperm meet the zona pellucida of the ova.

Although a simple sperm wash commonly is used to prepare sperm for intrauterine insemination, this technique generally is not applied in cases of MESA. For in vitro fertilization techniques, clean samples without numerous nonmotile sperm are desired; therefore, alternative processing techniques usually are employed. The swim-up technique is one of the most commonly used methods for standard in vitro fertilization. This technique involves centrifugation of the sperm followed by removal of the supernatant and layering of a clean media on top of the pellet. Motile sperm are allowed to swim into the supernatant and the supernatant subsequently is aspirated. Poor yields often are obtained with the swim-up technique and, therefore, it usually is not used for MESA, since the numbers of motile sperm often are a limiting factor. Sperm sedimentation attempts to increase yields by allowing a resuspended pellet to sit. Nonmotile sperm often will fall to the bottom, leaving a fraction of highly motile sperm in the supernatant.[43]

Percoll consists of a suspension of colloidal silica that may be used to prepare a gradient. Sperm are layered on top of the gradient, and centrifugation is performed. Motile sperm will form a pellet at the bottom of the gradient and may be collected. Discontinuous gradients are employed most frequently, but there is much variation in the number and percentages of Percoll used for these gradients. A commonly used preparation in non-MESA settings involves the use of a 45%/90% Percoll gradient.[44] Most recently, mini-Percoll centrifugation has been used in cases of MESA.[45] This technique involves layering 0.3 mL of washed epididymal sperm on top of a discontinuous Percoll gradient consisting of 0.3-mL layers of 50%, 70%, and 95% isotonic Percoll. Following centrifugation, the 95% layer is removed, washed, and resuspended in culture media. Using this procedure, Silber and coworkers recovered 1.1 to 34 million sperm with motilities of 1% to 60%. Again, the majority of postprocessed sperm had low motilities of 30% or less, somewhat higher than preprocessed samples.[36]

Fertilization

There are multiple assisted reproductive techniques in use today. The simplest of these involves manipulation of sperm, which then are placed inside the female, where fertilization occurs. Intrauterine insemination involves the placement of processed sperm inside the female reproductive tract. Although this is used commonly for male and female factor infertility, due to the low numbers of sperm obtained from patients with BCAV, this technique is generally not applied in MESA. In vitro fertilization involves the in vitro insemination of human eggs with sperm. Following fertilization, the embryo may be placed into the woman's uterus, as with standard in vitro fertilization-embryo transfer, or into the fallopian tube, as in zygote interfallopian transfer. Using these techniques, fertilization rates (the number of ova fertilized divided by the total number of ova inseminated) have ranged from 6% to 35%, averaging about 30%.[46, 47] This rate is significantly below the 90% fertilization rates that are obtained routinely with in vitro fertilization couples with female factor infertility. In an initial series of 28 men undergoing 32 treatment cycles, a per-cycle pregnancy rate of 31% was obtained, with a 22% live birth rate.[36] Subsequent reports have documented lower pregnancy rates of 4% to 20% per cycle.[46, 47] Although in vitro fertilization-embryo transfer and zygote interfallopian transfer remain the primary assisted reproductive techniques used in these cases, pregnancies have been reported with the use of gamete intrafallopian transfer.[48]

Attempts to increase fertilization rates and, therefore, subsequent pregnancy rates have involved the use of in vitro chemical stimulation of sperm or micromanipulation. Ord and coworkers[47] incubated sperm in pentoxifylline followed by a mini-Percoll centrifugation and subsequent incubation in 2-deoxyadenosine. They compared fertilization and pregnancy rates in this group with those achieved by couples being treated with a standard mini-Percoll processing technique or a standard sperm wash or swim-up technique. In the original sperm wash/swim-up group, a 6.5% fertilization rate was achieved as compared to a 16% rate in the mini-Percoll group and a 35% rate in the mini-Percoll chemically stimulated group. Interestingly, in the swim-up/wash group, 24% of couples achieved fertilization of at least some ova, whereas in the mini-Percoll and mini-Percoll chemically stimulated groups, fertilization was achieved in 59% and 57% of cases, respectively. Thus, it appeared that the mini-Percoll technique with or without chemical additives resulted in more couples fertilizing ova as compared with the sedimentation-swim-up techniques. The addition of pentoxifylline or 2-deoxyadenosine did not increase the number of couples who fertilized ova; however, it did increase the fertilization rates in those couples who did achieve fertilization. Thus, in those couples achieving fertilization of at least one ova, the mini-Percoll treatment alone yielded a 25% fertilization rate as compared to a 58% fertilization rate in the mini-Percoll/chemical stimulant group. This increase in the fertilization rate in couples who achieve fertilization resulted in more embryos available for transfer. To avoid multiple gestations, no more than 3 to 6 embryos generally are transferred into the female, and the excess embryos may be frozen and reimplanted in a subsequent cycle. Although this may result in additional pregnancies, none have been reported from the implantation of frozen embryos in the partners of patients with BCAV.

Micromanipulation of gametes has been used to increase fertilization rates in couples with male factor infertility. Two techniques currently being used are partial zona dissection[49] and para-vitelline injection.[50] Partial zona dissection involves tearing a hole in the zona pellucida of the human ova using a sharpened micropipette. Sperm then may travel through the tear to reach the oolemma. In para-vitelline injection, sperm are aspirated into a micropipette, the zona pellucida is punctured, and the sperm are injected into the space between the oolemma and the zona pellucida. These micromanipulative techniques are being used in some centers, but the experiences remain anecdotal and unpublished. Most recently, lasers have been used to drill holes in the zona pellucida to allow improved fertilization rates.[51] Although this approach holds promise, it has yet to be used in human patients with BCAV.

Future Advances

The current treatment of choice for patients with BCAV remains MESA combined with in vitro fertilization-embryo transfer or zygote interfallopian transfer. Current pregnancy rates average 5% to 20%, with low sperm recovery and poor fertilization rates remaining a problem. Advanced processing techniques such as in vitro chemical stimulation and micromanipulation procedures hold much promise for improving these rates. Further research is needed, however, to determine which drugs at what doses, and which micromanipulative procedures will offer the best fertilization and pregnancy rates.

It is important that the urologist adequately counsel patients with BCAV. These couples face the option of therapeutic donor insemination, adoption, or entrance into a MESA program. Both partners should be screened and counseled regarding the correlation with CF. With costs for a combined MESA and in vitro fertilization procedure averaging $10,000 to $15,000 per cycle, it is important that the couple have realistic expectations regarding pregnancy rates. It is possible to undergo more than one cycle of MESA, since the testes can be reoperated upon and, often, only one testis is used at each procedure. However, financial constraints often limit the number of cycles through which a couple will proceed. As advances are made in these techniques, we can expect more widespread use of this technology.

References

1. Hellinga G, Ultee WA, Ruward R: Bilateral and unilateral congenital anomalies of the Wolffian ducts. *Andrologia* 1971; 3:81.
2. Michelson L: Congenital anomalies of the ductus deferens and epididymis. *J Urol* 1949; 61:384.
3. Arce B, Padron RS, Perez-Plaza M: Sterility caused by functional absence of ejaculatory ducts. *Reproduccion* 1981; 5:105–111.
4. Jequier AM, Ansell ID, Bullimore NJ: Congenital absence of the vasa deferentia presenting with infertility. *J Androl* 1985; 6:15–19.
5. Goldstein M, Schlossberg S: Men with congenital absence of the vas deferens often have seminal vesicles. *J Urol* 1988; 140:85–86.
6. Lewis FT: The course of the Wolffian tubules in mammalian embryos. *Am J Anat* 1920; 26:423.
7. Van Wingerden JJ, Franz I: The presence of a caput epididymis in congenital absence of the vas deferens. *J Urol* 1984; 131:764–766.
8. Itrihi A, Abulfadl MAM, Girgis SM, et al: Bilateral congenital absence of the vas deferens: Diagnostic features of seminal picture in 42 new cases. *J Egypt Med Assoc* 1972; 55:184–191.
9. Rubin SO: Congenital absence of the vas deferens. *Scand J Urol Nephrol* 1975; 9:94–99.
10. Camatini M, Franchi E, Faleri M: Ultrastructure of spermiogenesis in men with congenital absence of the vasa deferentia. *Arch Androl* 1979; 3:93–99.
11. Girgis SM, Ekladious EM, Iskander R, et al: Sperm antibodies in serum and semen in men with bilateral congenital absence of the vas deferens. *Arch Androl* 1982; 8:301–305.
12. Amelar RD, Dubin L, Schoenfeld CY: Circulating sperm-agglutinating antibodies in azoospermic men with congenital bilateral absence of the vasa deferentia. *Fertil Steril* 1975; 26:228–231.
13. Patrizio P, Moretti-Rojas I, Ord T, et al: Low incidence of sperm antibodies in men with congenital absence of the vas deferens. *Fertil Steril* 1989; 52:1018–1021.
14. Maungman V: Absence of vasa deferentia. *J Med Assoc Thai* 1978; 61:364.
15. Kleczkowska A, Fryns JP, Steeno O, et al: On the familial occurrence of congenital bilateral absence of vas deferens. *Clin Genet* 1989; 35:268–271.
16. Petit P, Fryns JP: Two pericentric inversions inv(7)(p15;q32) and inv(9)(p11;q13) in a male with absence of vas deferens. *Hum Genet* 1983; 64:303.
17. Leiba SA, Ber H, Joshua J, et al: A case of XY/XXY mosaicism and bilateral absence of the vas deferens. *Acta Endocrinol (Copenh)* 1969; 62:498–504.
18. Fuse H, Shiseki Y, Shimazaki J, et al: A case of Klinefelter's syndrome with bilateral absence of the vas deferens. *Urol Int* 1990; 45:181–182.
19. Knowlton RG, Cohen-Haguenauer O, Van Cong N, et al: A polymorphic DNA marker linked to cystic fibrosis is located on chromosome 7. *Nature* 1985; 318:380.
20. White R, Woodward S, Lepper M, et al: A closely linked genetic marker for cystic fibrosis. *Nature* 1985; 318:382.
21. Wainwright BJ, Scambler PJ, Schmidtke J, et al: Localization of cystic fibrosis locus to human chromosome 7cen-q22. *Nature* 1985; 318:384.
22. Rommens JM, Iannuzzi MC, Kerem B, et al: Identification of the cystic fibrosis gene: Chromosome walking and jumping. *Science* 1989; 245:1059–1065.

23. Holsclaw DS, Perlmutter AD, Jockin H, et al: Genital abnormalities in male patients with cystic fibrosis. *J Urol* 1971; 106:568–574.
24. Rigot JM, Lafitte JJ, Dumur V, et al: Cystic fibrosis and congenital absence of the vas deferens. *N Engl J Med* 1991; 325:64–65.
25. Anguiano A, Oates RD, Amos JA, et al: Congenital bilateral absence of the vas deferens: A primarily genital form of cystic fibrosis. *JAMA* 1992; 267:1794–1797.
26. Hanley HG: Pregnancy following artificial insemination from epididymal cyst. *Proc Soc Study Fertil* 1956; 8:20.
27. Schoysman R: La creation d'un spermatocele artificial das les agenesis du conal deferent. *Bull Soc R Belge Gynecol Obstet* 1968; 38:307.
28. Ludvik W: Artificial spermatocele persisting for fourteen years. *J Urol* 1990:144:992–994.
29. Turner TT: On the development and use of alloplastic spermatoceles. *Fertil Steril* 1988, 49:387–395.
30. Belker AM, Jimenez-Cruz DJ, Kelami A, et al: Alloplastic spermatocele: Poor sperm motility and intraoperative epididymal fluid contraindicates prosthesis implantation. *J Urol* 1986; 136:408–409.
31. Pryor J, Parsons J, Goswamy R, et al: In vitro fertilization for men with obstructive azoospermia. *Lancet* 1984; 2:762.
32. Temple-Smith PD, Southwick GJ, Yates CA, et al: Human pregnancy by in vitro fertilization (IVF) using sperm aspirated from the epididymis. *J In Vitro Fert Embryo Transf* 1985; 2:119–122.
33. Silber S, Ord T, Borrero C, et al: New treatment for infertility due to congenital absence of vas deferens. *Lancet* 1987; 2:850–851.
34. Honig SC, Dubay A, Oates, RD: Successful microscopic sperm aspiration and pregnancies in patients with obstructive azoospermia/severe oligoasthenospermia. *Presented at the 87th Annual Meeting of the American Urological Association, Washington, DC, May 1992.*
35. Schlegel P, Gilbert B, Alikani M, et al: Micropuncture of the human epididymis: Therapeutic applications of infertile men (abstract). Presented at the American Urological Associatoin Annual Meeting, Toronto, Canada, June, 1991.
36. Silber SJ, Ord T, Balmaceda J, et al: Congenital absence of the vas deferens. The fertilizing capacity of human epididymal sperm. *N Engl J Med* 1990; 323:1788–1792.
37. Davis RO, Overstreet JW, Asch RH, et al: Movement characteristics of human epididymal sperm used for fertilization of human oocytes in vitro. *Fertil Steril* 1991; 56:1128.
38. Bearer EL, Friend DS: Modifications of anionic-lipid domains preceding membrane fusion in the guinea pig. *J Cell Biol* 1982; 92:604.
39. Singer SL, Lamberton H, Cross ML, et al: Alteration of the human sperm surface during in vitro capacitation as assessed by lectin-induced agglutination. *Gamete Res* 1985; 12:291.
40. Yamagimachi R: Calcium requirement for sperm-egg fusion in mammals. *Biol Reprod* 1978; 19:949.
41. Hyne RV, Garbers DL: Calcium-dependent increase in adenosine 3′, 5′-monophosphate and induction of the acrosome reaction in guinea pig spermatozoa. *Proc Natl Acad Sci U S A* 1979, 76:5699.
42. Cruss NL, Morales P, Overstreet JW, et al: Induction of acrosomal reaction by the human zona pellucida. *Biol Reprod* 1988; 38:235.

43. Cohen J, Edwards R, Fehilly C, et al: In vitro fertilization: A treatment for male infertility. *Fertil Steril* 1985; 43:422.
44. McClure RD, Nunes L, Tom R: Semen manipulation: Improved sperm recovery and function with a 2-layer percoll gradient. *Fertil Steril* 1989; 51:874.
45. Ord T, Patrizio P, Marello E, et al: Mini-percoll: A new method of semen preparation for IVF in severe male factor infertility. *Hum Reprod* 1990; 5:987–989.
46. Southwick G, Yates C, Temple-Smith PD: Treatment of obstructive azoospermia by sperm microaspiration retrieval technique for IVF smart-IVF. Presented at the 46th Annual Meeting of the American Fertility Society, Washington, DC, October 1990.
47. Ord T, Marello E, Patrizio P, et al: The role of the laboratory in the handling of epididymal sperm for assisted reproductive technologies. *Fertil Steril* 1992; 57:1103.
48. Oates RD, Oskowitz SP, Crane RJ: Epididymal sperm aspiration (ESA) in conjunction with gamete intrafallopian transfer (GIFT) to achieve pregnancy. Presented at the 85th Annual Meeting of the American Urologic Association, New Orleans, May 1990.
49. Malter HE, Cohen J: Partial zona dissection of the human oocyte: A non-traumatic method using micromanipulation to assist zona pellucida penetration. *Fertil Steril* 1989; 51:139.
50. Sakkas D, Lacham O, Gianaroli L, et al: Subzonal sperm microinjection in cases of severe male factor infertility and repeated in vitro fertilization failure. *Fertil Steril* 1992; 57:1279.
51. Blanchet G, Roussel JB, Fincher CR, et al: Laser micromanipulation in the mouse embryo: A novel approach to zona drilling. *Fertil Steril* 1992; 57:1337.

The Methodology for Evaluating the Subjective Outcomes of Treatment for Benign Prostatic Hyperplasia*

Michael J. Barry, M.D.

Director, Health Services Research, Henry J. Kaiser Family Foundation Faculty Scholar in General Internal Medicine, Department of Medicine, Harvard Medical School; Medical Practices Evaluation Center, Massachusetts General Hospital, Boston, Massachusetts

Floyd J. Fowler, Jr., Ph.D.

Senior Research Scientist, Center for Survey Research, University of Massachusetts, Boston, Massachusetts

Benign prostatic hyperplasia (BPH) is a common disease of older men that imposes a tremendous burden on patients and health care systems worldwide.[1] In the United States alone, about 400,000 prostatectomies were performed for this condition in 1987,[2] making prostatectomy the second most common major operation performed on older men, after cataract extraction.[2, 3] The development and dissemination of transurethral prostatectomy, the surgical procedure most commonly used to treat this condition actively in the United States, is a true success story of modern medicine.[4] In recent years, however, many forces have combined to focus strong interest on the study of treatment outcomes in BPH.

BPH can produce complications, such as refractory urinary retention, bleeding, infection, and obstructive uropathy. When men show signs of these complications, active intervention is necessary to prevent further progression that may limit life expectancy. In the United States, the great ma-

*This project was supported in part by grant number HSO6336 from the Agency for Health Care Policy and Research, and by the American Urological Association, Inc. The American Urological Association's Measurement Committee includes, in addition to the authors, Winston K. Mebust, M.D. (Chair), University of Kansas Medical Center; Jerry G. Blaivas, M.D., College of Physicians and Surgeons of Columbia University; Reginald C. Bruskewitz, M.D., University of Wisconsin at Madison; Abraham T. K. Cockett, M.D., University of Rochester School of Medicine; H. Logan Holtgrewe, M.D., Johns Hopkins University School of Medicine; Michael P. O'Leary, M.D., M.P.H., Tufts-New England Medical Center; and Alan J. Wein, M.D., University of Pennsylvania School of Medicine

jority of prostatectomies are performed primarily to improve bothersome symptoms of prostatism that often accompany BPH.[5] These procedures are done primarily to improve the *quality*, rather than the *quantity*, of patients' lives. Although some observers have misinterpreted this fact as suggesting that most prostatectomies performed in this country are unnecessary,[6] the truth is that improving quality of life is perhaps *the* most important goal of medicine.[7, 8] The nation's urologists, who performed an average of 67 prostatectomies apiece in 1986,[9] all have grateful patients who will attest to the importance of this procedure for improving their conditions.

Given this background, why is there such focus on the outcomes of treatment for BPH? Therapy of BPH has been caught up in an "outcomes research movement" that has been brought about by recognition of the generally weak scientific underpinnings of many common medical treatments, realization that resources for health care are limited even in countries that are as well off as the United States, and growing awareness on the part of patients of their need to participate actively in the process of health care decision-making.[10]

The Outcomes Research Movement

Many common medical treatments evolved before there was a strong ethic for using randomized trials to define the efficacy of new therapeutic technologies. Furthermore, older efficacy assessment studies tended to focus on physiologic outcomes that were seen as "hard" and "objective," but in fact are only "intermediate" outcomes on the road to the kinds of results that most interest patients, such as symptom level and functional status. Finally, many clinical studies have focused on defining the *efficacy* of a therapy in tightly controlled experiments with narrow spectra of patients, which provides clinicians with little sense of the *effectiveness* that treatment will have in the less controlled setting of clinical practice with a broad spectrum of patients.[11, 12]

Lack of information about treatment outcomes often is combined with insufficient information about the untreated natural history of a disease. This deficit in high-quality clinical research has created many "knowledge gaps" in medicine, particularly for diseases for which patients are treated predominantly to improve their quality of life. Prostatectomy certainly is such a treatment, but many other surgical interventions fit this description also; many hysterectomies and most coronary artery bypass procedures (other than those performed on men with left main coronary or three-vessel disease with impaired left ventricular function) are performed primarily to reduce symptoms and improve quality of life. The natural history of untreated BPH, which is of critical importance in determining the optimal point for intervention, is a particularly good example of an understudied area in medicine. For instance, in several small studies of men with symptoms of BPH who were untreated over time, the rate of acute retention varies tenfold.[13, 14] This lack of knowledge about the natural history of BPH is particularly ironic given epidemiologic data that suggest that, worldwide, literally millions of men are following a strategy of "watchful waiting" for their condition.[1, 15, 16]

When there is uncertainty about the science underlying the use of a procedure, variability in its use can result, as different physicians quite reasonably adopt different thresholds for offering the therapy. Such uncertainty likely underlies the threefold to fourfold variations seen when rates of prostatectomy among different communities are analyzed,[17] the 1.7-fold variations noted when larger regions of the country are compared,[18] and the equally dramatic variations observed among different developed countries.[19] It must be emphasized that these practice variations are not unique to urology or even to surgery. When indications for an intervention in a condition are uncertain, rates of hospitalization vary greatly for many surgical and medical problems. On the other hand, when indications for a treatment are relatively straightforward, such as internal fixation for a fractured hip or hospitalization for an acute myocardial infarction, remarkably stable rates of utilization are seen when areas are compared.[20]

These differences in practice styles among geographic areas have huge implications for medical care costs. For example, in 1982, Medicare recipients in the Boston area, where hospital use is high, generated annual per capita costs to Medicare of $2647, compared to $1561 for the New Haven area, which uses hospital beds more conservatively.[21] In the United States, medical care costs are consuming more than 13% of the gross national product, and continue to rise steadily out of proportion to inflation despite all attempts to put brakes on the system.[22] Clearly, if outcomes research can identify which treatments really are effective and which are not effective or are only marginally effective, this information would help greatly in obtaining maximum health benefits from limited health care funds.

Increasingly, patients are becoming better informed about their medical problems and are insisting on playing a more active role in their treatment. This tendency has been fueled in part by reports of the practice variation phenomenon in the popular press[23, 24] and by concerns about treatment choices being influenced unduly by pharmaceutical companies and device manufacturers.[25] Hundreds of "self-help" guides have been designed to help patients educate themselves about many medical problems, including prostate disease.[26, 27] Certainly, when a prostatectomy is aimed primarily at reducing a patient's symptoms and improving his quality of life, the patient's perspective on whether the small but finite risks of the procedure are worth the expected benefits are a key factor in making a good treatment decision.

The outcomes research movement, then, has evolved to stimulate the collection of data on the natural history and treatment results of a disease in order to fill the knowledge gap that exists for many common conditions.[12, 28] This information should help direct health care dollars toward interventions that have the highest impact, and should provide patients with the information necessary to participate in decision-making. For both purposes, the emphasis is on collecting data on the outcomes that are most important to patients.

Instruments developed to describe the natural history of a disease and to measure the effectiveness of different treatments in research studies may have applications in clinical practice as well. These instruments might be used in individuals to help decide which patients need intervention at what time, and to measure objectively both baseline condition and treatment response.

In regard to BPH, this measurement task includes capturing data on symptoms and higher levels of health status. The need to obtain information on these relatively subjective outcomes requires that the instruments used to do so should be developed carefully and validated rigorously. It should be emphasized that outcomes research, with its emphasis on effectiveness data and patient-centered outcomes, is meant to *complement*, rather than *substitute for*, tightly controlled clinical efficacy research focusing on anatomic and physiologic outcomes. In fact, in most cases, the more basic research needs to be done before it is appropriate to perform outcomes studies.

Levels of Health in Benign Prostatic Hyperplasia

BPH can be defined at a basic level as a histologic process that, over time, may result in both anatomic and then physiologic changes in the prostate and entire lower urinary tract.[29] These changes eventually can cause symptoms of prostatism (as can other pathologic processes in this anatomic area, such as urethral stricture or primary bladder instability). Symptoms are changes in urination that patients can perceive, such as increased urinary frequency or hesitancy. In turn, these individual symptoms can bother, or be seen as a problem by, the person who has the condition to varying degrees. At the same time, the patient may perceive that his prostate condition affects specific domains of his health status, such as his level of physical activity, mental health, or general health. At this level, a sense of the patient's "disease-specific" health status can be obtained. Finally, a description of the patient's overall health status, including all of his health problems, provides a complete overview of his health. In the rest of this chapter, the more specific term "health status" will be used in preference to the more comprehensive (but commonly used term) "quality of life,"[30] which also conceptually includes dimensions not clearly related to health, such as economic well-being. Figure 1 provides a schematic illustration of the levels of health status that might be considered in patients with BPH.

Paradoxes in Relationships Among Levels of Health in Benign Prostatic Hyperplasia

In a simpler world, the rudimentary hierarchical diagram in Figure 1 would represent fully the biology and psychology of BPH, with close interrelation-

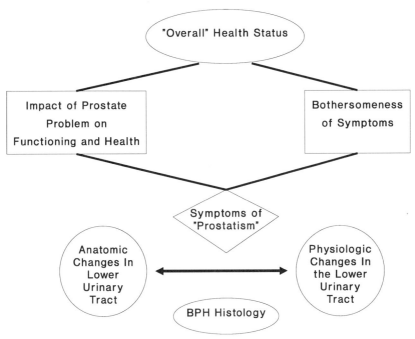

FIG 1.
A proposed conceptual model of different levels of health in men with benign prostatic hyperplasia *(BPH)*.

ships among the different levels of health represented. In reality, these levels are related much more loosely than one might hope, loosely enough to present a number of paradoxes that are important in the area of outcomes research in BPH[10]; two of these will be discussed in this article. The first paradox is the loose relationship between the severity of BPH at the anatomic/physiologic level and the severity of symptoms. The next paradox is at the level of the relationship between symptom severity and the higher levels of BPH-specific health status.

One might expect a close correlation between prostate size and severity of symptoms of prostatism, and between physiologic parameters of the severity of obstruction and symptom severity. Interestingly, many studies have suggested that these levels are related loosely, if at all. Prostate size has not correlated well with either symptoms reported by patients or peak urinary flow rates.[31, 32] In turn, peak urinary flow rates have been shown to be either not correlated, or at best modestly correlated, with symptom severity as reported by patients, even if only symptoms classically considered to be "obstructive," as opposed to "irritative," are examined.[32–35] For that matter, the so-called irritative symptoms have correlated only modestly with cystometric evidence of bladder instability among men with BPH.[32, 33, 35]

In fact, urinary flow rates alone may be poor proxies for measuring the true physiologic severity of BPH, which many experts believe can be derived only from more invasive studies of voiding pressure-flow relationships.[36–38] Even variables derived from studies using invasive measures of bladder pressure, however, have correlated relatively poorly with reported symptoms.[31, 33–35] Finally, and most surprisingly, although flow rates and symptoms both are improved by prostatectomy, the size of the changes on these measures have been correlated quite weakly.[39, 40]

These data challenge the traditional notions that increasing physiologic obstruction accounts for worsening "obstructive" symptoms, whereas progressive secondary bladder instability completely explains worsening irritative symptoms. Although both obstructive and irritative symptoms are ameliorated (albeit the former more efficiently) by relieving physiologic obstruction with a prostatectomy, mechanisms that still are understood poorly must link the underlying physiology with the symptoms patients report. In addition, these results dictate that studies of the outcomes of treatment for BPH must include measurements at multiple levels; the physiologic results of a treatment do not indicate the symptomatic results, and vice versa.

Symptom severity, in terms of the frequency of symptoms, also has an interesting relationship with the higher-order levels of patient-reported prostatic health. These higher-order levels clearly are related more closely to symptom severity than to physiologic and anatomic measures. The fact that the correlations are far from perfect, however, has interesting implications for making optimal treatment decisions. Patients may have completely different reactions to their symptom complexes. An actively working businessman with a relatively low tolerance for urinary symptoms given his social role and personality may be bothered extremely by only moderate symptoms, whereas a retired man with a higher tolerance may be unconcerned about even relatively severe symptoms.

Table 1 displays the relationship between symptom severity, broken into mild, moderate, and severe categories based on a symptom frequency score, and patient answers to questions designed to elicit the level of annoyance caused by the condition.[10, 41, 42] These responses were from a statewide study of men scheduled for elective prostatectomy by urologists in Maine.[41] Although about 25% of patients with mild symptoms found their condition to be at least somewhat limiting, uncomfortable, or worrisome, about half of those with severe symptoms were limited little or not at all, and 18% of these experienced little or no discomfort. These results reinforce the example of the two men given previously. Prostatectomy actually might be more appropriate for the man with moderate symptoms who is bothered extremely by them than for the man with severe symptoms who is not bothered. Without some understanding of the higher levels of "prostatic health," these choices might seem inconsistent.

TABLE 1.
Effects of the Severity of Prostatism on Some Answers to Questions About the Overall Impact of the Symptoms as Reported by the Patient*

Presurgical Responses ↓	Symptoms, %		
	Mild (N = 36) ↓	**Moderate (N = 104)** ↓	**Severe (N = 86)** ↓
Limited day-to-day by prostatism			
A lot or some	25	26	49
Little or none	75	74	51
Discomfort from prostatism			
A lot or some	28	52	82
Little or none	72	48	18
Worry about health due to prostatism			
A lot or some	28	37	57
Little or none	72	63	43

*From Fowler FJ, Wennberg JE, Timothy RP, et al: *JAMA* 1988; 259:3018. Used by permission.

Questionnaires for Quantifying Subjective Outcomes of Treatment

Given the need to quantify symptoms, annoyance of symptoms, disease-specific health status, and overall health status to get a full picture of the natural history of BPH and its response to different treatments, measures need to be taken by communicating with patients about these issues. Discussions with clinical experts and patients with the condition, either individually or in groups, are essential in questionnaire development. Responses are designed to be perceived by patients as mutually exclusive and collectively exhaustive, so that each patient can select only one response to describe his situation. Often, questions with scales of 5 to 7 responses are preferred, especially to detect changes over time.[43] The involvement of patients and experts is an iterative process in questionnaire development. Patients in particular can provide feedback on the clarity of questions, the comprehensiveness of the overall set of items, and the adequacy of the response frame.

An early choice in the methodology of questionnaire administration is whether the instrument will be administered by an interviewer (either in person or over the telephone) or self-administered by the research subject. An interviewer can help patients through complicated questionnaires and perhaps obtain more valid answers.[44] This mode of administration is always more expensive, however, and can produce biases in results when different interviewers administer a questionnaire or interpret patient responses differently. If an instrument is relatively simple, it can ideally be administered in multiple modes, depending on the need. The goal of the initial phase of questionnaire development is to generate a set of questions that is comprehensive and appropriate from the viewpoint of both the physician and the patient, as well as consistently understood and easy to answer.

Questionnaires: Reliability, Validity, and Sensitivity

Once an initial questionnaire is developed that seems to cover the intended concepts with clarity in the opinion of the experts and patients who participated in its development, studies are necessary to document that the questionnaire meets a set of psychometric and clinimetric standards. These standards often are grouped under the headings of reliability, validity, and sensitivity. In reality, no one health status measurement instrument is likely to be optimal for every possible use; different properties need to be maximized depending on the purpose for which the instrument is intended. Several excellent reviews on the topic of survey design and validation are available.[43, 45–47] In this article, an overview will be provided of the concepts of reliability, validity, and sensitivity, which often are considered in designing practical, parsimonious instruments that may be adaptable to many different outcomes research settings.

Two components of reliability usually are measured. First, individual questions, as well as groups of questions that might be combined into an index to generate an overall score, should yield similar answers when asked at different times to individuals whose disease status has not changed. Practically, this property commonly is measured by readministering the questionnaire after a short period to the same individuals, timing the interval so that it is brief enough that few patients would be expected to have had an important change in disease status. This psychometric property is known as test-retest reliability, and is analogous to the concept of precision in diagnostic testing. Test-retest reliability can be examined simply by correlating time one and time two results, or more elegantly by using statistics that reflect agreement corrected for chance agreement, like the kappa statistic.[48] Short-term test-retest reliability, along with sensitivity (a property that will be discussed shortly), are particularly important for indices that will be used to monitor patients over time. The more reliable the instrument, the more likely it is that changes observed are due to a true change in disease status rather than to random fluctuation, or "noise," in the measurement.

Another type of reliability refers to groups of questions that are assembled to measure the same concept. A group of related questions usually can give a better picture of that concept than can a single question, but the psychometric basis for combining questions into an index is strongest when the questions actually are related. This property of a group of questions is referred to as "internal consistency reliability," and can be examined with Cronbach's alpha statistic.[49] Higher values (Cronbach's alpha can range from 0 to 1) indicate a greater relatedness of the component items in an index. For example, questions about eye color, shoe size, and quality of urine stream would be expected to have a low value for Cronbach's alpha, whereas questions about intermittency, hesitancy, and quality of urine stream would be expected to have a high value if they all are symptoms of prostatism.

Diagnostic tests can be precise (repeatable), but completely inaccurate. Similarly, reliability of a questionnaire does not guarantee its validity, which is whether the questionnaire is measuring what it is intended to measure. Validity often is more difficult to ensure than reliability in evaluating health status measures. The principal problem often is the lack of a "gold standard" against which to evaluate a measure. More often, validity must be assessed more indirectly. Frequently, correlations are sought with other measures that should be related to the new measure at a conceptual level. Such tests assess "construct" validity. "Discriminant" validity, on the other hand, can be assessed by measuring how well the new measure discriminates between groups that should be different, such as patients who have been determined clinically either to have or not to have BPH. The discriminating ability of a measure can be described by calculating the area under that measure's "receiver-operating characteristic curve."[50] Receiver-operating characteristic curves are constructed by examining the true-positive (sensitivity) and false-positive (1-specificity) rates of the measure in a test population composed of diseased and healthy persons, using different cutpoints to designate the point at which the score is considered abnormal. The true- and false-positive rate pairs generated by moving the normal-abnormal cutpoint describe a receiver-operating characteristic curve. Conceptually, the area under this curve (which ranges from 0.5 for a worthless measure to 1.0 for a perfect measure) represents the probability that the measure will be more abnormal for a randomly selected diseased person than for a randomly selected healthy person from the test population.[51]

Another important property for some indices is sensitivity, or responsiveness. Sensitivity is particularly important when the measure will be used to follow patients over time, either to study the natural history of a disease or to describe its response to treatment. Insensitive instruments may miss clinically important changes in patient condition, particularly if small differences are perceptible to patients (many times, they are not). Generally, responsiveness is assessed by examining how the measure changes when patients undergo a change (often, with treatment) that should be detectable.

Reliability vs. Sensitivity

One particular problem with the overall health status measures is that they may be insensitive to changes in patient status related to a single disease, since they conceptually represent the overall impact of many diseases and other factors on patient health. On the other hand, such measures may be very valuable in health policy research for comparing the impact of the treatment of different diseases. In addition, when a treatment is studied that can have not only therapeutic effects on a diseased body system, but also potentially serious side effects on other systems, overall health status measures may be used to measure the net benefit of the treatment across all systems in a common currency.

Measuring Symptoms of Prostatism

A number of questionnaires have been designed to capture the symptom status of men with BPH in a standard way. Two of the best-known symptom scoring systems are the Boyarsky[52] and Madsen-Iversen[53] systems. Although widely used, these instruments, which are designed to be interviewer-administered, have not been validated formally. Recently, a measurement committee was appointed by the American Urological Association to develop outcome measures for a large randomized trial of BPH treatment outcomes, a study that is designed to measure the effectiveness of both old and new therapeutic technologies for this disease. The measurement committee reviewed existing instruments and concluded that there was no one optimal scoring system that met all the needs of the planned trial. Therefore, the committee decided to follow the steps outlined previously in this chapter to develop and validate a new symptom index as an outcome measure for this study.

An item list was developed by an expert panel by reviewing preexisting questionnaires and interviewing patients. Several questions were designed to cover each of the concepts of day frequency, nocturia, hesitancy, intermittency, weak stream, urgency, dysuria, postvoid dribbling, and incomplete emptying. Questions and their response frames were refined with the input of both the experts and the patients. Three sequential validation studies have been conducted to examine carefully the reliability, validity, and sensitivity of the proposed index.

First, the long instrument was administered to a group of patients with BPH (defined clinically) and to control subjects (who had no history of BPH) to assess the questionnaire's clarity and comprehensiveness, with a formal "debriefing" of all research subjects. The test-retest reliability of individual questions and potential indices were examined by readministering the questionnaire to all research subjects about 1 week after the initial encounter. The internal consistency reliabilities of potential indices were assessed as well. Correlations were sought with patients' global assessments of the degree of urinary problems they were having (a test of construct validity), and the ability of symptom scores derived from the questionnaire to discriminate patients with BPH from control subjects was examined. Alternative weightings of questions were explored for different indices, to see if some questions were more important than others in predicting patients' ratings of their overall urinary difficulties, or in discriminating patients with BPH from control subjects.

Next, a shortened, refined questionnaire was administered to similar patients to revalidate prospectively the core questionnaire and to test several variations in wording. Finally, the responsiveness of the proposed index was examined in a third study of men undergoing transurethral prostatectomy for symptomatic BPH. All men completed the questionnaire before and 1 month after surgery to assess the sensitivity of individual items and the overall score. Analysis of the data from these validation studies still is ongoing. Based on preliminary results, however, a seven-item version of the symptom index developed for the American Urological Association's BPH treatment outcomes study (Fig 2) was recommended by a recent World Health Organization consensus conference on BPH as potentially useful in clinical research and practice in urology.[54]

	not at all	less than 1 time in 5	less than half the time	about half the time	more than half the time	almost always
1. Over the past month or so, how often have you had a sensation of not emptying your bladder completely after you finished urinating?	0	1	2	3	4	5
2. Over the past month or so, how often have you had to urinate again less than two hours after you finished urinating?	0	1	2	3	4	5
3. Over the past month or so, how often have you found you stopped and started again several times when you urinated?	0	1	2	3	4	5
4. Over the past month or so, how often have you found it difficult to postpone urination?	0	1	2	3	4	5
5. Over the past month or so, how often have you had a weak urinary stream?	0	1	2	3	4	5
6. Over the past month or so, how often have you had to push or strain to begin urination?	0	1	2	3	4	5

7. Over the last month, how many times did you most typically get up to urinate from the time you went to bed at night until the time you got up in the morning?

    0 none   1 1 time   2 2 times   3 3 times   4 4 times   5 5 or more times

AUA Symptom Score = sum of questions A1–A7 = ___ ___.

FIG 2.
The American Urological Association Symptom Index.

The measurement committee hopes that the use of this instrument may bring some much-needed standardization to both clinical practice and clinical research in BPH. However, the committee recognizes that much more work should be done in this area. Modifications may be necessary in this instrument to make it useful in broad spectra of patients with BPH, especially internationally. Furthermore, additional symptom questions may be needed in either practice or research, depending on the specific purpose. Finally, symptom status is just one measure of the severity of BPH that needs to be considered in clinical research and practice, albeit a very important one from the patient's perspective. Information about other higher-order levels of health status in patients with BPH is important, as are practical tests of lower urinary tract physiology and renal function, to get a more complete picture of BPH severity.

Measuring Benign Prostatic Hyperplasia–Specific Health Status

BPH causes morbidity in most patients through its associated symptoms, which may bother only some and in turn cause them problems in physical functioning, mental health, social and role functioning, and perceptions of general health. Several measures have been proposed that, alone or integrated with symptoms scores, may provide information at these higher levels of health status.[55–57] The American Urological Association's measurement committee also is working on the development and validation of several indices that measure disease-specific health status in BPH. These measurements will focus on the annoyance of a man's individual symptoms of BPH, as well as on the degree to which his overall BPH problem is affecting various aspects of his life. These questions are being validated in the same populations described previously. One important hope for indices of this kind is that they will help provide a better understanding of how BPH affects overall health. In addition, these instruments may be sensitive enough to measure the impact of therapies on higher orders of health status in BPH without the very large sample sizes necessary to demonstrate changes in the less responsive measures of overall health status.

Measuring Overall Health Status in Benign Prostatic Hypertrophy

Many investigators have developed measures of health status that are applicable across diseases. Several excellent reviews of these instruments are available[47, 58, 59] These instruments often have subscales to measure different domains of health status, such as the following domains characterized by John Ware and colleagues: physical functioning, mental health, social and role functioning, general health perceptions, and pain.[60] Several of these instruments have been used to assess overall health status in men with BPH.[41, 42, 61]

Urologists might worry that, when they treat BPH, they are only treating a "bounded" urinary problem; they are not treating a patient's other problems or his social situation. Therefore, the benefits of treatment might not be reflected in improvements in these non–disease-specific indices. However, these studies have suggested that BPH is an intrusive disease; increasing severity of symptoms is associated with decrements in health status measurable on these instruments. Furthermore, when men undergo prostatectomy, statistically significant improvements have been observed in measures at this broad level, particularly for men with severe disease (Table 2).

Summary

The 1990s will be an exciting time for both basic and clinical research in BPH. The pace of research activity in this area already has escalated dramatically. Although the etiology of this condition is still unclear, important therapeutic advances are being made based on a better understanding of the disease and its complications at a basic level.[62, 63] Furthermore, the outcomes research movement has added impetus for the study of this

TABLE 2.
Changes in Symptoms and Health Status Measures When Men With Symptomatic Benign Prostatic Hyperplasia Undergo a Prostatectomy*

Presurgical Symptom Index ↓	Number of Patients	Symptom index† ↓	Activity Index ↓	General Health ↓	Mental Health ↓
Mild (5–8)					
Before surgery	62	6.7	12.4	14.3	24.9
After surgery		6.6	13.0	15.3‡	25.7
Moderate (9–12)					
Before surgery	129	10.3	11.7	14.1	24.3
After surgery		7.3§	12.7st	14.7‡	25.1‡
Severe (13+)					
Before surgery	129	16.0	11.0	13.4	23.2
After surgery		7.7§	12.2§	14.2§	24.3§

*From Fowler FJ, Wennberg JE, Timothy RP, et al: *JAMA* 1988; 259:3018. Used by permission.
†Lower symptom index score indicates lower symptom frequency; higher scores on other indices indicate better quality of life. *Includes only patients for whom complete data were available.*
‡*P* < .05.
§*P* < .01.

common, but heretofore underinvestigated, disorder at the clinical level. This broad basic and clinical approach will help ensure that fundamental advances in the understanding of the disease will translate relatively rapidly into improved patient outcomes that are measurable in terms that are most meaningful to men with the condition.

Already, careful symptom measurements and higher-level health status assessments are being incorporated into natural history studies and clinical trials of new therapies for BPH. Increasingly, policy-making groups, such as the U.S. Food and Drug Administration and the Medicare program, are paying close attention to health status data when making decisions about new treatment technologies. And now, groups of clinicians who are developing practice policies are considering how simple health status measures can improve the quality of day-to-date care for men with urologic disease. Much work remains to be done, however, before these tools can achieve their full potential.

References

1. Barry MJ: Epidemiology and natural history of benign prostatic hyperplasia. *Urol Clin North Am* 1990; 17:495–507.
2. Graves EJ: Detailed diagnoses and procedures, National Hospital Discharge Survey: 1987. *Natl Center Vital Health Stat* 1989; 13:295.
3. U.S. Bureau of the Census: *Statistical Abstract of the United States, 1989,* 109th ed. Washington, DC, US Government Printing Office, 1989.
4. Mebust WK: Transurethral prostatectomy. *Urol Clin North Am* 1990; 17:575–585.
5. Mebust WK, Holtgrewe HL, Cockett AT, et al: Transurethral prostatectomy: Immediate and postoperative complications. A cooperative study of 13 participating institutions evaluating 3,885 patients. *J Urol* 1989; 141:243–247.
6. Cotton P: Case for prostate therapy wanes despite more treatment options. *JAMA* 1991; 266:459–460.
7. Cluff LE: Chronic disease, function, and the quality of care. *J Chronic Dis* 1981; 34:299–304.
8. Deyo RA: The quality of life, research, and care. *Ann Intern Med* 1991; 114:695–697.
9. Holtgrewe HL: American Urological Association survey of transurethral prostatectomy and the impact of changing Medicare reimbursement. *Urol Clin North Am* 1990; 17:587–593.
10. Barry MJ: Medical outcomes research and benign prostatic hyperplasia. *Prostate Suppl* 1990; 3:61–74.
11. Institute of Medicine: *Assessing Medical Technologies.* Washington, DC, National Academy Press, 1985.
12. Salive ME, Mayfield JA, Weissman NW: Patient outcomes research and the Agency for Health Care Policy and Research. *Health Serv Res* 1990; 25:697–708.
13. Birkhoff JD, Wiederhorn AR, Hamilton ML, et al: Natural history of benign prostatic hypertrophy and acute urinary retention. *Urology* 1976; 7:48–52.
14. Ball AJ, Feneley RC, Abrams PH: The natural history of untreated "prostatism." *Br J Urol* 1981; 53:613–616.

15. Boyle P, McGinn R, Maisonneuve P, et al: Epidemiology of benign prostatic hyperplasia: Present knowledge and studies needed. *Eur Urol* 1991; 20(suppl 2):3–10.
16. Garraway WM, Collins GN, Lee RJ: High prevalence of benign prostatic hypertrophy in the community. *Lancet* 1991; 338:469–471.
17. Wennberg JE: Dealing with medical practice variations: A proposal for action. *Health Aff (Millwood)* 1984; 3:6–32.
18. Chassin MR, Brook RH, Park RE: Variations in the use of medical and surgical services by the Medicare population. *N Engl J Med* 1986; 314:285–290.
19. McPherson K, Wennberg JE, Hovind OB. Small area variations in the use of common surgical procedures: An international comparison of New England, England, and Norway. *N Engl J Med* 1982; 307:1310–1314.
20. Wennberg J, Gittelsohn A: Variations in medical care among small areas. *Sci Am* 1982; 246:120–134.
21. Wennberg JE, Freeman JL, Culp WJ: Are hospital services rationed in New Haven or over-utilized in Boston? *Lancet* 1987; 1:1185–1189.
22. Eddy DM: What do we do about costs? *JAMA* 1990; 264:1161–1170.
23. Maynard F: When to say no to surgery. *Readers Digest* 1988; pp 29–34.
24. Ray RD, Rogers PG: There's too much uncertainty in medical care. *The Wall Street Journal* October 13, 1987.
25. Pushing drugs to doctors. *Consumer Reports* Feb 1992; pp 87–94.
26. Rous S: *The Prostate Book: Sound Advice on Symptoms and Treatment.* New York, Norton Publishing, 1988.
27. Cunningham C: *Your Prostate: What Every Man Over 40 Needs to Know . . . Now!* Leucadia, California, United Research Publishers, 1990.
28. Mulley AG: Applying effectiveness and outcomes research to clinical practice, in Heithoff KA, Lohr KN (eds): *Effectiveness and Outcomes in Health Care.* Washington, National Academy Press, 1990, pp 179–189.
29. Sterling AM, Ritter RC, Zinner NR: The physical basis of obstructive uropathy, in Hinman F (ed): *Benign Prostatic Hypertrophy.* New York, Springer-Verlag, 1983, pp 433–442.
30. Bergner M: Quality of life, health status, and clinical research. *Med Care* 1989; 27:S148–S156.
31. Andersen JT, Nordling J, Walter S: Prostatism. I. The correlation between symptoms, cystometric, and urodynamic findings. *Scand J Urol Nephrol* 1979; 13:229–236.
32. Frimodt-Moller PC, Jensen KM, Iversen P, et al: Analysis of presenting symptoms in prostatism. *J Urol* 1984; 132:272–276.
33. Jensen KM: Clinical evaluation of routine urodynamic investigations in prostatism. *Neurology and Urodynamics* 1989; 8:545–578.
34. Bruskewitz R, Jensen KM, Iversen P, et al: The relevance of minimal urethral resistance in prostatism. *J Urol* 1983; 129:769–771.
35. Neal DE, Styles RA, Ng T, et al: Relationship between voiding pressures, symptoms, and urodynamic findings in 253 men undergoing prostatectomy. *Br J Urol* 1987; 60:554–559.
36. Abrams PH, Griffiths DJ: The assessment of prostatic obstruction from urodynamic measurements and from residual urine. *Br J Urol* 1979; 51:129–134.
37. Schafer W: The contribution of the bladder outlet to the relation between pressure and flow rate during micturition, in Hinman F (ed): *Benign Prostatic Hypertrophy.* New York, Springer-Verlag, 1983, pp 470–496.
38. Blaivas JG: Multichannel urodynamic studies in men with benign prostatic hy-

perplasia: Indications and interpretation. *Urol Clin North Am* 1990; 17:543–552.

39. Bruskewitz RC, Christensen MM: Critical evaluation of transurethral resection and incision of the prostate. *Prostate Suppl* 1990; 3:27–38.
40. Lepor H, Rigaud G: The efficacy of transurethral resection of the prostate in men with moderate symptoms of prostatism. *J Urol* 1990; 143:533–537.
41. Fowler FJ, Wennberg JE, Timothy RP, et al: Symptom status and quality of life following prostatectomy. *JAMA* 1988; 259:3018.
42. Fowler FJ: Patient reports of symptoms and quality of life following prostate surgery. *Eur Urol* 1991; 20(suppl 2):44–49.
43. Kirshner B, Guyatt G: A methodologic framework for assessing health indices. *J Chronic Dis* 1985; 38:27–36.
44. Anderson JB, Bush JW, Berry CC: Classifying function for health outcome and quality-of-life evaluation. *Med Care* 1986; 24:454–470.
45. Guyatt GH, Bombadier C, Tugwell PX: Measuring disease-specific quality of life in clinical trials. *Can Med Assoc J* 1986; 134:889–895.
46. Fowler FJ: *Survey Research Methods.* Newbury Park, California, Sage Publications, 1984.
47. McDowell I, Newell C: *Measuring Health: A Guide to Rating Scales and Questionnaires.* New York, Oxford University Press, 1987.
48. Rosner B: *Fundamentals of Biostatics.* Boston, Duxbury Press, 1986.
49. Cronbach LJ: Coefficient alpha and the internal structure of tests. *Psychometrika* 1951; 16:297–334.
50. Hanley JA, McNeil BJ: The meaning and use of the area under a receiver operating characteristic (ROC) curve. *Radiology* 1982; 143:29–36.
51. Centor RM: Signal detectability: The use of ROC curves and their analyses. *Med Decis Making* 1991; 11:102–106.
52. Boyarsky S, Jones G, Paulson DF, et al: A new look at bladder neck obstruction by the Food and Drug Administration regulators: Guide lines for investigation of benign prostatic hypertrophy. *Trans Am Assoc Genitourinary Surgeons* 1977; 68:29–32.
53. Madsen PO, Iversen P: A point system for selecting operative candidates, in Hinman F (ed): *Benign Prostatic Hypertrophy.* New York, Springer-Verlag, 1983, pp 763–765.
54. Cockett AT, Aso Y, Denis L, et al: World Health Organization Consensus Committee Recommendations. *Progrés en Urologie* 1991; 1:957–972.
55. Boyarsky S, Woodward RS: Prostatic health status index, in Hinman F (ed): *Benign Prostatic Hypertrophy.* New York, Springer-Verlag, 1983, pp 766–770.
56. Epstein RS, Deverka PA, Chute CE, et al: Urinary symptom and quality of life questions indicative of obstructive benign prostatic hyperplasia. *Urology* 1991; 38(suppl):20–26.
57. Hald T, Nordling J, Andersen JT, et al: A patient weighted symptom score system in the evaluation of uncomplicated benign prostatic hyperplasia. *Scand J Urol Nephrol Suppl* 1991; 138:59–62.
58. Nelson EC, Berwick DM: The measurement of health status in clinical practice. *Med Care* 1989; 27:S77–S90.
59. Brook RH, Ware JE, Davies-Avery A, et al: Overview of adult health status measures fielded in Rand's health insurance study. *Med Care* 1979; 17(suppl 7):1–131.
60. Stewart AS, Hays RD, Ware JE: The MOS short-form general health survey: Reliability and validity in a patient population. *Med Care* 1988; 26:724–735.

61. Flood AB, Black NA, McPherson K, et al: Assessing symptom improvement following elective prostatectomy for benign prostatic hypertrophy. *Arch Intern Med* 1992; 152:1507–1512.
62. McConnell JD: The pathophysiology of benign prostatic hyperplasia. *J Androl* 1991; 12:356–363.
63. Schroder FH: Changing approaches in the treatment of benign prostatic hyperplasia. *Eur Urol* 1991:20(suppl 2):63–67.

Immunotherapy of Renal Cell Carcinoma: Experience of the Surgery Branch, National Cancer Institute

Richard B. Alexander, M.D.

Senior Investigator, Division of Urologic Oncology, Surgery Branch, National Cancer Institute, Bethesda, Maryland

McClellan M. Walther, M.D.

Senior Investigator, Division of Urologic Oncology, Surgery Branch, National Cancer Institute, Bethesda, Maryland

W. Marston Linehan, M.D.

Chief, Division of Urologic Oncology, Surgery Branch, National Cancer Institute, Bethesda, Maryland

Steven A. Rosenberg, M.D., Ph.D.

Cheif, Surgery Branch, National Cancer Institute, Bethesda, Maryland

Immunotherapy of cancer is defined broadly as the use of the immune system as a therapy for human malignancy. The central questions of cancer immunotherapy are whether human tumors are immunogenic and can be recognized as non-self by the human immune system, and whether this recognition can be exploited to bring about a therapeutic response. Immunotherapy of cancer can be classified into two major strategies for treatment: (1) the adoptive transfer of components of the host immune system, such as cytokines or immune cells; and (2) attempts to boost or augment the immune response of the host to the tumor. Many fundamental observations about how the immune system and, in particular, the cellular immune system, functions recently have come to light. A basic understanding of the immune system is essential to an appreciation of immunotherapy. This chapter will review new insights into how the immune system recognizes foreign antigens, and how this information has been used in the past and might be used in the future as a therapy for cancer. The development and current status of immunotherapy at the Surgery Branch of the National Cancer Institute will be reviewed, with particular emphasis on renal cell carcinoma.

Brief Review of Cellular Immunology

A remarkable feature of the mature human immune system is its ability to recognize non-self. The immune system has the capability to recognize nonself epitopes of a very diverse nature, from soluble protein molecules to non-self human cells, such as occurs during transplantation. Besides this exquisitely specific recognition function, the immune system also contains a broad array of anticellular effector functions that have the capability to lyse and destroy non-self or altered-self cells. It is the goal of cancer immunotherapy to bring this specificity and powerful anticellular function to bear upon human cancers.

The immune system is made up of a variety of cells with different and overlapping functions, as outlined in Table 1. Cells of the immune system interact with one another both by direct contact and through a complex set of secreted products called cytokines, which can interact and signal immune cells by autocrine, paracrine, and endocrine mechanisms. Lymphocytes play a central role in the recognition of non-self antigens and are classified as B (bone marrow–derived) and T (thymus-derived) cells. B

TABLE 1.
Cells of the Immune System

Type of Cell	Characteristics*
Lymphocytes	
T lymphocytes	Antigen-specific recognition; MHC-restricted; highly proliferative; cytokine secretion; IL-2 is a growth factor
B lymphocytes	Antigen-specific recognition; not MHC-restricted; highly proliferative; antibody secretion; antigen presentation
Natural killer (NK) cells	Nonspecific recognition; not MHC-restricted; limited proliferation; IL-2 "activates"
Monocytes	Antigen presentation; cytokine secretion; pinocytosis
Macrophages	Antigen presentation; cytokine secretion; phagocytic
Dendritic cells	Antigen presentation; clustering with T cells; accumulation of antigens

*MHC = major histocompatibility complex; IL-2 = interleukin-2.

cells have on their surface immunoglobulin molecules that bind to a specific epitope, such as a foreign protein. This signals the B cell to enter the activation cycle, maturing into a plasma cell that secretes the same immunoglobulin located on its surface. Hence, B cells recognize soluble foreign material. Recognition of non-self cells, however, such as virally infected cells or transplanted tissues, is a function of T cells. T lymphocytes originate in the bone marrow, but then are processed within the thymus to form the mature T cell repertoire. Unlike B cells, T cells do not recognize soluble antigens. Instead, T cells recognize small peptide fragments of antigenic proteins presented on the surface of other cells. The structure on the surface of T cells that confers this antigen specificity is the T cell receptor (TCR), which is the distinguishing characteristic of T cells.[1]

The TCR is composed of two protein chains. These two chains span the membrane with an intracellular signaling area and an external constant region, and then, similar to immunoglobulins, a hypervariable region. The dimeric chain of the TCR is associated with the CD3 complex of proteins that is involved in signal transduction, the process by which binding of the TCR is communicated to the T cell.[2, 3] It is this TCR complex that is responsible for the specificity of antigen recognition by T lymphocytes.

For many years, there was great controversy as to whether specificity of T cells was an inherent property of T cells established during passage through the thymus or whether specificity could be acquired by the cell once it entered the periphery. It now is very clear that T cell specificity is established very early in the life of the T lymphocyte, and that each T lymphocyte can have only a single TCR conformation.[1] There is tremendous variation in TCRs during growth of the T cell precursors in the bone marrow. This occurs by a mechanism shared by the immunoglobulin gene superfamily. Basically, there are several regions in the genes coding for the TCR, and these regions can recombine to form an astonishing diversity, almost at random, of different TCR configurations. Each T lymphocyte, however, has only one particular TCR, but because of the large number of recombinational events that are possible, a large diversity of TCR complexes is generated from T cell to T cell. The process of becoming a mature peripheral T cell occurs in the thymus, beginning early in fetal life. One of the major functions of the thymus is to delete T cells that bear a TCR that reacts with self epitopes. Deletion of these cells occurs in the thymus, as does a complex series of maturation steps that ultimately leads to release of the mature T cell repertoire into the periphery.

What is the nature of the antigen recognized by the TCR? T cells, unlike B cells, do not recognize antigens in soluble form, such as foreign proteins. The antigen engaged and recognized by the TCR consists of short peptide fragments of proteins presented in the context of self major histocompatibility complex (MHC) antigens.[4, 5] An understanding of TCR antigens requires a brief review of the MHC system.

The MHC was named as it is because the products of MHC genes, expressed on the surface of cells, appear to be of overwhelming importance to the survival of skin grafts or other transplanted tissues. There are two families of MHC molecules expressed on the surface of cells. These are termed broadly class I and class II, and are shown in Figure 1. Class I molecules are expressed on the surface of all nucleated cells. These glycoprotein molecules are encoded by the human leukocyte antigen A, B, and C regions located on chromosome 6, and are associated noncovalently with β_2-microglobulin on the cell surface. The MHC region is highly polymorphic, meaning that there are many different alleles at each of these genetic loci. It is these class I molecules on the surface of cells that are the classic transplantation antigens principally responsible for the rejection of tissues transplanted from one individual to another. Class II MHC molecules have a different structure, as shown in Figure 1. Class II molecules are expressed on the surface of lymphocytes and other accessory cells of the immune system and are defined in the human mostly by mixed lymphocyte reaction.

Antigens presented to T cells do not consist of whole proteins, but rather of small peptide fragments that are bound noncovalently to a groove in the outer portion of MHC molecules (Fig 2).[5] The association of peptides with the MHC complex is the result of what is termed antigen processing. Antigen processing and presentation appear to occur in all nucleated cells that express class I MHC molecules. The peptide antigens in this case arise from inside of the cell in the cytoplasm and associate with class I MHC molecules during their formation before being transported to the cell surface. MHC class II expression, on the other hand, is limited mostly to cells of the immune system. A high level of MHC class II expression is a characteristic feature of specialized antigen-presenting cells such as B cells, monocytes, and dendritic cells. Antigens associated with MHC class II in such cells arise outside of the cell, are endocytosed, undergo degradation to peptides in the endosomal compartment, and then are associated with newly synthesized class II molecules before being transported to the sur-

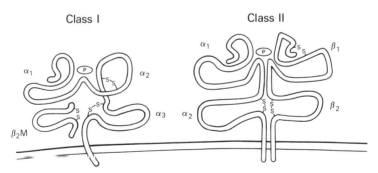

FIG 1.
Schematic drawing of class I and class II MHC molecules. P = peptide antigen; β_2M = β_2-microglobulin. 5–5 = disulfide bond. (From Restifo N: Antigen processing and presentation: An update, in DeVita VT, Hellman S, Rosenberg SA (eds): *Biologic Therapy of Cancer Updates*, vol 2. Philadelphia, Lippincott, 1992. p3. Used by permission.)

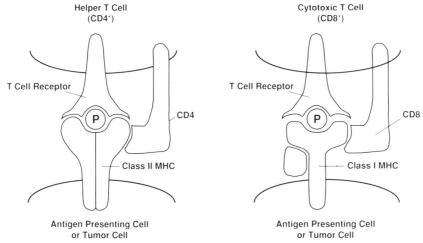

FIG 2.
Schematic drawing of CD4$^+$ and CD8$^+$ T cells interacting via the T cell receptor with antigenic peptide *(P)* presented by major histocompatibility complex *(MHC)* class II and class I on the antigen-presenting cell surface.

face. Thus, there appear to be two major antigen processing and presentation pathways—an endogenous one in which the peptides arise within the cytoplasm and are presented in the context of class I, and an exogenous one in which the antigens arise from outside of the cell, and are endocytosed, processed, and presented in the context of Class II.

The final dichotomy of this evolving story is the separation of the peripheral T cells into two different types depending upon whether they recognize antigens in the context of class I or class II MHC molecules. There are two major subsets of peripheral T lymphocytes, those expressing the surface marker CD4, which are termed helper T cells, and those expressing the surface marker CD8, which are known as cytotoxic T cells. CD4 helper T cells recognize antigens presented in the context of MHC class II, whereas CD8 T cells recognize antigens presented in the context of MHC class I.[5]

Engagement of the TCR by MHC-peptide complexes results in the initiation of a sequence of events in the T cell generally known as T cell activation. The binding of the specific epitope recognized by the TCR is signaled to the nucleus of the cell by a complex series of events, including increases in intracellular calcium concentration, activation of protein kinase C, and phosphorylation of internal proteins of the cell membrane.[3] These events ultimately signal the cell to initiate transcription of messenger RNAs, secrete cytokines, and enter into the cell cycle to begin proliferation. Since each T cell has a unique TCR, entry into this pathway by a T cell would result in proliferation and expansion of the clones of cells that have reactivity against the antigen presented in the context of MHC. Once the antigen is destroyed, the response abates. Just as is seen with B cells, however, there clearly are memory T cells that remain following resolution of the immune response, and these cells are capable of a secondary or anamnestic response if the host is rechallenged with the same antigen at a later time.[6]

It can be inferred that nucleated cells of the host constantly are assembling and presenting to the T cell repertoire around them components of their inner self for examination. Since self-reactive T cell clones are deleted in the thymus, the body is able to recognize cells that are self, and no T cell response is initiated. Should a cell become infected with virus, for example, viral proteins would be processed by this system and presented to the T cell repertoire, and T cells bearing the appropriate TCR would be stimulated to become activated and initiate the immune response against virally infected cells. Similarly, macrophages and other antigen-presenting cells (e.g., B cells, which are class II–positive) take up antigen in the extracellular compartment and present to the T cell repertoire in a similar fashion. Thus, the system is able to recognize foreign materials of many different forms and to initiate an appropriate immune response against it. What might be the function of such a highly polymorphic MHC system? It is becoming clear that the interaction between MHC and peptide is not simply a passive one in which any peptide randomly can be associated into the MHC complex. Rather, different MHC isotypes have different abilities to bind to different peptides.[7] Perhaps the evolution of the MHC system has been influenced by the ability of different alleles to present different antigenic peptides and the population of humans is more vigorous when this diversity is maintained.

Cancer and the Immune System

Do human tumors contain non-self antigens that could be recognized by the immune system? How might this powerful cellular system be exploited as a therapy for human cancer? Two fundamental approaches to cancer immunotherapy are (1) to try to increase the immune response of the host against the cancer, and (2) to administer components of the immune system in pharmacologic doses in an attempt to bring about a therapeutic response. This latter approach, known as adoptive immunotherapy, was the initial approach studied in the Surgery Branch of the National Cancer Institute.

Adoptive Immunotherapy

Given the central role played by T lymphocytes in the recognition and destruction of foreign cells, the early emphasis within the Surgery Branch of the National Cancer Institute was to attempt to produce T cells with specific reactivity against cancer and to try to develop methods to expand these cells to large numbers for therapy. Early efforts were hampered by an incomplete understanding of the factors required for T cell growth and the availability of such factors only as impure and heterogeneous mixtures of factors contained in conditioned supernatants. The discovery of the T cell growth factor, now called interleukin-2 (IL-2),[8] and its cloning and availability in large quantities as recombinant material were of critical importance to the development of immunotherapy. IL-2, secreted by helper T lymphocytes, plays an essential role in mediating T cell proliferation during the developing immune response and was the first soluble factor discovered that could result in the proliferation of T cells in vitro.

The initial hope was that IL-2 would support the in vitro growth of T cells that would have specific antitumor reactivity. Evidence of specific antitumor reactivity was sought in the peripheral blood mononuclear cells of patients with cancer and mice bearing experimental tumors. Peripheral blood mononuclear cells were cultured in vitro in IL-2 and were used as effector cells in short-term ^{51}Cr release assays with cultured and fresh tumor targets. Such cells never manifested activity specific for the autologous tumor, but substantial and reproducible lytic activity against a variety of tumor targets was found. This activity was named "lymphokine-activated killer," or LAK.[9, 10] Despite the fact that LAK cells are produced by culture of a heterogeneous group of cells in a T cell growth factor (IL-2), the cells that appear to manifest LAK activity are not T cells, but are derived from the natural killer line of immune cells. Natural killer cell precursors can be activated by culture in IL-2, and it is these cells that appear to mediate LAK activity.[11]

Preclinical Studies in Mouse Tumor Models

Before the initiation of human clinical trials, extensive studies of IL-2 and LAK were carried out in murine tumor models. These studies were designed to answer a fundamentally important question: Could a regimen based upon IL-2 have impact upon established experimental metastatic cancer in mice? This was a crucial question, since many previous studies of immunotherapy regimens were designed only to prevent the development of metastases or the establishment of growing tumors at challenged sites. This clearly does not mimic the clinical situation in which patients with established metastatic cancer present for therapy.

The murine tumor models studied at the Surgery Branch of the National Cancer Institute fulfilled a strict set of criteria designed to maximize the chance that these tumors would mimic the clinically relevant situation. First, the tumors were induced newly in mice by the injection into muscle of the carcinogen methylcholanthrene. This chemical carcinogen resulted in the development of a panel of murine sarcomas that were excised from the initial mouse and maintained by serial passage through syngeneic animals. These original tumors never were placed into tissue culture for the murine studies. The tumors were cryopreserved after a few very early passages through mice. After between 6 to 8 in vivo passages of the tumor, an early cryopreserved vial from passage 2 to 3 was thawed, injected into mice, and used for subsequent passages of that tumor. Hence, tumors used as a source of study in this model never had gone through more than eight passages in animals before observations were made about their immunogenicity or potential for immunotherapy. In this way, we were able to maintain a well-defined and reproducible set of tumors with a variety of immunogenic and nonimmunogenic properties.

To establish experimental metastases in mice, single-cell suspensions of fresh tumors serially passaged in the subcutaneous space of animals were prepared. When these tumor cells were injected intravenously, lung metastases were induced reliably. In addition, hepatic metastases could be induced by injection of single-cell suspensions of tumors into the spleen with subsequent splenectomy.

A large number of studies of IL-2 and LAK cells were carried out in these experimental murine tumor models.[12] A brief summary of these murine studies is presented in Table 2. It became quite clear at the outset of these studies that recombinant human IL-2 alone had antitumor activity when administered to mice bearing established experimental murine metastases.[13] IL-2 had this effect not through any direct toxic effect upon tumor cells, but through the recruitment and growth of immune cells within the animal. Murine studies also clearly demonstrated that LAK cells could be produced from murine splenocytes by culture in high-dose IL-2 for 3 to 5 days. Such cells, especially when combined with IL-2, demonstrated substantial efficacy in the treatment of both immunogenic and nonimmunogenic experimental metastases in mice.[14] An example of this phenomenon is shown in Figure 3. The mechanism of this combination therapy was suggested by the finding that systemic IL-2 resulted in the continued pro-

TABLE 2.
Systemic Interleukin-2 (IL-2)
Used Alone in Experimental
Murine Tumors

Hepatic and pulmonary experimental metastases can be inhibited significantly by IL-2

The antitumor effect and toxicity of IL-2 are dose dependent

IL-2 leads to the proliferation of lymphoid cells in mice and these cells can manifest lymphokine-activated killer activity in vitro

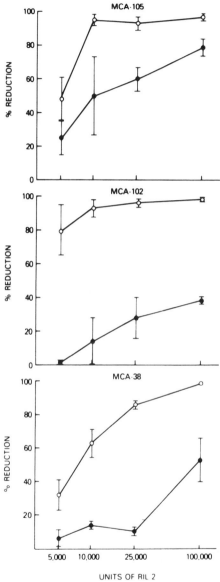

FIG 3.
Mice bearing established hepatic metastases of an immunogenic sarcoma *(MCA-105)*, a nonimmunogenic sarcoma *(MCA-102)*, and a colonic adenocarcinoma *(MC-38)* were treated with recombinant interleukin-2 (RIL-2) alone *(closed circles)* or RIL-2 plus LAK cells *(open circles)*. The reduction in number of metastases was greater in every instance for LAK cells plus RIL-2 compared to RIL-2 alone. (From Lafreniere R, Rosenberg SA: *J Immunol* 1985; 135:4273–4280. Used by permission.)

liferation of the transferred LAK cells in vivo for a limited period of time.[15] These murine studies were the basis for human trials of IL-2 and LAK in the treatment of metastatic cancer in patients.

Clinical Studies of Interleukin-2

The availability of recombinant IL-2 in large amounts led to the testing of this therapy in patients with cancer. Patients treated at the Surgery Branch of the National Cancer Institute since the initiation of IL-2–based immunotherapy have fulfilled several strict criteria. They must have metastatic cancer that has failed to respond to all standard therapy or for which no standard therapy exists. They must be in otherwise good health and have objectively evaluable metastatic lesions.

Phase I trials of recombinant IL-2 used alone were carried out. Twenty patients with metastatic carcinoma received bolus injections of recombinant IL-2 ranging from 10,000 units/kg weekly to 300,000 units/kg nine times a week. Dosages administered by continuous infusion ranged from 100 units/kg/hr to 3,000 units/kg/hr given for up to 7 days. Dose-limiting toxicity was seen at levels about 1 million units/kg given as a bolus or 3,000 units/kg/hr given by continuous intravenous administration.[16]

Morbidity related to IL-2 infusion included chills and fever within 4 hours of administration (100%), malaise (100%), weight gain (95%), nausea and vomiting (75%), headache (45%), diarrhea (45%), and a rash with pruritus (15%). Reasons for stopping therapy included hypotension, ascites, and marked fluid retention. Patients gained from 1 to 20 kg over a 3-week treatment period. Many of the side effects could be ameliorated by premedication with acetaminophen and indomethacin. These toxicities all reversed spontaneously after cessation of recombinant IL-2. No tumor regressions were seen at these dose levels.

As experience with recombinant IL-2 increased, it became clear that responses to IL-2 given alone could be observed at higher doses, albeit with greater toxicity. A phase I study was performed, treating 15 patients who had metastatic carcinoma with high-dose IL-2 (greater than 30,000 Cetus units/kg, three times daily) given as a bolus parenterally.[17] Three patients received 10,000 Cetus units/kg of recombinant IL-2 parenterally, three times daily, followed by escalation to 100,000 Cetus units/kg three times daily, until limiting toxicity was achieved.

Patients generally were treated on the ward, but as IL-2–related toxicity occurred, they were transferred to the intensive care unit for monitoring. Only 2 patients received 300,000 Cetus units/kg, as severe hypotension prohibited escalation beyond this dosage.[17] Treatment with IL-2 was based on clinical assessment, including evaluation of urine output, hypoxia, confusion, and agitation. Patients were examined prior to each dose, and a decision was made at that time whether to administer an additional dose.[17]

Medications helpful during treatment included antipyretics, antipruritics, and antacids. Nausea and vomiting, agitation, and confusion also occurred and required treatment. Patients required hydration to maintain urine output and systemic perfusion, receiving as much as 2 to 5 L/day. Administration of dopamine and phenylephrine was used to decrease fluid requirements. Central venous pressure and arterial pressure monitoring often were helpful. Diuretics also were used to maintain urine output. Similar toxicity was seen with intravenous and intraperitoneal administration of IL-2.

Patients were evaluated at least 2 months after treatment. A partial response was defined as more than a 50% decrease in the perpendicular diameter of all measurable lesions combined with the appearance of no new lesions. A complete response was defined as resolution of all measurable disease. Of the 15 patients treated, 1 patient with renal cell carcinoma had a complete response and 5 patients with melanoma had a partial response.[17]

The standard recombinant IL-2 schedule at the Surgery Branch of the National Cancer Institute is 100,000 Cetus units/kg every 8 hours by intravenous bolus. This dose in the now-standard international units is 720,000 IU/kg every 8 hours. Treatment is continued for up to 15 doses, until toxicity and the patient's tolerance preclude further doses. This constitutes one "cycle" of high-dose IL-2. Therapy consists of multiple cycles given with a 1-week rest period between cycles.

Interleukin-2 and Lymphokine-Activated Killer Cells

Before combination therapy with recombinant IL-2 and LAK cells (which animal models predicted would have significant antitumor efficacy) were performed in human patients, phase I trials of LAK cells used alone were carried out in individuals with metastatic cancer.[18] LAK cells were produced by culturing lymphocytes from peripheral blood or thoracic duct cannulation in recombinant IL-2 (1,000 Cetus U/mL) for 3 to 5 days. Such cells had nonspecific, non–MHC-restricted lytic activity against a variety of fresh and cultured human tumor target cells. Patients received 1.5 to 9.9 $\times$ 10^{10} total LAK cells intravenously. There was minimal toxicity associated with the infusions, and there were no favorable responses.[18]

Once phase I trials had defined the toxicity of IL-2 and LAK cells administered separately, these two modalities were combined. The first 25 patients treated with recombinant IL-2 and LAK were reported in 1985.[19] Patients were treated with a cycle of recombinant IL-2 followed by daily leukopheresis for 5 days (Fig 4). LAK cells were produced by culturing 5 $\times$ 10^9 to 5 $\times$ 10^{10} peripheral blood mononuclear cells in 1,000 units/mL of recombinant IL-2 for 3 to 4 days. The cells were washed and reinfused into the patients, along with intravenous recombinant IL-2.

In this early study, a 44% (11 of 25 patients) objective response rate was seen. These responses were seen in patients with metastatic malignant melanoma, colorectal cancer, renal cell carcinoma, and lung adenocarcinoma. The metastatic sites experiencing regression included the lung, liver,

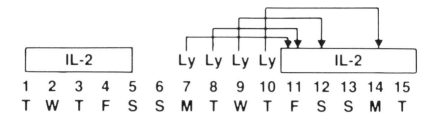

IL-2				Ly	Ly	Ly	Ly		IL-2				
1	2	3	4	5	6	7	8	9	10	11	12	13	14	15
T	W	T	F	S	S	M	T	W	T	F	S	S	M	T

Ly: lymphocytapheresis
IL-2: intravenously every 8 hours
LAK: intravenous infusion of cells

FIG 4.
Diagram of therapy with lymphokine-activated killer *(LAK)* cells plus interleukin-2 (IL-2) . (From Rosenberg SA: Adoptive cellular therapy: Clinical applications, in DeVita VT, Hellman S, Rosenberg SA (eds): *Biologic Therapy of Cancer.* Philadelphia, Lippincott, 1991, pp 214–236. Used by permission.)

and subcutaneous tissues.[19] Significant responses were seen in patients with metastatic renal cell carcinoma and melanoma. In some cases, these responses included the complete disappearance of bulky metastatic renal cell carcinoma in lung, liver, and bone (Fig 5).

Further experience with LAK and IL-2 in patients with metastatic renal cell carcinoma was reported in 1987.[20] The overall objective response rate (complete responses plus partial responses) was 33% in 36 evaluable patients with metastatic renal cell carcinoma (Table 3).

Toxicity related to the LAK cells in combination with IL-2 was similar to that seen with the infusion of IL-2 alone. Patients experienced fever and chills soon after infusion of the LAK cells. IL-2–related toxicity included fluid retention, pulmonary edema, fever, chills, and malaise, similar to that described previously. Subsequent treatment of large numbers of patients further characterized the toxicity of high-dose IL-2 used alone and in combination with LAK cells[20, 21] (Table 4). Four deaths were seen in 180 courses given to 157 patients. Two patients died with a myocardial infarction and 2 with pulmonary insufficiency related to sepsis. Experience with these patients has led to careful selection criteria that exclude patients with brain metastases, cardiac ischemia, or significant compromise of pulmonary, renal, or hepatic function. This selection process, in combination with the experience gained in treating patients, has led to the elimination of treatment related deaths in the last 150 patients treated. Overall treatment-related mortality for the Surgery Branch of the National Cancer Institute (1.3% in 1,023 patients) and the National Cancer Institute IL-2 Working Group (3.5% in 515 patients) has been 2.0% in 1,538 patients.

Because significant and durable responses were seen with high-dose IL-2 given alone as well as in combination with LAK cells, a prospective

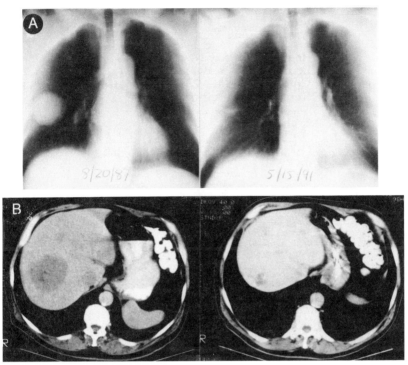

FIG 5.
Example of responses to immunotherapy with high-dose IL-2–based regimens in two patients with metastatic renal cell carcinoma. **A,** complete response of bulky pulmonary metastasis of renal cell carcinoma. **B,** partial response of large liver metastasis of renal cell carcinoma. In both panels, the left images are before therapy and the right images are after IL-2–based immunotherapy.

randomized trial of 181 patients comparing these two therapies was performed.[22] The majority of patients randomized under this protocol had metastatic renal cell carcinoma or melanoma. The data from this trial are mature, with 5-year follow-up, and the overall survival of patients with renal cell carcinoma is shown in Figure 6. There was no difference in survival between the two groups. Thus, in patients with metastatic renal cell carcinoma, LAK cells did not increase the efficacy of high-dose IL-2 given alone. However, the overall survival of both groups was in the range of 30%. It was these survival data and the overall response rates from the Surgery Branch of the National Cancer Institute, the National Cancer Institute extramural trial, and patients treated by Cetus Corporation that resulted in the approval of IL-2 in 1992 by the U.S. Food and Drug Administration for the treatment of metastatic renal cell carcinoma. These response rates are shown in Table 5; the overall objective response rates. (partial and complete) to high-dose IL-2 used alone in patients with meta-

TABLE 3.
Response to Interleukin-2 Plus
Lymphokine-Activated Killer
Cells in Patients With Metastatic
Renal Cell Carcinoma*†

Evaluable Patients	CR	PR	CR + PR
36	4	8	12 (33%)

*Data from Rosenberg SA, Lotze MT, Muul LM, et al: N Engl J Med 1985; 313:1485–1492. Used by permission.
†CR = complete response of all tumor; PR = at least 50% reduction in the sum of the perpendicular diameters of all lesions.

static renal cell carcinoma is 15% in this group evaluated by the U.S. Food and Drug Administration.

The optimum schedule and dosage of IL-2 in renal cell carcinoma remains to be determined. We have initiated a randomized trial of standard high-dose IL-2 (720,000 IU/kg intravenously every 8 hours) vs. a dose tenfold lower given on the same schedule (72,000 IU/kg intravenously every 8 hours) in patients with metastatic renal cell carcinoma. Responses have been seen in both groups, with a substantial decrease in toxicity noted in the low-dose IL-2 group, but it is too early to draw any conclusions (J. Yang, unpublished results, 1992). Many such trials will be required to optimize the administration of IL-2; high-dose bolus IL-2 must be considered standard therapy in such trials, as this is the only regimen with established efficacy for metastatic renal cell carcinoma.

Interleukin-2 Plus α Interferon

α-Interferon given alone has been shown to have antitumor activity against melanoma and renal cell carcinoma. α-Interferon also has a broad range of immunostimulatory effects. Murine studies demonstrated synergy of recombinant IL-2 and α-interferon, which led to phase I trials in humans.[23] Ninety-four patients were treated with 1, 3, or 4.5 × 10^6 Hoffmann-LaRoche units/m² of IL-2 and 3 × 10^6 to 6 × 10^6 units/m² of α-interferon, administered intravenously every 8 hours for 5 days. After a 1- to 2-week rest, the 5-day cycle was repeated.

Side effects were similar to those seen when α-interferon or IL-2 was used alone, and included malaise, nausea, vomiting, diarrhea, chills, fluid

TABLE 4.
Toxicity of Interleukin-2 (IL-2) and Lymphokine-Activated Killer (LAK) Cells Plus IL-2 Administration*

Toxicity	LAK + IL-2	IL-2	Total
	Number of Courses		
Total	127	53	180
Chills	101	20	120
Pruritus	57	30	87
Anaphylaxis	0	0	0
Mucositis (requiring liquid diet)	7	0	7
Nausea and vomiting	107	46	153
Diarrhea	106	47	153
Hyperbilirubinemia (highest level)			
2.1–6.0 mg/dL	61	24	85
6.1–10.0 mg/dL	29	16	45
≥10.0 mg/dL	16	7	23
Hepatitis A (due to LAK-cell infusion)	5	—	5
Oliguria			
<80 mL/8 hr	32	19	51
<240mL/24 hr	3	9	12
Weight gain (% body weight)			
2.1–6.0	38	15	53
6.1–10.0	35	17	52
10.1–14.0	25	13	38
14.1–18.0	6	4	10
≥18.1	9	1	10
Elevated creatinine (highest level)			
2.1–6.0 mg/dL	88	34	122
6.2–10.0 mg/dL	12	8	20
≥10.0 mg/dL	2	2	4
Hematuria (gross)	0	0	0
Edema (symptomatic nerve or vessel compression)	2	1	3
Respiratory distress			
No intubation	13	5	18
Intubation	10	6	16
Bronchospasm	2	0	2
Pleural effusion (requiring thoracentesis)	5	0	5
Somnolence	17	9	26
Coma	5	4	9
Disorientation	48	16	64
Hypotension (requiring pressors)	89	34	123
Myocardial infarction	1	3	4
Arrhythmias			
Atrial	19	5	24
Ventricular	1	0	1

(Continued.)

TABLE 4 (cont.).

Anemia (number of units transfused)			
1–5	51	25	76
6–10	35	12	47
11–15	14	3	17
≥16	10	0	10
Thrombocytopenia (lowest level)			
≤20,000/mm^3	17	7	24
21,000–60,000 mm^3	42	17	59
61,000–100,000/mm^3	31	12	43
Central-line sepsis	20	3	23
Death	1	3	4

*From Rosenberg S, Lotze MT, Muul LM, et al: *N Engl J Med* 1987; 316:889–897. Used by permission.

retention, and weight gain. Toxicity was more severe at higher doses, and three particular side effects were more severe than expected: elevated liver transaminase levels, confusion, and mild to moderate disorientation. The liver abnormalities were temporary and spontaneously reverted to normal (median, 10 days). One patient of 94 died (1.1%) of aspiration pneumoni-

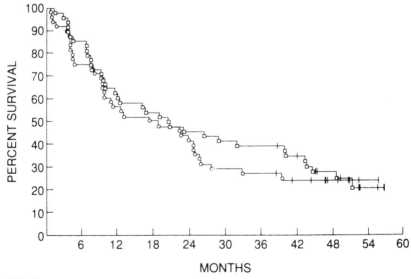

FIG 6.
Survival of patients with metastatic renal cell carcinoma randomly assigned to receive high-dose IL-2 alone *(open circles)* or IL-2 plus LAK cells *(open squares)*. No difference in survival was seen (P = .55). (From Rosenberg SA: *J Clin Oncol* 1992; 10:180–199. Used by permission.)

TABLE 5.
U.S. Food and Drug Administration Review of Patients With Metastatic Renal Cell Carcinoma Treated With High-Dose Interleukin-2*

Center	Number of Patients	CR	PR
Surgery Branch, NCI	68	5	9
NCI extramural phase II studies	124	3	11
Cetus Corporation, phase II studies	63	1	8
Total	255	9	28

*CR = complete response; PR = partial response; NCI = National Cancer Institute.

TABLE 6.
Response to α-Interferon (α-INF) and Interleukin-2 (IL-2) Combination Therapy in Renal Cell Carcinoma*

Response ↓	Dose ($\times 10^6$ units/m^2)			
	α-INF 3 + IL-2 1	α-INF 3 + IL-2 3	α-INF 3 + IL-2 4.5	α-INF 6 + IL-2 4.5
Total number of patients	4	11	7	13
Number with a partial response	0	2	2	3
Number with a complete response	1	1	0	2
Percent partial and complete response	25	27	29	38

*Data from Rosenberg SA, Lotze MT, Yang JC, et al: *J Clin Oncol* 1989; 7:1863–1874. Used by permission.

tis following treatment. Autopsy study of this patient demonstrated dense lymphocytic infiltrates in all organs examined, including tumor sites. The median number of doses received for each escalating dosage was 25, 20, 18, and 15, respectively. Thirty-nine patients received more than one course of treatment. Since the maximum number of doses in one course is

30, it is apparent that, even at low doses, significant dose-limiting transient toxicity occurred.

Seven of the 91 patients treated had complete tumor regression and 18 had partial regression. The responses in patients with metastatic renal cell carcinoma are listed in Table 6. Responses were seen most commonly in patients with melanoma or renal cell carcinoma. They appeared to be associated with patients receiving the highest dosages (43% and 38%, respectively), although the difference was not statistically significant ($P = .12$). Responses were seen in multiple sites, as was observed with IL-2 and LAK cells. These sites included the lung, lymph nodes, adrenal glands, and subcutaneous tissues. The remissions appeared to be clinically significant, lasting as long as 14 months at the time of the last evaluation.

Role of Nephrectomy

We generally have removed the primary renal tumor in patients who are candidates for immunotherapy.[24] This approach was selected for several reasons. First, many of our patients presented for immunotherapy having undergone nephrectomy either for palliation of symptoms or because they presented with metastases following nephrectomy in the past. Hence, nephrectomy of all patients before immunotherapy maintained a more uniform population of patients. Second, we have made extensive studies of the nephrectomy specimens, both the tumor cells and the infiltrating lymphocytes, which is possible only if nephrectomy is performed before immunotherapy. It is by no means clear that this is the best way to proceed, however. For example, in our patient population with metastatic renal cell carcinoma who were undergoing nephrectomy prior to immunotherapy, 40% of patients never received immunotherapy, principally because of progression of cancer (M. Walther, unpublished observations, 1992). Hence, a criticism of this approach is that most patients undergo surgery unnecessarily, since a substantial number of those operated upon are unable to receive immunotherapy, and most of those who do receive immunotherapy do not respond to it.

Because of this, we carried out a pilot study of initial immunotherapy in patients with newly diagnosed metastatic renal cell carcinoma and with the primary tumor in place.[25] A total of 12 such patients received α-interferon and IL-2. There was one complete response of all metastatic disease, and this patient was rendered tumor-free with a subsequent nephrectomy. In other patients, mixed responses were seen, but no responses were observed in the primary tumor. Thus, responses can be seen in patients having their primary tumor in place and, in this instance, nephrectomy can be reserved for those patients who respond to immunotherapy. However, as we never have seen a response to immunotherapy in the renal primary tumor, it theoretically is possible that its presence could inhibit responses at distant sites. The answer to this question can come only from prospective randomized trials.

Tumor-Infiltrating Lymphocytes

The continued search for specifically reactive antitumor T cells led back to the tumor itself, in which tumor-infiltrating lymphocytes (TILs) first were described in 1986.[26] Histologic examination of tumors frequently demonstrates a lymphocytic infiltrate. TILs are produced by culture of single-cell suspensions from human and murine tumors in IL-2. Such cultures yield growing lymphocyte populations that, in both mice and humans, consist mainly of cells with T lymphocyte markers. TILs differ fundamentally from LAK cells in many ways. TILs are largely T lymphocytes and exhibit many of the properties associated with T lymphocytes in antiviral or transplantation models. A summary of observations concerning TILs is shown in Table 7.[27-30] Most studies of human TILs in the Surgery Branch of the National Cancer Institute have involved patients with melanoma. Other tumor types, such as renal cell carcinoma, have been studied; however, most observations relevant to TILs in patients have been demonstrated clearly only in melanoma.

The most important observation with regard to TILs is that they can be produced from both murine and human tumors, which specifically recognize the autologous tumor of origin, but not other tumors.[27, 28] This tumor recognition is MHC-restricted and antigen-specific, and appears to be mediated by T cell receptor/CD3 complex signal transduction. Tumor specificity is of fundamental importance, because it supports the belief that at least some human tumors contain antigens that can be recognized as non-self or

---

TABLE 7.
Characteristics of Tumor-Infiltrating Lymphocytes (TILs)

TILs contain T lymphocytes (CD3$^+$, CD8$^+$, or CD4$^+$)

TILs from some murine and human tumors can manifest specific recognition of tumor antigens

Specific recognition of tumor antigens is restricted by major histocompatibility complex

TILs proliferate under the influence of interleukin-2 in vitro and in vivo

TILs are more potent than lymphokine-activated killer cells in mediating antitumor effects in mice

TILs can survive long term and mediate memory T cell functions

altered-self by the T cell repertoire. The nature of such tumor antigens, how they are expressed, and how the response to them might be suppressed by the tumor or augmented as a therapeutic attempt are crucial questions that must be addressed if specific adoptive immunotherapy ever will have general application to patients with cancer.

Recognition by TILs of autologous tumors has been measured principally by cytolytic activity of T cells. In melanoma, the majority of TIL cultures contain substantial numbers of CD8+ cytotoxic T cells, which recognize tumor-associated antigens in the context of MHC class I molecules on the surface of the tumor cell. The majority of cultured human tumor lines obtained from patients with melanoma express class I MHC markers and when these tumor lines are mixed with TILs, autologous tumor-specific lysis of tumor cells can be observed in about 30% of TIL cultures.[28] Not only is this autologous tumor-specific lysis MHC-restricted, but there appear to be antigen(s) shared among melanomas from different patients.[31] This suggests that these antigens represent melanoma-associated aberrant or altered proteins, and that these proteins are processed and presented to the TILs by the tumor cells. Thus, CD8+ TILs that recognize this antigen in the context of self MHC also will recognize other melanomas expressing the same MHC class I isotype, either naturally occurring or transfected into the tumor cell.[32] The actual antigenic moiety recognized by TILs remains unknown. A family of oncofetal proteins recently has been cloned and appears to represent a melanoma-associated antigen.[33]

In addition to lytic activity, TILs also can secrete lymphokines specifically after exposure to autologous tumor.[34] This has been demonstrated in melanomas and other tumors. Such cytokine secretion appears to be critical to the in vivo function of the TILs. In murine tumor models, in vivo efficacy of TILs correlates more closely with cytokine secretion than with lysis.[35] Finally, TILs manifest a rapid and sustained increase in intracellular calcium after conjugation to autologous tumor cells.[36] This signal transduction pathway is typical of that mediated by the TCR. These studies demonstrate that TILs can recognize antigens associated with human melanoma in a way analogous to that which is well-known to occur in other systems of T cell recognition of viral or transplantation antigens. This observation is important, first, because such tumor-specific antigens exist and, second, because TILs can be produced in large numbers for trials as a therapeutic agent for patients with cancer.

Immunotherapy With Tumor-Infiltrating Lymphocytes and Interleukin-2

Murine studies demonstrated that TILs alone or in combination with IL-2 had substantial antitumor activity against established pulmonary and hepatic metastases.[26, 37] TILs are up to 100 times more potent than LAK cells in such models.[26, 37] In addition, the use of cyclophosphamide pretreatment increased the efficacy of TILs and IL-2; cyclophosphamide was required for TILs to be effective against bulky experimental metastases.[26]

Based upon the animal data, a preliminary trial of cyclophosphamide, TILs, and IL-2 was carried out in 12 patients.[38] Patients received cyclophosphamide, 25 to 50 mg/kg intravenously, with parenteral hydration. At least five half-lives later (cyclophosphamide plasma half-life = 6.5 hours), TIL infusions were begun. Patients received 8×10^9 to 2.3×10^{11} cells. A maximum of 6×10^{10} cells were infused per treatment. Recombinant IL-2 was administered intravenously at 10,000, 30,000, or 100,000 Cetus units/kg intravenously every 8 hours, beginning with completion of the first infusion of TILs. IL-2 administration was continued to dose-limiting toxicity, similar to the procedure used in patients treated with IL-2 alone, but was limited to one course of treatment.

In 4 of 12 (33%) patients, TIL growth was not sufficient for the target dosage for infusion of 10^{10} TILs per patient. In subsequent studies with larger groups of patients, about one third also did not have growth of their TILs. The time needed to grow TILs ranged from 19 to 48 days, with an average of about 4 weeks. TIL growth in vitro did not correlate with tumor type, site of metastatic lesion harvested, or amount of lymphoid infiltrate in the tumor when harvested. Toxicity related to TIL infusion was minimal, usually including chills, which responded to meperidine. Toxicity appeared to be related closely to IL-2 administration. These toxicities were self-limited following cessation of therapy. Neutropenia and thrombocytopenia were most severe in patients receiving cyclophosphamide, but were not significantly worse than in patients not receiving cyclophosphamide. One patient with metastatic melanoma and 1 with metastatic renal cell carcinoma achieved a partial response.[38]

Following demonstration of the safety of administering IL-2 in combination with TILs, 20 patients with metastatic malignant melanoma were treated with high-dose IL-2 (100,000 Cetus units/kg every 8 hours) and TILs (median dosage, 2×10^{11} cells) following pretreatment with cyclophosphamide (25 mg/kg).[39] Toxicity was similar to that described previously. One patient achieved a complete response and 10 patients achieved partial responses (11 of 20, 55%). These responses lasted a minimum of 2 months to more than 13 months. Regression of cancer was observed in multiple sites, as described with IL-2 and LAK cells.

The mechanism of cyclophosphamide's effect in this therapy is unknown. Previous studies suggested that pretreatment with cyclophosphamide was needed to remove suppressor T cells from the host.[40] Another possibility is that cyclophosphamide directly decreases the tumor burden. This latter prospect was supported by the observation in mice that TILs, IL-2, and tumor irradiation had synergistic antitumor activity, but only if the treated tumor was preirradiated.[41] Synergistic antitumor effects of TILs and IL-2 were not seen if the entire animal except for the tumor was preirradiated.[41] Such an observation is inconsistent with suppressor cell inactivation as the mechanism of cyclophosphamide's activity in TIL therapy.

To determine if TILs could localize specifically to tumor sites, localization studies were performed using [111]Indium oxine–labeled TILs in patients with metastatic malignant melanoma.[42] These patients were pretreated with cyclophosphamide. [111]Indium TILs were seen to traffic to lung, liver, and spleen within 2 hours after intravenous infusion, with clearance from the lung in 24 hours. Labeled TILs were seen to localize in sites of metastatic disease by 24 hours. Biopsies of tumor tissue demonstrated 3 to 40 times greater [111]Indium activity than is found in normal tissue. These studies demonstrate that TILs could traffic specifically to tumor sites in patients with melanoma. Interestingly, patients treated under later TIL protocols without cyclophosphamide pretreatment had specific trafficking to tumor demonstrated less frequently.[43] The fact that pretreatment with cyclophosphamide improves tumor trafficking by TILs may explain the synergistic antitumor effects of the combination therapy.[43]

Tumor-Infiltrating Lymphocytes From Renal Cell Carcinoma

TILs can be grown readily from the majority of patients with renal cell carcinoma. This has been demonstrated both for the primary tumor as well as for metastatic sites. TILs from patients with renal cell carcinoma differ from those found in melanoma, principally in that specific antitumor reactivity is seen much less frequently with renal cell carcinoma. TILs from renal cell carcinoma typically are enriched for cells of the helper (CD4) phenotype rather than the cytotoxic (CD8) phenotype. Although specific antitumor reactions in patients with renal cell carcinoma mediated by TILs have been observed less frequently, they clearly do occur.[44, 45]

In preliminary studies at the Surgery Branch of the National Cancer Institute, patients with metastatic renal cell carcinoma have received treatment with IL-2 and TILs. Responses have been observed, including two unequivocal responses in patients who failed to respond to high-dose IL-2 alone. This suggests that TILs from patients with renal cell carcinoma can exhibit antitumor activity (J. Yang, unpublished results, 1992). However, the number of patients treated is small.

Current Studies and Future Plans

We are attempting to develop methodologies to detect T cells with specific reactivity to renal cell carcinoma tumor antigens, analogous to those found in melanoma. We also are trying to devise methods to grow such cells to large numbers while maintaining their specific reactivity. We are examining T cells obtained not only from lymphocytes infiltrating tumors, but also from regional lymph nodes and peripheral blood. We have developed a method to detect T cell reactivity in individual T cells,[36] and have begun to study different types of antigen-presenting cells in order to stimulate tumor-reactive T cells. In murine tumor models, dendritic cells, which are very potent antigen-presenting cells, can present tumor antigens to T cells and can stimulate the proliferation of tumor-specific CD4[+] T cells.[46] Such studies are being extended to patients with metastatic renal cell carcinoma.

Such specifically reactive T cells could be used to define the antigen(s), if present, expressed by renal cell carcinoma cells and also may have potential for therapy of patients.

References

1. Weiss A, Imboden J, Hardy K, et al: The role of the T3/antigen receptor complex in the T cell activation. *Annu Rev Immunol* 1986; 4:593–619.
2. Krensky AM, Weiss A, Crabtree G, et al: T-lymphocyte antigen interactions in transplant rejection. *N Engl J Med* 1990; 322:510–517.
3. Weiss A, Imboden JB: Cell surface molecules and early events involved in human T-lymphocyte activation. *Adv Immunol* 1987; 41:1–38.
4. Gotch F, Rothbard J, Howard K, et al: Cytotoxic T lymphocytes recognize a fragment of influenza virus matrix protein in association with HLA-A2. *Nature* 1987; 326:881–882.
5. Restifo NP: Antigen processing and presentation: An update, in DeVita VT, Hellman S, Rosenberg SA (eds): *Biologic Therapy of Cancer Updates,* vol 2. Philadelphia, Lippincott, 1992, p 1–10.
6. Swain SL, Bradley LM: Helper T cell memory: More questions than answers. *Semin Immunol* 1992; 4:59–68.
7. Matsumura M, Fremont DH, Peterson PA, et al: Emerging principles for the recognition of peptide antigens by MHC class I molecules. *Science* 1992; 257:927–934.
8. Morgan DA, Ruscetti FW, Gallo RG: Selective in vitro growth as T lymphocytes from normal bone marrow. *Science* 1976; 193:1007–1008.
9. Grimm EA, Mazumder A, Zhang HZ, et al: Lymphokine activated killer cell phenomenon: Lysis of natural-killer resistant fresh solid tumor cells by interleukin-2 activated autologous human peripheral blood lymphocytes. *J Exp Med* 1982; 155:1823–1841.
10. Yang JC, Mulé JJ, Rosenberg SA: Murine lymphokine activated killer cells. *J Immunol* 1985; 137:715–722.
11. Phillips JH, Lanier LL: Dissection of the lymphokine activated killer phenomenon. *J Exp Med* 1986; 164:814–825.
12. Yang JC, Rosenberg SA: Adoptive cellular therapy: Preclinical studies, in DeVita VT, Hellman S, Rosenberg SA (eds): *Biologic Therapy of Cancer.* Philadelphia, Lippincott, 1991, pp 197–213.
13. Mulé JJ, Rosenberg SA: Interleukin-2: Preclinical trials, in DeVita VT, Hellman S, Rosenberg SA (eds): *Biologic Therapy of Cancer.* Philadelphia, Lippincott, 1991, pp 142–158.
14. Lafreniere R, Rosenberg SA: Adoptive immunotherapy of murine hepatic metastases with lymphokine activated killer (LAK) cells and recombinant interleukin-2 (rIl-2) can mediate the regression of both immunogenic and nonimmunogenic sarcomas and an adenocarcinoma. *J Immunol* 1985; 135: 4273–4280.
15. Ettinghausen SE, Lipford EH, Mulé JJ, et al: Recombinant interleukin-2 stimulates in vivo proliferation of adoptively transferred lymphokine activated killer (LAK) cells. *J Immunol* 1985; 135:3623–3635.
16. Lotze MT, Matory YL, Ettinghausen SE, et al: In vivo administration of purified human interleukin-2. II. Half life, immunologic effects, and expansion of peripheral lymphoid cells in vivo with recombinant IL-2. *J Immunol* 1985; 135:2865–2875.

17. Lotze MT, Chang AE, Seipp CA, et al: High-dose recombinant interleukin-2 in the treatment of patients with disseminated cancer. JAMA 1986; 256: 3117–3124.
18. Rosenberg SA: Immunotherapy of cancer by systemic administration of lymphoid cells plus interleukin-2. J Biol Response Mod 1984; 3:501–511.
19. Rosenberg SA, Lotze MT, Muul LM, et al: Observations on the systemic administration of autologous lymphokine activated killer cells and recombinant interleukin-2 to patients with metastatic cancer. N Engl J Med 1985; 313:1485–1492.
20. Rosenberg SA, Lotze MT, Muul LM, et al: A progress report on the treatment of 157 patients with advanced cancer using lymphokine-activated killer cells and interleukin-2 or high-dose interleukin-2 alone. N Engl J Med 1987; 316:889–897.
21. Rosenberg SA, Lotze MT, Yang JC, et al: Experience with the use of high-dose interleukin-2 in the treatment of 652 cancer patients. Ann Surg 1989; 210:474–484.
22. Rosenberg SA, Yang JC, Topalian SL, et al: Prospective randomized trial of high dose interleukin-2 alone or with lymphokine activated killer cells for the treatment of patients with advanced cancer. J Natl Cancer Inst, in press.
23. Rosenberg SA, Lotze MT, Yang JC, et al: Combination therapy with interleukin-2 and alpha-interferon for the treatment of patients with advanced cancer. J Clin Oncol 1989; 7:1863–1874.
24. Robertson CN, Linehan WM, Pass HI, et al: Preparative cytoreductive surgery in patients with metastatic renal cell carcinoma treated with adoptive immunotherapy with interleukin-2 or interleukin-2 plus lymphokine activated killer cells. J Urol 1990; 144:614–618.
25. Spencer WF, Linehan WM, Walther MM, et al: Immunotherapy with interleukin-2 and alpha-interferon in patients with metastatic renal cell cancer with in situ primary cancers: A pilot study. J Urol 1992; 147:24–30.
26. Rosenberg SA, Spiess P, Lafreniere R: A new approach to the adoptive immunotherapy of cancer with tumor infiltrating lymphocytes. Science 1985; 233:1318–1321.
27. Barth RJ Jr, Block SN, Mulé JJ, et al: Unique murine tumor associated antigens identified by tumor infiltrating lymphocytes. J Immunol 1990; 144: 1531–1537.
28. Topalian SL, Solomon D, Rosenberg SA: Tumor-specific cytolysis by lymphocytes infiltrating human melanomas. J Immunol 1989; 142:3714–3725.
29. Alexander RB, Rosenberg SA: Long term survival of adoptively transferred tumor infiltrating lymphocytes in mice. J Immunol 1990; 145:1615–1620.
30. Alexander RB, Rosenberg SA: Adoptively transferred tumor infiltrating lymphocytes can cure established metastatic tumor in mice and persist long-term in vivo as functional memory T lymphocytes. J Immunother 1991; 10: 389–397.
31. Hom SS, Topalian SL, Simonis T, et al: Common expression of melanoma tumor-associated antigens recognized by human tumor infiltrating lymphocytes: Analysis by human lymphocyte antigen restriction. J Immunother 1991; 10:153–164.
32. Kawakami Y, Zakut R, Topalian SL, et al: Shared human melanoma antigens. Recognition by tumor infiltrating lymphocytes in HLA-A2.1-transfected melanomas. J Immunol 1992; 148:638–643.
33. van der Bruggen P, Traversari C, Chomez P, et al: A gene encoding an antigen recognized by cytolytic T lymphocytes on a human melanoma. Science 1991; 254:1643–1647.

34. Schwartzentruber DJ, Topalian SL, Mancini MJ, et al: Specific release of gran-ulocyte-macrophage colony-stimulating factor, tumor necrosis factor alpha, and IFN-γ tumor stimulation. *J Immunol* 1991; 146:153–164.

35. Barth RJ Jr, Mulé JJ, Spiess PJ, et al: Interferon-γ, and tumor necrosis factor have a role in tumor regressions mediated by murine CD8+ tumor-infiltrating lymphocytes. *J Exp Med* 1991; 173:647–658.

36. Alexander RB, Bolton ES, Koenig S, et al: Detection of antigen specific T lym-phocytes by determination of intracellular calcium concentration using flow cy-tometry. *J Immunol Methods* 1992; 148:131–141.

37. Spiess PJ, Yang JC, Rosenberg SA: In vivo antitumor activity of tumor-infil-trating lymphocytes expanded in recombinant interleukin-2. *J Natl Cancer Inst* 1987; 79:1067–1075.

38. Topalian SL, Solomon D, Avis FP, et al: Immunotherapy of patients with ad-vanced cancer using tumor infiltrating lymphocytes and recombinant interleu-kin-2. A pilot study. *J Clin Oncol* 1988; 6:839–853.

39. Rosenberg SA, Packard BS, Aebersold PM, et al: Use of tumor-infiltrating lym-phocytes and interleukin-2 in the immunotherapy of patients with metastatic melanoma. A preliminary report. *N Engl J Med* 1988; 319:1676–1680.

40. Greenberg PD, Cheever MA: Treatment of disseminated leukemia with cyclo-phosphamide and immune cells: Tumor immunity reflects long term persis-tence of tumor-specific donor T cells. *J Immunol* 1984; 133:3401–3407.

41. Cameron RB, Spiess PJ, Rosenberg SA: Synergistic antitumor activity of tu-mor infiltrating lymphocytes, interleukin-2 and local tumor irradiation: Studies on the mechanism of action. *J Exp Med* 1990; 171:249–263.

42. Fisher B, Packard BS, Read EJ, et al: Tumor localization of adoptively trans-ferred indium-111 labeled tumor infiltrating lymphocytes in patients with met-astatic melanoma. *J Clin Oncol* 1989; 7:250–261.

43. Pockaj BA, Sherry R, Wei J, et al: Localization of [111]indium-labelled tumor in-filtrating lymphocytes to tumor in patients receiving adoptive immunotherapy: Augmentation with cyclophosphamide and association with response. Submit-ted for publication.

44. Finke JH, Rayman P, Edinger M, et al: Characterization of a human renal cell carcinoma specific cytotoxic CD8+ T cell line. *J Immunother* 1992; 11:1–11.

45. Belldegrun A, Kasid A, Uppenkamp M, et al: Lymphokine mRNA profile and functional analysis of a human CD4+ clone with unique antitumor specificity isolated from renal cell carcinoma ascitic fluid. *Cancer Immunol Immunother* 1990; 31:1–10.

46. Cohen PJ, Cohen PA, Rosenberg SA, et al: Murine epidermal Langerhans cells and splenic dendritic cells process and present tumor-associated antigens to primed T cells. Submitted for publication.

Chemotherapy for Bladder Cancer

Malcolm Moore, M.D.

Assistant Professor, Department of Medicine and Pharmacology, Princess Margaret Hospital and University of Toronto, Toronto, Ontario, Canada

Ian Tannock, M.D., Ph.D.

Professor and Chairman, Department of Medicine, Princess Margaret Hospital and University of Toronto, Toronto, Ontario, Canada

Of patients who present with muscle-invasive bladder cancer, about one third are cured with local therapy, whereas the remainder develop pelvic recurrence or distant metastases. Almost all of these patients will die of their disease and, although symptomatic care and the use of radiation therapy may provide palliation, any major improvement in symptom control or prognosis is likely to derive from improvements in chemotherapy.

When patients with bladder cancer develop distant metastases, these usually become clinically apparent within 3 years after local treatment. Since growth from a single cell or a small cluster of cells to form a clinically evident metastasis usually requires a longer period, it is probable that these distant sites are seeded prior to treatment of the primary tumor. Thus, improvements in local therapy have only a limited potential to increase the probability of long-term survival for patients with muscle-invasive bladder cancer. Rather, a substantial improvement in outcome requires the use of effective adjuvant systemic therapy to eradicate micrometastatic disease.

In this chapter, we provide an overview of the current status of chemotherapy for muscle-invasive and metastatic bladder cancer. Since the evaluation of chemotherapy requires critical examination of clinical trials, we will outline initially the essential components of the design, analysis, and reporting of trials. A review of selected clinical trials that meet reasonable criteria then will allow assessment of the current status of chemotherapy in the treatment of metastatic bladder cancer and as an adjunct to surgery, radiation therapy, or both for the treatment of localized muscle-invasive disease.

Clinical Trials

Types of Clinical Trial

Clinical trials of chemotherapy may be separated conveniently into phase 1, 2, and 3 trials, depending on the goals of investigation. The design and analysis of each type of trial is quite different.

The major goal of a phase 1 trial is to determine the toxicity of a new treatment and to devise a dose schedule that can be tested further. Such trials usually are performed on new drugs that have antitumor activity in tissue culture and in animals, but have not been tested in patients yet. A dose schedule of the drug that would be expected to have minimal toxicity based on experiments in animals is given to a small group of patients with cancer for whom no known effective treatment is available. These patients are monitored for toxicity and pharmacokinetics of the drug. If there are no severe side effects, successive groups of patients receive gradually increased doses until a maximal tolerated dose is found. Any response to treatment is recorded, but this is not a major aim of the study. Responses usually are infrequent,[1, 2] because most participants in phase 1 trials already have shown tumor progression after treatment with standard agents.

Phase 2 trials evaluate a new drug or drug combination for antitumor activity in a group of patients with a given type of cancer. In bladder cancer, this could involve testing in patients who no longer are responsive to standard treatment or in those who have not received prior chemotherapy. The patients should have measurable soft-tissue lesions, and the study end point is tumor shrinkage. A new drug is considered worthy of further study only if it causes shrinkage in at least 20% of patients. Since the probability of a 20% response rate is small (<5%) if there are no responses in the first 14 patients, it is common to accrue only about 14 to 16 patients initially. The assessment of tumor response is subject to error and depends on the criteria of response that are used.[3, 4] It is important to recognize that tumor response does not imply benefit to patients, and that any drug or combination that causes tumor shrinkage needs further evaluation to determine whether it is useful in palliation.

Ideally, any new treatment showing promise in phase 2 studies should be evaluated in a trial in which patients are randomized to receive the new or standard treatment. These randomized phase 3 trials are appropriate when evaluating new treatments for metastatic disease (e.g., methotrexate, vinblastine, doxorubicin [Adriamycin], and cisplatin [M-VAC] vs. cisplatin) or for local disease (e.g., cystectomy alone vs. cystectomy and chemotherapy). The appropriate end points for such trials are those that evaluate benefit to patients (i.e., survival and quality of life); other measures, such as tumor response, are less important.

Unfortunately, because of the cost, the large numbers of patients required, and difficulties of organization, only a small number of experimental clinical strategies can be tested in a randomized trial against standard treatment. Investigators may believe so strongly in their approach that they consider testing against standard treatment unnecessary. Although this may be true for major advances such as the treatment of metastatic testicular cancer with cisplatin, improvements in the treatment of bladder cancer are expected to be more modest. The true benefits can be assessed only with a standardized comparison against other treatment approaches. Instead of performing randomized studies, many investigators enter patients into a larger single-arm trial that uses a uniform treatment policy, and then report their results (e.g., the large series of patients treated with the M-VAC regimen at Memorial Hospital).[5] These trials also usually are referred to as phase 2, although their goals are quite different than those of a phase 2 trial of a new agent, in which the aim is simply to establish whether the drug has sufficient evidence of biologic activity to warrant further study. In the larger, nonrandomized studies, it already is established that the treatment produces an effect, and the (often unstated) aim is to evaluate benefit to patients.[6]

Nonrandomized Control Patients

The outcome of patients receiving a new form of treatment often is compared with a historical series from the same institution or a concurrent series from a different center. Frequently, such comparisons are accompanied by a statement that the control and experimental populations have a similar distribution of prognostic factors such as age, stage, grade, and location of metastatic sites. Such comparisons usually are subject to considerable bias, often in favor of the group who receive the newer, experimental treatment.[7, 8] The medical literature contains numerous examples of highly promising results from single-arm studies that were not confirmed when compared to standard treatment in a randomized, controlled trial.[9, 10] Some of the reasons for this are discussed following.

Selection of Patients

Patients with bladder cancer frequently have complicating factors such as abnormal renal function or cardiovascular or pulmonary disease. Drugs that are active against bladder cancer often are quite toxic, and not all patients are able to tolerate them. Thus, single-arm series of patients who receive aggressive chemotherapy for metastatic disease or adjuvant chemotherapy for locally advanced disease, usually are selected from a larger group. This selection may take place within an institution or prior to referral to an academic center, so that even treatment of a "consecutive series" of patients does not exclude selection bias. It is not surprising that a series of patients selected for a new treatment on the basis of higher performance status and lack of other medical problems will have better survival than an unselected group of patients, even if the new therapy conferred little benefit.

Comparison of Poorly Defined End Points

Comparisons frequently are made between reported response rates from single-arm series that have evaluated different protocols of chemotherapy. Even if the patients were comparable, the determination of response rate depends on the response criteria used, which may vary, and on errors of assessment.[3, 4] Demonstration models have been used to show that analysis of a data set can lead to marked differences in estimates of response rate, depending on the methods used.[11, 12] This effect probably contributes to the lower response rates that usually are seen in multi-institution group studies (where there is careful review and stringent standards are applied) as compared to those from single institutions.[13]

Publication Bias

Publication bias refers to the tendency for investigators to submit, and for journal editors to accept, apparently "positive" trials, as compared to those that suggest no improvement in outcome.[14, 15] Publication bias also may apply to randomized studies, but large randomized studies usually are published even if there is no difference in outcome between their arms, albeit often in a less prominent journal than positive studies. A related effect, which has been termed "continuation bias," also may contribute to distortion of the literature.[8] Many investigators may initiate single-arm studies of combined modality treatment. Those studies in which (by chance alone) the first few patients do well are likely to be continued, and eventually published, whereas those in which the first few patients do not respond to treatment may be abandoned. It has been shown that publication bias (or rather "presentation bias") also leads to the preferred acceptance of apparently positive studies for presentation at medical meetings.[16]

Stage Migration

Stage migration produces bias in the stage-by-stage comparison of current patients with those treated previously.[17, 18] As new diagnostic techniques are introduced, smaller foci of disease may be detected than was possible previously. The effect is to upstage some patients (Fig 1). Thus, patients categorized as having stage 2 disease with current diagnostic technology may include a group who, a few years earlier, would have been classified as stage 1, and may exclude a group that now has been upstaged to stage 3. The net result is an apparent stage-by-stage improvement for the most recent series, even if there has been no change in therapy, since each stage grouping now contains patients with lower-volume disease (see Fig 1).

Survival as a Function of Response

If chemotherapy is given to patients with bladder cancer, a proportion of patients will have tumor shrinkage and will be designated responders to therapy. Regardless of whether treatment is given for metastatic disease or prior to local therapy for localized disease, it usually is found that patients who respond to chemotherapy have a better outcome than those who do

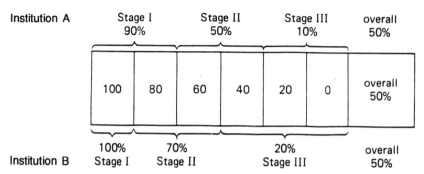

FIG 1.
Stage migration.

not respond[19, 20]; this should not be taken to imply a cause-and-effect relationship. Patients might have a better outcome *because* they responded to chemotherapy, but equally plausible is the hypothesis that those who were destined to do well (independent of the type of treatment used) also are those whose disease is most likely to respond to chemotherapy. Experience with neoadjuvant chemotherapy for head and neck cancer has shown that the latter hypothesis is correct for that disease: responders to chemotherapy almost always have better survival than do nonresponders, but randomized trials have shown no overall improvement in survival when compared to standard therapy with surgery, radiotherapy, or both.

Randomized Trials

Randomized, controlled trials offer the only rigorous method for comparing different schedules of chemotherapy in the treatment of metastatic bladder cancer and for evaluating the potential benefit from adjunctive chemotherapy. They are expensive, require collaboration between institutions, and, for studies of adjuvant chemotherapy, necessitate cooperation between different specialties. Only a very small number of new treatments for bladder cancer can be evaluated in randomized trials and, in North America, such trials have met with poor accrual. Attempts to mount simultaneous trials, in either the metastatic or adjuvant setting, have not been successful because of failure to agree on a protocol. It is unlikely that smaller individual trials will provide definitive answers.

Although randomized trials represent the only rigorous method for providing a valid comparison between two treatments, they also are subject to problems of interpretation. Some of these problems are outlined as follows.

Sample Size

Before initiating a clinical trial, it is important to specify its primary end point (usually survival), and to determine the magnitude of the difference in that end point that should be detected (if it truly exists) or excluded (if it does not exist) by the clinical trial. Ideally, this difference should be the smallest that is judged to warrant the introduction of the new treatment into clinical practice. In practice, it also will be influenced by the number of patients that can be accrued in the trial in a reasonable period of time. Tables are provided in most textbooks[21] providing estimates of the numbers of patients required to detect or exclude a given difference in survival between two arms of a trial. This estimate depends on the expected outcome with standard treatment, and the degree of certainty that is required. For example, a trial of adjuvant chemotherapy plus cystectomy as compared to cystectomy alone that seeks to detect or exclude an improvement in 5-year survival from 35% to 50% will require about 480 patients; this is likely to allow 95% certainty that a positive result is real (i.e., $\alpha = .05$) and 90% certainty (power, $1-\beta = 0.9$) that a negative result is valid. A trial designed to detect or exclude a 10% difference in 5-year survival with similar values of α and β would require more than 1,000 patients. It is sobering to reflect that the largest published trial of adjunctive chemotherapy for muscle-invasive bladder cancer accrued 376 patients,[22] and that no published North American trial has accrued more than 100 patients. Only one trial evaluating different regimens in treating metastatic disease in more than 100 patients has been completed.[23]

The results of small randomized trials sometimes are reported as showing no difference in outcome. A theoretic example is as follows: Fifty patients with T3 bladder cancer are randomized to receive either cystectomy (24 patients) or chemotherapy followed by cystectomy (26 patients). Five-year survival is 42% for patients receiving cystectomy alone (N = 24) and 50% for those receiving both chemotherapy and cystectomy (N = 26). The difference in outcome is not significant ($P \sim .6$). Similar trials have been reported to demonstrate that there is no difference between the two arms; this is not a valid conclusion. The trial has a very high probability of missing a clinically important result. The 95% confidence limits on the recorded values for 5-year survival are 22% to 63% for cystectomy alone, and 30% to 70% for combined treatment. The trial results are consistent with substantial benefit from either arm. The power of the study is much too low for its results to be meaningful, and it has a 60% probability of failing to detect a real difference in survival of 25% or greater. This magnitude of difference would have major clinical implications.

Repeated Analysis and Analysis of Subgroups

The aforementioned estimates of sample size that are required for a given randomized trial are based on comparison of one major end point between two groups of randomized patients. It is quite common, however, for investigators to analyze their trials repeatedly, after different periods of follow-up, and to divide their patients into subgroups (e.g., male patients with positive nodes) that then are compared between the two treatment arms. Both of these analyses can lead to invalid conclusions. Permutations of even a small number of categories (e.g., male vs. female, visceral vs. bone vs. soft-tissue metastases, grade of disease) can lead to a very large number of subgroups, and will generate a large number of potential comparisons. One in every 20 *P* values will be less than .05 by chance alone, so that statistical variation can lead to false-positive (or false-negative) results among subgroups. There is a tendency to believe results that appear plausible (e.g., adjuvant chemotherapy improves survival for node-positive bladder cancer) and to reject those that are nonsensical (e.g., adjuvant chemotherapy improves survival in divorced women). The first example may have no more validity than the second. In general, (1) only one or two analyses should be undertaken to prevent a chance result occurring from frequent reanalyses of data, and these should be done at predetermined times; and (2) subgroup analyses should be performed only to generate new hypotheses that can be tested in future trials.

Generalizability of Trials

Although a randomized trial may provide a valid comparison between the two enrolled groups of patients, its results will be generalizable only if they can be applied to the larger group of patients who present with similar stages of bladder cancer. Factors that may limit generalizability include the use of very toxic treatment that requires specialized support that is available only in highly specialized cancer centers, and a high degree of selection of enrolled patients. In particular, results may not be generalized if a trial enrolls only a small proportion of eligible patients, as may be the case for the current intergroup study of cystectomy vs. M-VAC followed by cystectomy for muscle-invasive bladder cancer. Problems of generalizability often are evident from comparisons of a pilot study in a single institution (with selected patients and highly specialized care) with the same treatment given in a multi-institutional study (with less selection, and often better quality-control and review of data). Poorer results (i.e., lower response rates, or smaller or no differences in end points, as compared to standard treatment) almost always are found in multi-institutional studies.

The previous discussion has outlined some important components of the design, analysis, and reporting of clinical trials that must be considered in evaluating any benefits of chemotherapy. In the subsequent sections, we apply these principles to analyze critically the current results of bladder cancer chemotherapy trials in the treatment of recurrent or metastatic disease, and as an adjuvant to local therapy in disease that is localized to the bladder and pelvis.

Chemotherapy of Metastatic Bladder Cancer

Metastatic bladder cancer is a rapidly fatal disease with a median survival of less than 9 months. Over 10,000 people in North America die from this disease each year. There has been increased interest in the use of more intensive systemic treatments for metastatic disease during the past 5 years. This has been stimulated in large part by the results from the use of M-VAC at Memorial Sloan-Kettering Cancer center in New York.[5]

Phase 2 Studies of Single-Agent Therapy

A large number of phase 2 studies of single-agent therapy have been performed during the last 20 years.[24] The largest experience is from Memorial Sloan-Kettering, where a systematic approach to the evaluation of anticancer drugs using well-defined eligibility and evaluation criteria was undertaken. One difficulty in the assessment of the results of all these phase 2 trials has been the variability in eligibility and response criteria between different studies. They often have included a mix of untreated and previously treated patients. The chance of a drug showing activity is significantly less in patients who are heavily pretreated. The most active drugs as single agents are cisplatin and methotrexate, with more modest activity seen with the use of vinblastine and doxorubicin. Some agents, such as 5-fluorouracil, mitomycin-C, and cyclophosphamide, have been reported as having moderate activity. This generally is based on small studies, performed around 1970 when the criteria for determining response were less stringent and the patient population studied was less well characterized.[25] A true evaluation of the activity of these drugs would require additional studies using modern clinical trial methods. Agents that have been demonstrated to have minimal activity against transitional cell carcinoma include etoposide, vincristine, mitoxantrone, and bleomycin.[24]

Cisplatin generally is given at a dosage of 60 to 100 mg/m^2 along with intravenous hydration every 3 to 4 weeks. Escalation of single doses beyond this level is limited by nephrotoxicity. Cumulative neurotoxicity, ototoxicity, and nephrotoxicity limits the number of cisplatin cycles that can be given. Cisplatin produces severe nausea and vomiting that can be controlled reasonably well with the new antiemetic regimens, including the 5-hydroxytryptamine blockers and steroids.

Although the effects of cisplatin on the kidney can be reduced through the use of intravenous hydration and mannitol, there are no known strategies to decrease the neurotoxicity and ototoxicity. Patients with renal dysfunction or preexisting high-frequency hearing loss are more sensitive to the effects of cisplatin. This drug presents problems in patients with bladder cancer, as many have compromised renal function on the basis of age, urinary obstruction, and/or infection. The overall response rate in 320 patients treated in a number of phase 2 studies was 30%,[26] although somewhat lower response rates have been recorded when cisplatin was given in the control arm of phase 3 trials (see subsequent section).

The cisplatin analogue, carboplatin, has a much lower incidence of adverse effects on the kidney, hearing, and peripheral nerves. The activity of carboplatin has been evaluated in a number of studies, it produced an overall response rate of 11% in 80 patients.[27] A direct comparison of the activity of cisplatin and carboplatin has not been made. The dose-limiting toxicity of carboplatin is myelosuppression. This renders it a poor substitute for cisplatin in combination regimens that include other myelosuppressive drugs, even if it did have equivalent activity.

Methotrexate is a folic acid analogue that can be given weekly as a single agent in dosages of 30 to 40 mg/m^2. The dose-limiting toxicity includes myelosuppression and stomatitis. The use of the reduced folate leucovorin decreases toxicity, but also may protect the tumor and, therefore, should be used routinely only in patients with renal dysfunction or third-space accumulations of fluid. Responses were seen in 10 of 33 patients (30%) treated weekly.[28] Many of these patients had received prior chemotherapy, and the response rate in previously untreated individuals was even higher. Some evidence of a dose-response relationship was demonstrated in studies in which responses were documented in 3 of 23 patients receiving 50 mg/m^2 every 2 weeks and in 12 of 22 patients receiving 100 mg/m^2.[29] Higher doses of methotrexate (>100 mg/m^2) require the coadministration of leucovorin 24 hours later. It is not known whether the use of high-dose methotrexate regimens plus leucovorin rescue provides better results than have been seen with maximally tolerated doses of methotrexate without leucovorin. Other antifolates are undergoing early clinical testing, but none has been demonstrated to have greater benefit than methotrexate.

Doxorubicin (Adriamycin) is given by bolus intravenous injection every 3 to 4 weeks in dosages ranging from 30 to 75 mg/m^2. The dose-limiting toxicity includes myelosuppression and stomatitis. Cardiomyopathy is seen at cumulative doses greater than about 500 mg/m^2, although this usually is not a problem with the schedules used in bladder cancer. This drug originally was reported to have significant activity against bladder cancer, with 30 of 87 patients (35%) achieving a response.[30] These data were based on the original trials done with the drug in the late 1960s, and more recent studies have shown lesser activity. The overall response rate in 223 patients treated in a number of phase 2 studies was 18%.

Vinblastine is an inhibitor of mitosis that can be given weekly in dosages of 0.1 to 0.15 m/kg. The dose-limiting toxicity includes myelosuppression and neuropathy, the latter occurring in only some patients. Responses were seen in 5 of 28 patients (18%) given weekly vinblastine as a single agent.[31] Two thirds of patients had been pretreated heavily. The duration of the responses was short.

Phase 2 Studies of Combination Chemotherapy

The combination of two active agents generally has not resulted in dramatic improvements in antitumor efficacy. The combinations of cisplatin with cyclophosphamide, doxorubicin, or methotrexate appear to give response rates of the same order as those of cisplatin alone.

Widely varying rates of tumor response have been obtained for combinations of two or more drugs, as is shown in Table 1. These results emphasize the fact that the reported response rates may depend as much on the selection of patients and the methodologic issues as on the drugs used. The most extensively studied combination has been cyclophosphamide, doxorubicin, and cisplatin, for which the reported response rates have ranged from 13% to 82%.[13] Restricting the analysis to trials with 30 patients or more still demonstrates a range of 17% to 64% (see Table 1).

TABLE 1.
Phase 2 Trials of Combination Chemotherapy in Advanced Bladder Cancer*

Treatment	Number of Patients	Response Rate, %	Complete Response %	References
Cisplatin, cyclophosphamide, doxorubicin	34	38	0	Troner et al., 1987[32]
	97	64	36	Logothetis et al., 1989[33]
	42	40	12	Mulder et al., 1981[35]
	96	17	4	Maru et al., 1987[36]
Cisplatin, methotrexate	43	46	23	Stoter et al., 1987[37]
Cisplatin, methotrexate, vinblastine (CMV)	50	56	28	Harker et al., 1985[34]
Cisplatin, doxorubicin, methotrexate, vinblastine (M-VAC)	133	72	25	Sternberg et al., 1989[5]
	30	40	13	Tannock et al., 1989[38]
Cyclophosphamide, doxorubicin, methotrexate	38	39	5	Tannock et al., 1983[39]
Doxorubicin, 5-fluorouracil	52	40	8	Smith et al., 1983[40]
Methotrexate, vinblastine	47	40	6	Ahmed et al., 1985[41]

*Reports from single trials with 30 or more evaluable patients. Variability in rates of response illustrates the dependence of response rate on selection of patients and criteria used to evaluate response.

The highest response rates reported are with the use of more intensive regimens that combine three or more active drugs at the maximally tolerated doses. These series were the first to report that a small proportion of patients achieve durable complete responses and possibly are cured of their disease. With the advent of aggressive combination chemotherapy and a higher proportion of patients achieving complete remission, the development of recurrence at atypical sites such as the central nervous system (including meningeal carcinomatosis) has been reported increasingly.[42] All of these regimens are associated with moderate to severe normal tissue toxicity.

The MD Anderson Cancer Center (Houston) has conducted pilot studies of the combination of cyclophosphamide 650 mg/m^2, doxorubicin 50 mg/m^2, and cisplatin 70 to 100 mg/m^2 (CISCA). A review of their experience in 97 patients treated over a period of 8 years reported an overall response rate of 64%, with 36% achieving a complete response.[33] About half of all patients achieving a complete response remained free of relapse after 2 years. The median survival still was less than 1 year (44 weeks), although about 10% were alive after 5 years. This review did not report any difference in response rate or survival between patients with nodal and visceral metastases, but did note a lower response rate in patients with mixed histology as opposed to those with pure transitional cell carcinoma.

The Northern California Oncology group treated 58 patients who had metastatic disease with cisplatin 100 mg/m^2, methotrexate 30 mg/m^2, and vinblastine 4 mg/m^2 given every 21 days (CMV).[34] They initially had tried slightly higher doses of methotrexate and vinblastine, but excessive hematologic toxicity was experienced. The overall response rate was 56%, with half of these being complete responses. At the most recent update of the study, only 4 patients remained in complete remission, and the median survival was 8 months. The main toxicity included nausea and vomiting, mucositis, and granulocytopenia.

The most renowned combination chemotherapy regimen for metastatic transitional cell carcinoma is that of methotrexate 30 mg/m^2 on days 1, 5, and 22; vinblastine 3 mg/m^2 on days 2, 15, and 22; cisplatin 70 mg/m^2 on day 2; and doxorubicin 30 mg/m^2 on day 2 (M-VAC). The largest series of patients is from Memorial Sloan-Kettering, where this protocol was developed.[5, 43] In their most recent update on 133 patients, they report an overall response rate of 72%, with 36% of patients achieving a complete response. About one third of patients who achieved a complete response did so only after surgical resection of residual disease; these patients had an outcome similar to that of patients achieving a complete response by chemotherapy alone. The median survival was 13 months and 18% of patients remained alive at 4 years. The major complication of treatment is myelosuppression, with 90% of patients experiencing neutropenia sepsis. Mucositis was seen in half the patients; other side effects were less frequent.

Other centers, including our own, also have reported on the use of M-VAC. In our initial experience, we observed responses in 12 of 30 patients (40%) with measurable disease, at the expense of quite severe toxicity.[38] Fifty-four percent of patients required hospitalization for a toxic complication, which most commonly was sepsis, and there was 1 drug-related death. Four patients achieved complete responses, and 2 of these were maintained at 3 years.

Phase 3 Trials in Advanced Bladder Cancer

A true assessment of the relative merits of single-agent vs. combination therapy, or of one combination regimen over another, requires a prospective, randomized study. The number of such studies performed in patients with advanced urothelial cancer is limited to five comparing single-agent cisplatin to combinations including cisplatin, and one comparing two different cisplatin-based combinations (Table 2). In only one study was combination therapy found to provide a survival benefit over that achieved with cisplatin alone.

The National Bladder Cancer Collaborative Group compared cisplatin as a single agent at a dosage of 70 mg/m^2 every 3 weeks to cisplatin at the same dosage plus cyclophosphamide 750 mg/m^2.[44] Toxicity was not a major problem in either arm, and the majority of patients were able to tolerate these doses. The response rate to the combination was 7 of 59 patients (12%), less than the 10 of 50 patients (20%) who responded to cisplatin alone. There were no differences in survival between the two arms.

The Eastern Cooperative Oncology Group performed a randomized study comparing cisplatin 60 mg/m^2 every 3 weeks to cisplatin 60 mg/m^2, doxorubicin 40 mg/m^2, and cyclophosphamide 400 mg/m^2.[45] The response rate achieved with cisplatin alone was 8 of 48 patients (17%), and that achieved with the combination was 15 of 45 patients (33%, $P = .09$), with median survival periods of 6.0 and 7.3 months, respectively (not significant). Only 4 patients remained in complete remission at 1 year, and only 1 of these did not relapse subsequently. The same two regimens also were compared in a Southeastern Cancer Study Group trial that included 91 evaluable patients.[32] Responses were seen in 7 of 45 cisplatin-treated patients (16%) and in 9 of 42 patients (21%) who received the three-drug combination. Median survival was 4.8 months for patients receiving cisplatin alone and 6.7 months for those receiving the combination therapy (not significant), with no long-term complete responses seen.

An Australian study of 108 patients compared cisplatin 80 mg/m^2 every 4 weeks to methotrexate 50 mg/m^2 on days 1 and 15 plus cisplatin 80 mg/m^2 on day 2.[46] The response rate to cisplatin alone was 31%, with a median survival of 7.2 months, and the response rate to the combination was 45% ($P = .18$), with a median survival of 8.7 months ($P = .7$). The addition of methotrexate to cisplatin increased the incidence of hematologic toxicity and mucositis, but 96% of patients were able to receive at least 85% of the desired doses of drugs. Only 8 patients remained alive and free of disease at 2 years. Although this study does show that there are no large improvements from the combined chemotherapy regimen, one cannot conclude that there is no benefit from the addition of methotrexate to cisplatin because the sample size was not adequate to rule out differences in response rate of less than 25%.

A study comparing M-VAC with CISCA was performed in 110 patients with metastatic urothelial tumors at MD Anderson Cancer Center.[48] This study was performed over a period of 3.5 years, with 82% of all potentially eligible patients being randomized. The trial was stopped early because of the superior results achieved with the use of M-VAC. Both of these regimens are intensive and their toxicity was similar. There was a 65% response rate for M-VAC, with 35% of patients achieving a complete response, as compared to 46% total and 25% complete response rates with CISCA ($P < .05$). The median survival with CISCA was 36 weeks and that with M-VAC was 48 weeks ($P < .005$), with the separation between the survival curves increasing over time.

TABLE 2.
Phase 3 Trials of Chemotherapy in Advanced Bladder Cancer

Treatments	Number of Patients	Response Rate (%)	Complete Response (%)	References
Cisplatin	50	20	10	Soloway et al., 1983[44]
Cisplatin plus cyclophosphamide	59	12	5	
Cisplatin	48	17	2	Khandekar et al., 1985[45]
Cisplatin plus cyclophosphamide plus doxorubicin	45	33	22	
Cisplatin plus cyclophosphamide	45	16	0	Troner et al., 1987[32]
Cisplatin plus cyclophosphamide plus doxorubicin	42	21	5	
Cisplatin	55	31	9	Hillcoat et al., 1987[46]
Cisplatin plus methotrexate	53	46	9	
Cisplatin plus cyclophosphamide plus doxorubicin	42	46	5	
M-VAC*	59	65	5	Logothetis et al., 1990[47]
Cisplatin	120	12	3	Loehrer et al., 1992[23]
M-VAC	126	39	13	

*M-VAC = methotrexate, vinblastine, doxorubicin (Adriamycin), and cisplatin.

The use of M-VAC was compared to cisplatin alone at a dose of 70 mg/m^2 given every 28 days in an intergroup trial. This was a cooperative effort of the Eastern Cooperative Oncology Group, the Southeastern Cancer Study Group, the Southwest Oncology Group, the National Cancer Institute of Canada, and the Australian Bladder Cancer Group, and 246 patients with measurable metastatic bladder cancer were randomized.[23] The overall response rates for evaluable patients were 12% for those given cisplatin alone and 39% for those treated with M-VAC ($P < .0001$), with complete responses seen in 3% of the former and 13% of the latter. The median survival times were 8.2 months for patients receiving cisplatin and 12.5 months for those given M-VAC, with a significant separation of the survival curves ($P < .005$). The 2-year survival of M-VAC–treated patients was twice as high. Of patients treated with M-VAC, 17% developed grade 3 or 4 mucositis and 10% had neutropenic fever, whereas neither of these complications was observed with the use of cisplatin. There were 5 drug-related deaths, mostly due to sepsis, all of which occurred in patients receiving M-VAC. Only 24% of patients were able to receive this combination chemotherapy without dosage reductions or treatment delays.

This intergroup trial is important because it was the first to demonstrate the benefits of intensive treatment of bladder cancer over single-agent therapy. It also provides a useful data base for understanding which patients are most likely to benefit from chemotherapy. Not surprisingly, a good performance status, the absence of weight loss, and metastases confined to nodal areas were factors associated favorably with response and survival. Patient age and a history of prior radiotherapy or radical cystectomy were not favorable prognostic indicators. The response rates achieved also are of interest. They demonstrate the effects that the standardization of response criteria, patient selection, and independent review of responses can have on the results. The overall response rate to M-VAC and the frequency of complete response rates were significantly less than initially reported by the group at Memorial Hospital. The response to cisplatin, which generally is considered to be the most active single agent against transitional cell carcinoma, was only 12%. In a phase 2 study, such a response rate would lead to the conclusion that cisplatin is an inactive agent. In five of the six randomized studies we have discussed, one of the treatments was single-agent cisplatin. The response rates to cisplatin ranged from 12% to 31%; overall, there were 56 responses in 318 evaluable patients (18%). This is in contrast to the reports in phase 2 nonrandomized studies, in which the average response rate was 30%.[26]

Other Issues

Pure squamous cell carcinoma of the bladder is uncommon and in other countries frequently is associated with bilharzial bladder. Some patients with transitional cell carcinoma have a mixed histology, with a significant squamous cell component in their tumors. These patients sometimes are excluded from chemotherapy studies, and the available evidence suggests that the response rate usually is lower than that in patients with pure transitional cell carcinoma.[23, 47] With a more detailed analysis, many patients with transitional cell carcinoma can be found to have mixed histology. This may account for the higher proportion of patients with squamous or mixed components being reported in some recent studies. Although the response rate may be lower, some patients with mixed-histology tumors do achieve meaningful remissions, and the presence of squamous metaplasia should not preclude the use of chemotherapy.

Patients with locally advanced tumors frequently have hydronephrosis. Since the toxicity from cisplatin and methotrexate is increased in the presence of renal dysfunction, percutaneous drainage or stenting should be performed prior to chemotherapy. Cisplatin dosage often is calculated based on glomerular filtration rate to limit further deterioration of renal function by the drug. As cisplatin is not cleared by the kidney, any reduction in dosage also will limit the exposure of the tumor to the drug and, thus, adversely affect response. Methotrexate is excreted in the kidney, and its clearance decreases proportionately with reduced creatinine clearance. Maintenance of methotrexate dosage in the presence of renal dysfunction will lead to excessive toxicity. A study that examined chemotherapy in the presence of ureteric obstruction reported a higher incidence of serious hematologic toxicity and a lower response rate if the urinary obstruction was not relieved.[49]

Future Directions

Transitional cell carcinoma is a chemosensitive tumor, and a dose-response relationship has been suggested by trials such as the intergroup study. Further escalations in the intensity of treatment are limited by normal tissue toxicity, particularly myelosuppression and mucositis. The hematopoietic growth factors, granulocyte colony-stimulating factor (G-CSF) and granulocyte-macrophage colony-stimulating factor (GM-CSF), are being evaluated for their ability to protect against hematologic toxicity and may allow for dose escalation.

Gabrilove and colleagues[50] compared the use of G-CSF with M-VAC on the first cycle of treatment with the use of M-VAC alone on the second. This strategy decreased the number of days during which the neutrophil count was less than 1,000 and reduced the antibiotic requirements. There also was a decrease in mucositis, and a larger percentage of patients could receive their planned day 15 chemotherapy. This early study suggested that the colony-stimulating factors may have a role in reducing the toxicity of M-VAC or allowing for the administration of higher doses of chemotherapy.

Logothetis and coworkers[48] treated 32 patients who had disease that was refractory to standard chemotherapy with escalated doses of M-VAC in combination with GM-CSF. Their escalated M-VAC regimen incorporated a 30% increase in vinblastine, a 100% increase in doxorubicin, and a 40% increase in cisplatin, but no increase in methotrexate. Hematologic toxicity remained a problem with 31 of 32 patients experiencing a granulocyte count less than 500×10^9/mL and 30 of 32 patients having platelet counts less than 25,000 during the first course of therapy. Of 30 evaluable patients, 12 (40%) achieved a partial or complete remission, which is more than expected in a pretreated population. The investigators currently are testing the merits of escalated M-VAC plus GM-CSF as compared to chemotherapy without growth factors in a randomized trial.

We have treated 21 patients who had advanced transitional cell carcinoma with a combination of standard M-VAC plus GM-CSF.[51] The use of GM-CSF is associated with significant toxicity in this population, with 6 patients having a first-dose reaction of hypotension and hypoxemia, and 8 patients having to discontinue GM-CSF because of side effects. There was evidence of protection against neutropenia in the first two courses of treatment, but this effect diminished with repeated treatment cycles. We did see responses in 8 of 11 patients with measurable disease.

Regimens such as M-VAC contain the most active of the currently available anticancer agents at a maximally tolerated dose. It is unlikely that minor alterations in drugs or dose schedules will lead to major improvements in outcome. One study used a modification of M-VAC in which mitoxantrone and carboplatin were substituted for doxorubicin and cisplatin.[52] The subjective toxicity was less, although myelosuppression remained a problem. Responses were reported in 21 of 33 evaluable patients. Approaches such as this might reduce some of the toxicity associated with chemotherapy and allow patients in poorer general condition to receive treatment. As the substituted drugs appear to have lower activity against the disease, this might be accomplished at the expense of effects against the cancer.

Gallium nitrate has shown some promise in two phase 1–2 studies done in patients with disease refractory to M-VAC. In the first, gallium was given by 5-day continuous infusion with escalating doses.[53] No patients responded at an infusion rate of less than 300 mg/m²/day, but 4 of 23 (17%) achieved a partial response at rates of 350 mg/m²/day or higher. Further dose escalation was limited by ocular toxicity. In a smaller study using a 7-day infusion schedule of 300 mg/m²/day, Seligman and associates[54] saw responses in 5 of 6 patients. This compound will require further study to evaluate its activity against bladder cancer. As the toxicity profile differs from that of conventional chemotherapy, it may be useful given in combination with current cytotoxic drugs.

The testing of new cytotoxic and biologic agents for activity against transitional cell carcinoma should be a high priority. If new drugs are to be incorporated with presently available agents, then those with a dose-limiting toxicity other than myelosuppression or mucositis would be preferable. Agents showing promise in early testing that should be studied in bladder cancer include taxol, the anthrapyrazoles, and the topoisomerase inhibitors.

The aggressive chemotherapy regimens have been shown to improve survival for patients with metastatic bladder cancer. There are always some unpleasant and potentially dangerous side effects associated with their use. The benefit is modest and can be measured in additional months of life. Patients who achieve complete remissions may have a more sustained benefit; unfortunately, these are a minority. As we understand more about the factors that predict good outcome, we should be better able to select those who will benefit from aggressive treatment and to use less intensive therapy in those with little chance of complete remission or prolonged survival. Complete responses and 2-year survival are seen most commonly in patients with low tumor volumes. The probability of tumor cells being resistant to therapy is lower in these patients and they are better able to tolerate aggressive treatment. The greatest potential for the use of chemotherapy may be as an adjunct to local therapy at a time when the systemic burden of disease is the smallest.

Chemotherapy as an Adjunct to Local Treatment

Chemotherapy may be administered during a course of radiation therapy, or before or after local treatment (or both). When chemotherapy is given prior to local treatment, it may be referred to as "neoadjuvant," "induction," or "preemptive"; chemotherapy given after surgery or radiation usually is referred to as adjuvant, following the sequence that has been used most often in other diseases, such as breast cancer (Table 3). Adjuvant chemotherapy also is used, however, as a generic term to indicate the use of chemotherapy with local treatment (in any sequence) for potentially curable disease.

TABLE 3.
Chemotherapy as an Adjunct to Local Treatment

Sequence	Descriptive Terms
Chemotherapy given before local treatment	Neoadjuvant, induction, preemptive
Chemotherapy given at the same time as local treatment (usually radiation therapy)	Concurrent
Local treatment given before chemotherapy	Adjuvant,* maintenance

*Adjuvant also is used generically to describe chemotherapy given with local treatment to any patient without overt metastatic disease, regardless of sequence.

End Points: Survival, Local Control, and Downstaging

In trials of adjunctive chemotherapy, it is important that the goals of treatment be set *a priori*, and that appropriate end points be defined. Chemotherapy might confer benefit by eradicating subclinical metastases or by improving the probability of local control after surgery or radiation therapy. The most important end point is survival and, in randomized trials, actuarial survival curves should be compared for patients receiving local treatment plus chemotherapy with those of patients receiving local treatment alone, using appropriate statistical methods.

The end points of local control and freedom from overt metastatic disease are important in providing clues to the possible mechanism(s) by which drugs might modify overall survival. These end points are more difficult to define, and an effect of chemotherapy to delay recurrence is not necessarily of therapeutic value if there is no subsequent improvement in survival.

Chemotherapy also might be beneficial if it improves the quality of survival. This could occur if chemotherapy were administered with radiation therapy, aggressive transurethral resection, or partial cystectomy and increased the probability of local control as a result of these procedures. Such an effect would increase the proportion of patients who might avoid cystectomy and retain a functional bladder.

Some investigators have used tumor shrinkage (or "downstaging") as a major end point in clinical trials in which chemotherapy is used initially. Chemotherapy is unlikely to confer benefit unless it leads to tumor shrinkage. In contrast, although there is no question that chemotherapy can lead to downstaging in some patients, occasionally to the point that no tumor can be detected by subsequent cystoscopy and imaging, this does not constitute proof that chemotherapy will improve survival or even lead to durable local control. As described previously, improved survival in responding patients is not proof of benefit from the therapy that produced the response.

Some investigators have found no evidence of bladder cancer in the resected bladders of a small proportion of patients who have received chemotherapy prior to cystectomy. In reporting this result, some investigators have implied that the cystectomy was unnecessary, and that the pathologic complete response indicates a high probability that the patient would have achieved local control with chemotherapy alone. Although this might apply to a small proportion of patients, it is instructive to consider the implications of pathologic complete response (Fig 2). At the start of treatment, a clinically evident tumor may weigh about 10 g and will contain about 10 billion (10^{10}) malignant cells. If the bladder is clinically clear after chemotherapy, the pathologist will examine sections carefully for the presence of malignant cells. A good pathologist might detect about 1 malignant cell among 1,000 normal cells; since 1 g of tissue contains about 10^9 cells, this sets a limit of detection of about 1 million (10^6) malignant cells per gram of normal tissue. Thus, a pathologic complete response should be taken to

Moving?

I'd like to receive my *Advances in Urology* without interruption.
Please not the following change of address, effective:

Name: _____

New Address: _____

_____

City: _____ State: _____ Zip: _____

Old Address: _____

_____

City: _____ State: _____ Zip: _____

Reservation Card

Yes, I would like my own copy of *Advances in Urology*. Please begin my subscription with the current edition according to the terms described below.* I understand that I will have 30 days to examine each annual edition. If satisfied, I will pay just $69.95 plus sales tax, postage and handling (price subject to change without notice).

Name: _____

Address: _____

City: _____ State: _____ Zip: _____

Method of Payment
○ Visa   ○ Mastercard   ○ AmEx   ○ Bill me   ○ Check (in US dollars, payable to Mosby, Inc.)

Card number: _____ Exp date: _____

Signature: _____

LS-0908

*Your *Advances* Service Guarantee:

When you subscribe to *Advances*, we'll send you an advance notice of future volumes about two months before they publish. This automatic notice system is designed to take up as little of your time as possible. If you do not want *Advances*, the advance notice makes it quick and easy for you to let us know your decision, and you will always have at least 20 days to decide. If we don't hear from you, we'll send you the new volume as soon as it's available. And, of course, *Advances* is yours to examine free of charge for 30 days (postage, handling and applicable sales tax are added to each shipment.).

BUSINESS REPLY MAIL
FIRST CLASS MAIL   PERMIT No. 762   CHICAGO, IL

POSTAGE WILL BE PAID BY ADDRESSEE

Chris Hughes
Mosby-Year Book, Inc.
200 N. LaSalle Street
Suite 2600
Chicago, IL 60601-9981

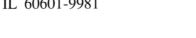

NO POSTAGE
NECESSARY
IF MAILED
IN THE
UNITED STATES

BUSINESS REPLY MAIL
FIRST CLASS MAIL   PERMIT No. 762   CHICAGO, IL

POSTAGE WILL BE PAID BY ADDRESSEE

Chris Hughes
Mosby-Year Book, Inc.
200 N. LaSalle Street
Suite 2600
Chicago, IL 60601-9981

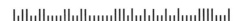

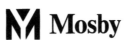

Dedicated to publishing excellence

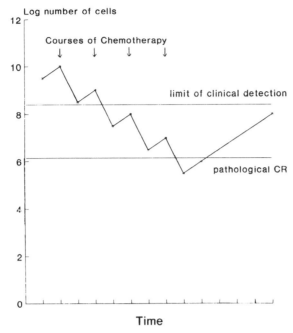

FIG 2.
Pathologic complete response *(CR)*.

imply the presence of from 0 to 10^6 malignant cells per gram of tissue—certainly no proof of curative therapy.

Lessons From Nonrandomized Studies

Based on the previous discussion of clinical trials, it is evident that nonrandomized trials of adjunctive chemotherapy are useful for (1) determining whether the added treatment has acceptable toxicity and is feasible, and (2) determining whether there is sufficient evidence of activity such that the protocol may be deemed worthy of evaluation in a randomized trial.

Evidence of biologic activity may be obtained most readily from pilot studies of neoadjuvant chemotherapy, in which the bladder can be examined by subsequent cystoscopy (or at cystectomy) for evidence of downstaging of disease. These studies have shown that several cisplatin-based regimens are capable of downstaging muscle-invasive bladder cancer, with a proportion of patients achieving complete clinical or pathologic response[55] (Table 4). The following comments may be made about the results of these trials.

In trials in which clinical staging (prior to cystectomy) has been compared to pathologic staging, there is a high probability of staging error from cystoscopy and examination under anesthesia. Thus, although there are a few patients who have refused local treatment after a complete clinical re-

TABLE 4.
Complete Pathologic Response in the Bladder Using Combination Chemotherapy*

Regiment	Number of Trials	Evaluable Patients	Complete Response at Cystectomy, % (95% Confidence Level)
CM	2	75	35 (24–45)
CMV	3	71	31 (20–42)
Cyclo/A/C	4	83	22 (13–31)
M-VAC	7	138	30 (23–38)

*Adapted from Scher HI: *Semin Oncol* 1990; 8:555–565.
†C = cisplatin; M = methotrexate; V = vinblastine; A = doxorubicin (Adriamycin); Cyclo = cyclophosphamide.

sponse to chemotherapy, and have remained disease-free, this strategy cannot be recommended.

Even achievement of pathologic complete response does not imply the absence of tumor cells.

Chemotherapy usually is administered after transurethral resection, and this procedure alone may render some patients with T2 tumors free of disease.

The probability of complete response is much higher for small T2 and T3a tumors than for more advanced lesions. In a recent trial at Princess Margaret Hospital in Toronto including patients with large T3b or T4b lesions, three courses of M-VAC were given prior to radiation therapy, and only 2 of 26 patients achieved clinical complete response after chemotherapy.[56]

The data in Table 4 suggest that any of the cisplatin-based regimens might be selected as appropriate for testing in randomized trials. The CMV and M-VAC regimens currently are being tested in controlled trials of neoadjuvant therapy, whereas the cisplatin, doxorubicin, cyclophosphamide (CAP) regimen has been studied as adjuvant treatment after cystectomy.[57] The experience from Princess Margaret Hospital with the use of neoadjuvant M-VAC for T3b and T4 tumors suggests that any therapeutic gains from this strategy in the larger tumors will be limited. At present, only 3 of the 26 patients remain alive and free of disease with a median follow-up of about 2.5 years.

Because nonrandomized studies have a limited ability to demonstrate efficacy, only two of the larger series will be discussed further. In one of these, 54 patients with stage T2 to T3b tumors were treated by as complete a transurethral resection as possible followed by eight doses of methotrexate (2 g intravenously followed by leucovorin rescue).[58] More recently, this strategy has been modified to include subsequent combination chemotherapy with CMV. This approach appears to be associated with reasonable rates of local control and survival, and might be evaluated appropriately against standard local therapy in a randomized trial.

In another study, Logothetis and colleagues[59] treated 71 patients with the CISCA regimen following cystectomy. Patients received chemotherapy if they had pathologic findings that predicted a high probability of relapse. The outcome of these treated patients was considerably better than that of a group of high-risk patients who did not receive chemotherapy (because of refusal, nonreferral, or medical contraindications), and closer to that of a group of lower-risk patients who also did not receive chemotherapy (Fig 3). The authors concluded that adjuvant CISCA chemotherapy conferred a therapeutic benefit. Although this might be true, and the study suggests that such a hypothesis is worthy of testing in a randomized trial, the result also might have been due to patient selection. The reasons for nonreferral, medical contraindications, or even patient refusal all may have conferred a relatively poor prognosis for those patients compared to the patients who received chemotherapy. Patients who agree to take part in clinical trials

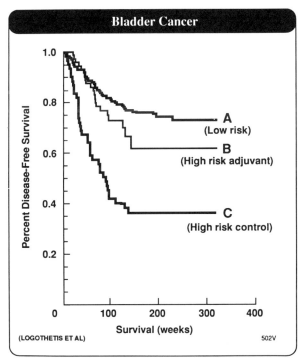

FIG 3.
Logothetis study. (From Logothetis CJ, et al: *J Clin Oncol* 1988; 6:1590. Used by permission.)

usually have a better outcome than those who do not, even if they are randomized to the control arm and receive identical treatment.[60, 61]

Randomized Trials of Adjunctive Therapy

There are four publications describing five published trials that have randomized patients with muscle-invasive bladder cancer to receive either local treatment alone or local treatment combined with chemotherapy. These trials are summarized in Table 5; two additional trials have been reported only in abstract form. None of the published trials has shown an improvement in patient survival, although in one, there is a nonsignificant trend toward improved survival and a significant increase in time to relapse. Of the two trials reported in abstract form, one shows an improved rate of local control and the other shows no improvement in any end point. These results should be regarded with caution until a full-length publication allows a critical review of the data. The results of the four published trials are discussed following.

The trial conducted by the Yorkshire Urology Cancer Research Group[62] accrued 129 patients with T3NXM0 bladder cancer. They were randomized to receive radical radiotherapy alone or radical radiotherapy followed by at least four courses of chemotherapy. Chemotherapy consisted of doxorubicin (50 mg/m^2) and 5-fluorouracil (500 mg/m^2) given intravenously at 3-week intervals for a maximum of 11 courses. Only 110 patients were available for analysis, with 91 patients receiving a radical course of radiation. Treatment appears to have been aborted in 19 others because of rapid progression of disease.

End points of the aforementioned study were overall survival, death from cancer, and relapse-free survival. There were no significant differences in any end point between the two arms, and the 3-year actuarial survival rates were 35% and 37%. The small sample size leads to very wide confidence limits, and the trial is consistent with chemotherapy causing any effect, from an absolute decrease of 22% in absolute (2-year) survival to a 12% increase.[62] The trial illustrates the limitations of a small sample size, but the lack of positive trends does not encourage further study of this type of chemotherapy, especially as studies of metastatic cancer have revealed much more active drug combinations.

A much larger study was conducted by the British Cooperative Urological Cancer Group, in which 423 patients with T3 bladder cancer were randomized and data were presented on 376 patients followed for at least 1 year.[22] Local treatment was radical radiotherapy in 304 patients, of whom 236 were aged 65 years and older; 72 patients under 65 years of age were treated with preoperative radiation therapy and cystectomy. Patients randomized to receive chemotherapy were given methotrexate 100 mg/m^2 intravenously weekly for three doses with leucovorin rescue, and radiotherapy was commenced 1 week later. Methotrexate also was given starting 1 month after the completion of radiation or surgery, with planned doses of methotrexate (100 mg) given at 2-week intervals for 3 months and then

TABLE 5.
Randomized, Controlled Trials of Adjunctive Chemotherapy for Muscle-Invasive Bladder Cancer[*]

Investigators	Number of Patients Randomized (Evaluable)	Local Treatment	Chemotherapy	Result
Richards et al.[62]	129 (110)	Radical RT	Doxorubicin plus 5-FU (≥4 courses after RT)	No difference
Shearer et al.[22]	423 (376)	Radical RT or preoperative plus cystectomy	MTX given pre- or post-RT	No difference
Raghavan et al.[42]	255 (combined from 2 trials)	Radical RT	Cisplatin ×2 or 3 pre-RT	No difference
Skinner et al.[57]	101 (91)	Cystectomy	CAP ×4 after cystectomy	Increased time to recurrence; trend toward improved survival
Studer et al.[63]	80 (77)	Cystectomy	Cisplatin for 3 courses after surgery	No difference (trend toward poorer survival)
Coppin et al.[64]	99 (99)	Radical RT or preoperative plus cystectomy	Cisplatin ×3 during RT	Decreased local relapse (trend toward improved survival)

[*]RT = radiation therapy; 5-FU = 5-fluorouracil; MTX = methotrexate; CAP = cisplatin, doxorubicin, cyclophosphamide.

monthly for a further 9 months. The methotrexate dose (and leucovorin rescue) was adjusted in patients with abnormal renal function.

The major end point in the trial was survival, and the survival curves were very similar. There were problems in administering methotrexate: the drug was not given in 13% of 188 patients assigned to receive it, and the dosage given prior to radiotherapy was reduced in 21%. Sixty-seven patients received no maintenance chemotherapy, and only 38 patients completed all chemotherapy as planned. This trial was sufficiently large to detect a 15% difference in overall survival. The authors appropriately concluded that future trials should concentrate on more active drug regimens.

Two similar trials from the Australian Bladder Cancer Study Group and from the British West Midlands Urological Research Group were combined in the report of Raghavan and associates.[65] The individual trials randomized patients with T2 to T4 bladder cancer to receive radical radiotherapy alone, or two or three courses, respectively, of cisplatin (100 mg/m^2 intravenously) given at 3-week intervals prior to radiotherapy. Radiotherapy was started at 10 days and at 3 weeks, respectively, after the completion of chemotherapy in the two trials. Neither trial met its projected accrual of 250 to 320 patients, largely because referring urologists began to opt for pilot studies of combination chemotherapy. The trials were combined to give a total sample of 255 patients.

The major end point of these trials was survival, and there was no significant survival difference between patients who did or did not receive chemotherapy; 3-year survival rates were 38% and 39%, almost identical to those reported in the earlier British trials. The overall odds ratio for survival was 1.13 (in favor of the control group), with 95% confidence limits of 0.80 to 1.57. Even the combined trials are not sufficiently large to rule out meaningful benefit from this type of chemotherapy, although the opposite trend makes this very unlikely.

The trial reported by Skinner and colleagues[57] has met with considerable controversy (see editorials following the paper), and a detailed critique by one of us has appeared elsewhere.[66] The trial randomized 101 patients (of 160 eligible) who had undergone cystectomy and were found to have pathologic T3, T4, and/or N+ disease; 91 with transitional cell carcinoma were analyzed. Forty-four patients were randomized to receive chemotherapy, but only 33 actually received treatment. Most, but not all, patients received cisplatin, doxorubicin, and cyclophosphamide, and only 23 patients received three or more cycles. The abstract of the paper is misleading because it reports a significant improvement in median survival with chemotherapy; an overall comparison of the survival curves does not show such improvement, although there is a trend in favor of chemotherapy at shorter intervals after treatment (Fig 4). The aforementioned trial contains many flaws, including a poorly defined protocol that is not adhered to well, a small sample of heterogeneous patients, and the performance of subgroup analysis without correction of P values. It does not prove the value of chemotherapy, but similar to the single-arm study of Logothetis and coworkers,[59] suggests that further testing of this schedule of adjuvant chemotherapy would be worthy of study in a large, controlled trial.

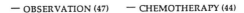

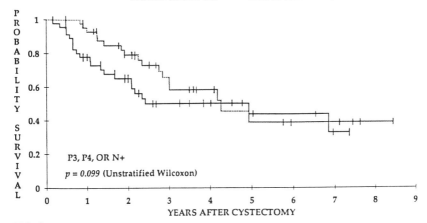

FIG 4.
Skinner study: effect of chemotherapy on survival. (From Skinner DG, et al: *J Urol* 1991; 145:459. Used by permission.)

Conclusions

There is no question that the systemic treatment of bladder cancer has advanced over the past 10 years. Intensive chemotherapy has been shown to improve the survival of patients with metastatic disease. The M-VAC regimen consistently has produced the best results and has been shown to be superior to single-agent and other combination therapy in randomized trials.

This improvement in survival is modest, with almost all patients still dying of their disease. Further increases in the intensity of treatment are not likely to improve the situation, as the majority of patients cannot receive full doses of currently prescribed regimens.

As new agents with activity against bladder cancer are identified, they will be combined with current agents in phase 2 studies, and the more promising combinations could be tested against M-VAC. Unless a new drug has dramatic activity against bladder cancer, the impact of combination chemotherapy on the death rate in patients with metastatic disease will be limited. No such new drugs currently are on the horizon.

Chemotherapy may have a much more substantial impact on mortality from bladder cancer when given in the adjuvant or neoadjuvant setting. In this setting, the systemic burden of disease is less and it possibly might be eradicated. Although neither breast nor colorectal cancer can be cured when metastatic disease is apparent, adjuvant therapy has been shown to improve survival. The true value of adjuvant chemotherapy should be demonstrated by two large trials that currently are ongoing. One compares M-VAC prior to cystectomy to cystectomy alone; the other compares CMV prior to cystectomy or radiation therapy to local treatment alone. Even a 10% improvement in survival from the use of such adjuvant therapy would translate into over 1,000 lives per year saved in North America alone.

References

1. Estey E, Hoth D, Simon R, et al: Therapeutic response in phase I trials of antineoplastic agents. *Cancer Treat Rep* 1986; 70:1105–1115.
2. Decoster G, Stein G, Holdener EE: Responses and toxic deaths in phase I clinical trials. *Ann Oncol* 1990; 1:175–181.
3. Warr D, McKinney S, Tannock IF: Influence of measurement error in assessment of response to anticancer chemotherapy: Proposal for new criteria of tumor response. *J Clin Oncol* 1984; 2:1040–1046.
4. Tonkin K, Tritchler D, Tannock IF: Criteria of tumor response used in clinical trials of chemotherapy. *J Clin Oncol* 1985; 3:870–875.
5. Sternberg CN, Yagoda A, Scher HI, et al: Methotrexate, vinblastine, doxorubicin, and cisplatin for advanced transitional cell carcinoma of the urothelium. Efficacy and patterns of response and relapse. *Cancer* 1989; 64:2448–2458.
6. Tannock IF, Warr D: Nonrandomized clinical trials of cancer chemotherapy. Phase II or III? *J Natl Cancer Inst* 1988; 80:800–801.
7. Arriagada R, Auquier A: Difficulties in evaluating non-randomized studies. *Radiother Oncol* 1989; 15:307–312.
8. Tannock IF: Combined modality treatment with radiotherapy and chemotherapy. *Radiother Oncol* 1989; 16:83–101.
9. Sacks H, Chalmers TC, Smith Jr H: Randomized versus historical controls for clinical trials. *Am J Med* 1982; 72:233–240.
10. Diehl LF, Perry DJ: A comparison of randomized concurrent control groups with matched historical control groups: Are historical controls valid? *J Clin Oncol* 1986; 4:1114–1120.
11. Yagoda A, Watson RC, Natale RB, et al: A critical analysis of response criteria in patients with bladder cancer treated with cis-diamminedichloride platinum II. *Cancer* 1979; 44:1553–1562.
12. Baar J, Tannock IF: Analyzing the same data in two ways: A demonstration model to illustrate the reporting and misreporting of clinical trials. *J Clin Oncol* 1989; 7:969–978.
13. Tonkin K, Tannock IF: Evaluation of response and morbidity following treatment of bladder cancer, in Rahgavan D (ed): *The Management of Bladder Cancer*. London, Edward Arnold, 1988, pp 228–244.
14. Simes RJ: Publication bias: The case for an international registry of clinical trials. *J Clin Oncol* 1986; 4:1529–1541.
15. Begg CB, Berlin JA: Publication bias and dissemination of clinical research. *J Natl Cancer Inst* 1989; 81:107–115.
16. DeBellefeuille C, Morrison CA, Tannock IF: The fate of abstracts submitted to a cancer meeting: Factors which influence presentation and subsequent publication. *Ann Oncol* 1992; 3:187–191.
17. Bush RS: *Malignancies of the Ovary, Uterus and Cervix*. London, Edward Arnold, 1979.
18. Feinstein AR, Sosin DM, Wells CK: The Will Rogers phenomenon. Stage migration and new diagnostic techniques as a source of misleading statistics for survival in cancer. *N Engl J Med* 1985; 312:1604–1608.
19. Anderson JR, Cain KC, Gelber RD: Analysis of survival by tumor response. *J Clin Oncol* 1983; 1:710–719.
20. Weiss GB, Bunce III H, Hokanson JA: Comparing survival of responders and nonresponders after treatment: A potential source of confusion in interpreting cancer clinical trials. *Controlled Clin Trials* 1983; 4:43–52.

21. Simon RM: Design and conduct of clinical trials, in DeVita VT Jr, Hellman S, Rosenberg SA (eds): *Cancer, Principles and Practice of Oncology*, ed 3. Philadelphia, Lippincott, 1989; pp 396–420.
22. Shearer RJ, Chilvers CED, Bloom HJG, et al: Cooperative Urological Cancer Group. Adjuvant chemotherapy in T3 carcinoma of the bladder: A prospective trial. A preliminary report. *Br J Urol* 1988; 62:558–564.
23. Loehrer PJ, Einhorn LH, Elson PI, et al: A randomized comparison of cisplatin alone or in combination with methotrexate, vinblastine and doxorubicin in patients with metastatic urothelial carcinoma. *J Clin Oncol* 1992; 10:1066–1073.
24. Whitmore WF, Yagoda A: Chemotherapy in the management of bladder tumours. *Drugs* 1989; 38:301–312.
25. Carter SK, Wasserman TH: The chemotherapy of urological cancer. *Cancer* 1975; 36:729–747.
26. Yagoda A: Chemotherapy for advanced urothelial cancer. *Semin Oncol* 1983; 1:60–74.
27. Wagstaff AJ, Ward A, Benfield P, et al: Carboplatin. *Drugs* 1989; 37:162–190.
28. Natale RB, Yagoda A, Watson RC, et al: Methotrexate: An active drug in bladder cancer. *Cancer* 1981; 47:1246–1250.
29. Turner AG, Hendry WF, Williams GB, et al: The treatment of advanced bladder cancer with methotrexate. *Br J Urol* 1977; 49:673–678.
30. Middleman E, Luce J, Frei E: Clinical trials with adriamycin. *Cancer* 1971; 28:844–850.
31. Blumenreich MS, Yagoda A, Natale RB, et al: Phase II trial of vinblastine sulfate for metastatic urothelial tract tumors. *Cancer* 1982; 40:435–438.
32. Troner M, Birch R, Omura GA, et al: Phase III comparison of cisplatin alone versus cisplatin, doxorubicin and cyclophosphamide in the treatment of bladder cancer. *J Urol* 1987; 137:660–662.
33. Logothetis CJ, Dexeus FH, Chong C, et al: Cisplatin, cyclophosphamide and doxorubicin chemotherapy for unresectable urothelial tumors. The MD Anderson experience. *J Urol* 1987; 141:33–37.
34. Harker WG, Meyers FJ, Freiha FS, et al: Cisplatin, methotrexate and vinblastine. An effective chemotherapy regimen for metastatic transitional cell carcinoma of the urinary tract. *J Clin Oncol* 1985; 3:1463–1470.
35. Mulder JH, Fossa SD, DePauw M, et al: Cyclosporin, doxorubicin and cisplatin chemotherapy in advanced bladder carcinoma. *Eur J Clin Oncol* 1982; 47:111–112.
36. Maru A, Akaza H, Isaka S, et al: Phase III trial of the Japanese Urological Cancer Research Group for doxorubicin. *Cancer Chemother Pharmacol* 1987; 20:44–48.
37. Stoter G, Splinter TAW, Child JA, et al: Combination chemotherapy with cisplatin and methotrexate in advanced transitional cell carcinoma of the bladder. *J Urol* 1987; 137:663–667.
38. Tannock IF, Gospodarowicz M, Connolly J, et al: M-VAC chemotherapy for transitional cell carcinoma: The Princess Margaret Hospital experience. *J Urol* 1989; 142:289–292.
39. Tannock IF, Gospodarowicz M, Evans WK: Chemotherapy for metastatic transitional carcinoma of the urinary tract. *Cancer* 1983; 51:216–219.
40. Smith PH, Child JA, Mulder JH, et al: Co-operative studies of systemic chemotherapy. *Cancer Chemother Pharmacol* 1983; 11:S25–S31.

41. Ahmed T, Yagoda A, Needles B, et al: Vinblastine and methotrexate for advanced bladder cancer. J Urol 1985; 133:602–605.
42. Raghavan D, Chye RWM: Treatment of carcinomatous meningitis from transitional cell carcinoma of the bladder. Br J Urol 1991; 67:438–440.
43. Sternberg CN, Yagoda A, Scher HI, et al: M-VAC (methotrexate, vinblastine, doxorubicin and cisplatin) for advanced transitional cell carcinoma of the urothelium. J Urol 1988; 139:461–469.
44. Soloway MS, Einstein A, Corder MP, et al: A comparison of cisplatin and the combination of cisplatin and cyclophosphamide in advanced urothelial cancer. Cancer 1983; 64:2448–2458.
45. Khandekar JD, Elson PJ, De Wys WD, et al: Comparative activity and toxicity of cisplatin and a combination of doxorubicin, cyclophosphamide, and cisplatin in disseminated transitional cell carcinomas of the urinary tract. J Clin Oncol 1985; 3:539–545.
46. Hillcoat BL, Raghavan D, Matthews J, et al: A randomized trial of cisplatin versus cisplatin plus methotrexate in advanced cancer of the urothelial tract. J Clin Oncol 1989; 7:706–709.
47. Logothetis CJ, Dexeus FH, Finn L, et al: A prospective randomized trial comparing MVAC and CISCA chemotherapy for patients with metastatic urothelial tumors. J Clin Oncol 1990; 8:1050–1055.
48. Logothetis CJ, Dexeus FH, Sella A, et al: Escalated therapy for refractory urothelial tumors: MVAC plus recombinant human granulocyte-macrophage colony stimulating factor. J Natl Cancer Inst 1990; 82:6670–6672.
49. MacNeil HF, Hall RR, Neal DE, et al: Systemic chemotherapy for urothelial cancer in patients with ureteric obstruction. Br J Urol 1991; 67:169–172.
50. Gabrilove JL, Jakubowski A, Scher HA, et al: Effect of granulocyte colony-stimulating factor on neutropenia and associated morbidity due to chemotherapy for transitional-cell carcinoma of the urothelium. N Engl J Med 1988; 318:1414–1422.
51. Moore MJ, Tannock IF, Iscoe N, et al: A phase II study of methotrexate, vinblastine, doxorubicin and cisplatin (MVAC) + GM-CSF in patients (Pts) with advanced transitional cell carcinoma. Proc ASCO, 1992; 11:611.
52. Waxman J, Abel P, James N, et al: New combination chemotherapy programme for bladder cancer. Br J Urol 1989; 63:68–71.
53. Seidman A, Scher H, Sternberg C, et al: Gallium nitrate (GaN): An active agent in patients (pts) with advanced refractory transitional cell carcinoma (TCC) of the urothelium (abstract). Cancer 1991; 68: 2561–2565.
54. Seligman PA, Crawford ED: Treatment of advanced transitional cell carcinoma (TCC) of the bladder with constant infusion gallium nitrate (GA-nitrate) (abstract). ASCO Proceedings 1991; 10:534.
55. Scher HI: Chemotherapy for invasive bladder cancer: Neoadjuvant versus adjuvant. Semin Oncol 1990; 8:555–565.
56. Gospodarowicz MK, Tannock IF, Moore MJ, et al: Phase I and II study of MVAC chemotherapy followed by radical radiation for locally advanced bladder cancer (abstract). J Urol 1991; 145:336A.
57. Skinner DG, Daniels JR, Russell CA, et al: The role of adjuvant chemotherapy following cystectomy for invasive bladder cancer: A prospective comparative trial. J Urol 1991; 145:459–467.
58. Hall RR, Newling DW, Ramsden PD, et al: Treatment of invasive bladder cancer by local resection and high dose methotrexate. Br J Urol 1984; 56:668–672.

59. Logothetis CJ, Johnson DE, Chong C, et al: Adjuvant chemotherapy of bladder cancer: A preliminary report. *J Urol* 1988; 139:1207–1211.
60. Antman K, Amato D, Wood W, et al: Selection bias in clinical trials. *J Clin Oncol* 1985; 3:1142–1147.
61. Davis S, Wright PW, Schulman SF, et al: Participants in prospective, randomized clinical trials for resected non-small cell lung cancer have improved survival compared with non-participants in such trials. *Cancer* 1985; 56:1710–1718.
62. Richards B, Bastable JR, Freedman L, et al: Adjuvant chemotherapy with doxorubicin (Adriamycin) and 5-fluorouracil in T3NxMo bladder cancer treated with radiotherapy. *Br J Urol* 1983; 55:386–391.
63. Studer UE, Hering F, Jaeger P, et al: Adjuvant cisplatinum chemotherapy following cystectomy for bladder cancer. *J Urol* 1991; 145:335A.
64. Coppin C, Gospodarowicz M, Dixon P, et al: Improved local control of invasive bladder cancer by concurrent cisplatin and preoperative or radical radiation. *Proc Am Soc Clin Oncol* 1992; 11.
65. Raghavan D, Wallace D, Sandeman T: First randomized trials of pre-emptive cisplatin for invasive transitional cell carcinoma of the bladder. *Proc Am Soc Clin Oncol* 1989; 8:516.
66. Tannock IF: The current status of adjuvant chemotherapy for bladder cancer. *Semin Urol* 1990; 8:291–297.

Prostate-Specific Antigen and the Clinician

M'Liss A. Hudson, M.D.

Assistant Professor, Division of Urologic Surgery, Washington University, School of Medicine, St. Louis, Missouri

History of Prostate-Specific Antigen

The discovery of prostate-specific antigen (PSA) has been attributed to M.C. Wang and associates,[1] who described and purified a unique antigen specific to prostate tissue. Before 1979, however, several different groups had reported the discovery of distinctive proteins in seminal plasma and human semen. Two groups in Japan independently reported on a protein component of seminal plasma that they called gamma-seminoprotein and protein E1 antigen, respectively.[2, 3] Sensabaugh[4] also characterized a semen-specific protein with a molecular weight of 30,000 daltons, which he designated p30. Subsequent studies using immunohistochemical, immunodiffusion, and immunoblotting techniques demonstrated that patterns of localization and distribution of PSA and gamma-seminoprotein are identical in both benign and cancerous human prostate sections.[5] Enzyme immunoassays for PSA and gamma-seminoprotein showed the two proteins to be immunologically identical. PSA and p30 produce an identical calibration curve to a PSA kit calibrator on a commercially available immunoassay for PSA.[6] Papsidero and colleagues[7] also identified PSA in human serum and verified this protein to be identical to the one purified from prostatic tissue.

Characteristics of Prostate-Specific Antigen

PSA is a single-chain glycoprotein monomer composed of 240 amino acid residues and four carbohydrate side chains. Its molecular weight is 34,000 daltons and it has an isoelectric point that varies from 6.8 to 7.2.[1, 8] PSA has been shown to be produced by the epithelial cells lining the acini and ducts of the prostate gland and the urethra. Normally, PSA is secreted into the lumen of the prostatic ducts and enters the seminal plasma in high concentrations. The production of PSA appears to be under the control androgen stimulation mediated through the androgen receptor.[9] Using LN CaP cells, a cell line derived from a human prostatic carcinoma metastasis, PSA messenger RNA (mRNA) can be induced by either the synthetic androgen, miberone, or the natural androgen, dihydrotestosterone, but not by glucocorticoids or estrogens. Moreover, in the presence of dihydrotestosterone, PSA mRNA production was depressed by the antiandrogen, hydroxyflutamide. This strongly suggests that the androgen receptor is a regulator of PSA production.[10, 11]

The normal physiologic function of PSA is believed to be to bring about the liquification of seminal coagulum by cleaving seminal vesicle–specific antigen and semenogelin into low–molecular weight proteins.[9] PSA functions like a serine protease of the kallikrein family. A high gene sequence homology has been noted between the PSA gene and the human glandular kallikrein (hGK-1) gene.[9, 12] PSA also has chymotrypsin-like, and possibly trypsinlike, activity. Killian and Chu[13] determined that PSA is a relatively stable molecule that can be maintained at room temperature for up to 48 hours without any apparent loss of biologic activity. No significant differences in PSA values were noted when samples were stored at $-20°C$ to $-80°C$ for up to 6 months. Inactivation of PSA occurs when there is cleavage of the carboxyterminal of Lys 1-45.[4, 5]

In serum, PSA may be detected in its monomeric form. When added to normal human plasma, active PSA forms stable complexes with both α_2-macroglobulin and α_1-antichymotrypsin. Complex formation with α_1-antichymotrypsin has been suggested to be a crucial determinant of the turnover of active PSA in vitro, with the major serum component of PSA existing in the form complexed to α_1-antichymotrypsin.[14] In patients with metastatic prostate cancer and very high levels of serum PSA, complexes with α_1-protease inhibitor also have been observed. In addition, low levels of PSA complexed to α_2-macroglobulin and interα-trypsin have been reported.[15]

The uniqueness of PSA lies in its specificity for prostatic tissue. PSA has been localized to the epithelial cells lining the acini and ducts of the normal prostate gland, in primary and metastatic prostate cancer, in benign hyperplastic tissue (BPH), and in other diseases of the prostate.[16, 17] Several studies have attempted to quantitate the relative amounts of PSA produced by normal, cancerous, and hyperplastic tissue. Early studies by Kuriyama and colleagues[18] suggested that the amount of PSA found in normal or hyperplastic tissue is similar to that found in malignant tissue. Bruce and Chloe[19] also reported that the concentration of PSA per gram of tissue is similar in the three types of tissue. More recent studies, however, report that there are differences in PSA production by benign and cancerous tissue. In a study by Qui and associates,[20] both PSA protein and PSA mRNA were measured in benign glandular epithelium and in malignant prostatic tissue using complementary DNA (cDNA) probe and immunohistochemical techniques, respectively. PSA protein production was noted to parallel PSA mRNA production. The benign epithelium demonstrated a uniformly high level of PSA production. Tumor specimens showed a heterogeneous expression of PSA, and both PSA protein and PSA mRNA were decreased significantly in malignant epithelium as compared with benign prostatic epithelium. Ersev and coworkers[21] correlated PSA immunoreactivity and tumor grade in 31 prostate cancers. In this study, a weak trend for less immunoreactivity to PSA was noted in higher-grade tumors. Gallee and colleagues[22] tested 55 radical prostatectomy specimens with four different monoclonal antibodies to PSA. Maximal staining intensity was found on BPH tissue sections. Irrespective of the antibodies used, these authors found PSA expression to be decreased consistently in cancerous tissue. A clear-cut relationship was demonstrated between the immunoreactivity for PSA and the degree of tumor differentiation. PSA expression was shown to be present, but in reduced concentrations, in most undifferentiated tumors. Stege and coworkers[23] correlated DNA ploidy and cellular PSA concentration in fine-needle biopsy specimens of prostatic carcinomas. Intracellular PSA concentration was less in high-grade and aneuploid tumors than in low-grade and diploid tumors. Northern and slot-blot analysis were used by Henttu and associates[12] to study PSA gene expression in tissue samples of BPH and adenocarcinoma of the prostate. No significant differences in PSA gene expression were found between BPH and cancer samples. The total amounts of PSA mRNA were similar in the BPH specimens, but up to a threefold variation in PSA mRNA levels was noted in the cancer specimens.

Detection of Prostate-Specific Antigen in Human Serum

Papsidero and coworkers[7] were the first to demonstrate that PSA is detectable in the serum of men. Virtually all men with functional prostatic tissue have been shown to have measurable serum PSA levels (in the absence of androgen deprivation therapy), whereas serum PSA usually is undetectable in women or in men in whom all prostatic tissue has been removed. Rare cases of cross-reacting antibodies for PSA have been reported in female sera; these nonspecific cross-reactions may be caused by rheumatoid factors.[24] Neither a diurnal nor a circadian rhythm has been demonstrated for serum PSA production. Stamey and colleagues[25] demonstrated that serum PSA levels are most reliable when they are collected from ambulatory patients in an outpatient setting as opposed to from hospitalized patients. In a study of 31 patients, these investigators found that the serum PSA level decreased by a mean of 18% in an inpatient hospital setting and, in some patients, it decreased by nearly 50% after admission to the hospital.

Effect of Prostatic Manipulation on Serum Prostate-Specific Antigen Levels

Several forms of prostatic manipulation have been suggested to produce transient elevations in serum PSA levels (Table 1). Because digital rectal examination (DRE) has been reported to increase serum prostatic acid phosphate levels, physicians empirically have assumed that a DRE also could cause an elevation in serum PSA values. In a series of 24 patients with prostate cancer, BPH, or prostatitis, Brawer[29] reported no significant

TABLE 1.
Effect of Prostatic Manipulation on Serum Prostate-Specific Antigen (PSA) Level

Test	Change in PSA Over Baseline
Digital rectal examination[26]	No significant change
Foley catheter[27]	No significant change
Transrectal ultrasound[28]	Occasional increase in PSA, primarily in patients with prostatitis
Prostatic massage[25]	At most, a mild, transient increase of 1.5 to 2 times over baseline, often resolved after 24 hours
Cystoscopy[25]	Increase of 4 times over baseline
Prostatic biopsy[26]	Marked increase over baseline and prolonged time (up to 6 weeks) to return to baseline
Transurethral resection of prostate[25]	Marked increase over baseline, presumed prolonged interval to return to baseline

difference in serum PSA levels (Tandem R) measured 40 and 10 minutes before or 5 and 30 minutes after DRE. In a similar study involving 43 men, Yuan and colleagues[26] confirmed that DRE rarely causes a significant change in serum PSA levels. In this study, no significant difference was detected between serum PSA levels obtained immediately before, and at 5 and 95 minutes after a DRE. A study by Brawn and associates[27] found that an indwelling Foley catheter had no effect on serum PSA levels. Transrectal ultrasonography (TRUS) did not appear to elevate serum PSA values in patients with prostate cancer or BPH in the study by Hughes and associates.[28] Patients with prostatitis were found to have a mild rise in serum PSA after a TRUS. Yuan and coworkers[26] noted a significant increase in serum PSA values in only 3 of 36 patients following TRUS. In a study of 60 patients who had serum PSA levels determined before and 1 minute after prostatic massage by Stamey and associates,[25] serum PSA levels (Pros-check) were noted to increase 1.5-fold to twofold after massage. Seven patients in Stamey's study who were undergoing cystoscopy in addition to prostatic massage were found to have even greater elevations to about four times the baseline level. However, el-Shirbiny and colleagues[30] found that serum PSA values did not increase appreciably in 19 men without prostatic disease after prostatic massage. Moreover, after 24 hours, levels returned to premassage values.

Procedures that disrupt the architecture of the prostate gland may allow direct entry of PSA into the bloodstream and result in greater, more prolonged elevations of serum PSA values. Stamey and coworkers[25] found that the serum PSA levels increased 57 times over the baseline value

(Pros-check) in seven men undergoing perineal core-needle biopsies of the prostate. Yuan and associates[26] found that TRUS-guided needle biopsy increased serum PSA values (Tandem R) an average of sevenfold over the prebiopsy values immediately after the procedure in 89 of 100 men. Stamey and his group[25] also found that transurethral resection of the prostate increased serum PSA values in eight men 53-fold over the baseline level. Although Stamey and colleagues[25] and Oesterling and associates[31] both calculated the metabolic clearance rate for serum PSA to be 2 to 3 days following radical prostatectomy, more prolonged elevations of serum PSA are seen after injury to the prostate, as with needle biopsy[26] or transurethral resection,[9] presumably due to continued leakage of PSA into the circulation.

Assays for Determination of Serum Prostate-Specific Antigen Values

A number of assays for determining serum PSA values have become available during the last several years. The following is an overview of the more commonly used assays in the United States.

Pros-check Prostate-Specific Antigen Assay

The Pros-check PSA assay was the first PSA assay developed in the United States. It is performed by incubating 0.2 mL of serum at room temperature for 18 hours with rabbit polyclonal antibodies directed against PSA. A second incubation then is performed using goat antirabbit antibodies, again at room temperature, for 30 minutes to precipitate the primary antibody-PSA complex. Seven calibrators with PSA at concentrations of 0, 0.5, 1, 2, 3, 8, 20, and 50 µg/L in a matrix of bovine serum albumin are used to construct a calibration curve. The reference interval was established using a total of 157 normal men without known prostatic disease using the mean PSA value plus two standard deviations. The normal range thus was established to be 0 to 2.5 ng/mL.

Tandem R Radioimmunoassay

The Tandem R radioimmunoassay is performed by incubating a 50-µL serum sample at room temperature for 2 hours with a 125-I–labeled monoclonal antibody directed against a different site on the PSA molecule. After the solid-phase PSA-radiolabeled antibody sandwich is formed, the beads are washed to remove unbound labeled antibody. The radioactivity remaining bound to the beads is measured. Six calibrators with PSA concentrations of 0, 2, 10, 25, 50 and 100 µg/L in human female serum are used to construct a calibration curve. The reference interval was established using a total of 472 men without known prostatic disease. All men less than 40 years of age and 97% of men over 40 years of age in this study group were found to have a serum PSA value between 0 and 4 ng/mL.

Tandem E Prostate-Specific Antigen Assay

Like its predecessor, the Tandem E assay used the same two murine monoclonal antibodies directed against the PSA molecule. Instead of using a radioactive-labeled antibody, the Tandem E assay has an enzyme, alkaline phosphatase, attached to the unbound antibody to measure serum PSA concentrations. The main advantages of this assay are that no radioactive materials are required and it is less expensive to perform. The reference interval also is 0 to 4 ng/mL.

IRMA-Count Prostate-Specific Antigen Assay

The IRMA-Count PSA assay is an amplified immunoradiometric assay based on ligand-coated tubes and three monoclonal anti-PSA antibodies, one 125-I–labeled, the other two linked to a ligand. The PSA calibrator or serum sample then is "sandwiched" between the monoclonal antibodies in a reaction proceeding with liquid-phase kinetics. Separation is achieved by the ligand-coated tube/antiligand bridge method.

IMx Assay

A newer, commercially available PSA assay for serum PSA levels is the Abbott IMx System, which is based on microparticle enzyme immunoassay technology. This assay has produced reliable and reproducible results at levels as low as 0.1 ng/mL.

Comparison of Prostate-Specific Antigen Assays

The Pros-check PSA assay and the Tandem R radioimmunoassay have been the most frequently compared assays. Both have been shown to have good precision and accuracy; there also is a close linear correlation in PSA values determined by the two assays.[32] The PSA values reported by the Pros-check assay are consistently 1.5 to 2 times higher on the same serum sample than those reported on the Tandem R assay. The difference may be due to the use of different standards in the kits. One criticism of the Tandem R assay is the "hook effect" seen at high concentrations of PSA, in which an artificially low value may be measured.[33] This effect may be avoided by using a two-step dilution of the sample with a high PSA concentration.[34] Further refinement in the performance technique for this assay has brought the clinical sensitivity to 0.1 ng/mL.

A comparison of the Tandem R and IRMA-Count assays showed that the PSA values obtained with each correlated well, and there were no differences in the detection limits.[35] Within-assay precision was better with the IRMA-Count assay in the upper part of the normal reference interval and above; however, a "hook effect" also has been observed with this assay.[35] When the IMx assay was compared to the Tandem E assay, the IMx assay proved to be accurate and precise, with intra-assay variations of less than 5%.[36]

Ultrasensitive Prostate-Specific Antigen Assays

Newer, ultrasensitive assays for the detection of serum PSA are being tested for usefulness in the management of patients with prostate cancer. Stamey and associates[37] recently reported the use of an ultrasensitive radioimmunoassay for PSA based on a 72-hour incubation (4°C) of the primary polyclonal antibody in the Pros-check assay. The minimally detectable PSA level with this assay was 0.012 ± 0.023 ng/mL. Using sera from selected men with an initially undetectable PSA level following radical prostatectomy, the ultrasensitive assay of a rising serum PSA value was reported to be detected earlier than by the standard Pros-check assay, by a mean of 310 ± 278 days. These results may have been influenced to some extent by the intervals of testing.

Villers and colleagues[38] also have reported the use of an ultrasensitive PSA assay for detection of PSA values below 0.1 ng/mL using a modification of the polyclonal (Pros-check) assay. All 25 patients with prostate cancer who had negative or equivocal surgical margins after radical prostatectomy had a serum PSA value less than 0.1 ng/mL, whereas all 15 patients with positive surgical margins had serum PSA levels greater than 0.1 ng/mL. An important issue in the use of ultrasensitive assays is their reproducibility and reliability over time when used in the serial monitoring of patients with cancer. In this regard, monoclonal antibodies are more consistent than polyclonal antibodies. It is important to be certain that changes observed over time are not due to variability in the assay in the range of these very low PSA levels.

Prostate-Specific Antigen and Benign Prostatic Hyperplasia

Although the production of PSA is specific to the prostate gland, elevations in serum PSA levels may be seen in both benign and malignant disorders of the prostate. As is summarized in Table 2, about 30% of men with clinical symptoms of prostatism and a palpably enlarged, benign-feeling prostate gland on DRE have an elevation of serum PSA level above the upper limit of normal using the Tandem R radioimmunoassay (reference interval, 0 to 4 ng/mL). The majority of patients with histologically confirmed BPH and an elevated PSA level have values between 4 and 10 ng/mL; only a small percentage have a PSA level greater than 10 ng/mL[31, 34, 39, 40, 42, 43] (see Table 2). Previous studies have shown that, irrespective of the DRE findings, the odds ratio for a patient having BPH is greater if the serum PSA value is between 0 and 10 ng/mL, whereas the odds are greater that the patient has prostate cancer if his serum PSA value is greater than 10 ng/mL. The early work of Yang,[44] and of Stamey and associates[25] using the Pros-check PSA assay showed a much higher percentage of men with BPH (62% and 86%, respectively) to have a PSA value above the reference interval of 0 to 2.5 ng/mL for this assay.

Empirically, it seems that a direct correlation may exist between increas-

TABLE 2.
Previous Reports of Elevated Prostate-Specific Antigen (PSA)
Values in Patients With Benign Prostatic Hyperplasia

Author	Number of Patients (%) With Elevated PSA Value	
	4 to 10 ng/mL	>10 ng/mL
Myrtle et al.[39]	63/352 (18)	7/352 (2)
Oesterling et al.[31]	34/72 (47)	7/72 (10)
Partin et al.[41]	33/72 (46)	5/72 (7)
Ercole et al.[40]	64/357 (18)	11/357 (3)
Hudson et al.[34]	32/168 (19)	3/168 (2)

ing serum PSA levels and increasing volume of the hyperplastic prostate gland. As previously suggested by Brawer,[45] there are several variables that may account for the elevated serum PSA levels associated with BPH. The histology of the prostate gland significantly influences both PSA production and its subsequent secretion into the circulation. One of the greatest limitations of examining serum PSA levels in men with presumed BPH is the number of cases diagnosed on clinical grounds alone[39] and the lack of histologic confirmation of the diagnosis. Even those studies demonstrating histologic confirmation of the diagnosis of BPH by simple prostatectomy may have included patients who harbored occult prostate cancer in the unsampled peripheral zone (the most common site in which prostate cancer arises). Although it has been suggested that the serum PSA level is elevated 0.3 ng/mL for each gram of hyperplastic tissue present,[25] this arbitrary value is unlikely always to be true due to the variable histologic features of BPH: at least five different patterns of BPH have been described and the ratio of stroma to epithelium may vary considerably from case to case.[46] Since only the epithelial cells of the prostatic acini and ducts produce PSA, hyperplastic glands with the same volume but differing proportions of glandular elements and stroma would be expected to produce different amounts of PSA. This concept is supported by the studies of Weber and colleagues,[47] who found as much as a threefold difference in PSA production by glandular and stromal elements in hyperplastic glands. These authors, as well as Partin and associates,[41] were unable to demonstrate a direct relationship between serum PSA levels and the volume of BPH tissue in the prostate.

Other histologic findings in the hyperplastic gland that may be responsible for elevated serum PSA levels include focal areas of prostatitis, prostatic infarction, prostatic intraepithelial neoplasia (PIN), and unsuspected adenocarcinoma. In their autopsy series of 105 untrimmed prostates from men without a history of prostate cancer and a DRE not suspicious for cancer, Brawn and coworkers[27] found that a significantly higher proportion of patients whose prostate had severe acute or chronic inflammation had PSA levels above 4 ng/mL (Tandem R, 50% vs. 22%), particularly those with smaller glands. Brawer,[45] studying 155 men undergoing TRUS-guided biopsy of the prostate, found that the mean PSA value was 5.9 ng/mL in patients with PIN as compared to 3.6 ng/mL in those with BPH alone. This author noted a mean PSA level of 17.9 ng/mL in men with adenocarcinoma detectable by TRUS-guided biopsy. In the autopsy series by Brawn and associates,[27] occult prostatic carcinomas less than 1 mL in volume usually did not elevate the serum PSA value, whereas those larger than 1 mL frequently elevated it above 4 ng/mL. Quantitative immunohistochemical stains previously have shown decreased immunoreactivity with PSA in both carcinoma and PIN when compared to BPH tissue. Brawer[45] interpreted these results as showing that it is not increased production of PSA in PIN and carcinoma tissue that is associated with increased serum levels, but rather increased disruption of the normal glandular architecture that leads to PSA leakage into the circulation.

Several authors have attempted to correlate serum PSA levels with prostatic volume. Littrup and colleagues[48] reported on patients without evidence of prostate cancer from DRE or TRUS who had statistically significant increases in mean PSA values; these patients had increasing gland volumes. Patients with PSA values above the volume-adjusted 95th percentile were estimated to have a risk of prostate cancer up to nine times that of those within the "normal" volume-adjusted range. Babaian and associates[49] also found a direct relationship between prostate volume as calculated by ultrasonography and serum PSA level. They determined a threshold value for predicting prostate cancer, which was 20 ng/mL (Tandem R). Veneziano and associates[50] calculated the volume of the prostate by TRUS in 108 patients and related it to the serum PSA value as a PSA/volume index (Fig 1). Histologic examination was performed and the mean serum PSA/volume index was 0.099 in patients with BPH in comparison to 1.73 in those with prostate cancer. This prompted the authors to conclude that this ratio may be useful in determining whether patients have benign or malignant diseases of the prostate. Benson and coworkers[51] used the same equation (serum PSA/prostatic volume) to define the term "PSA density," which is really a misnomer, because the ratio does not measure the density of PSA in the prostate. Rather it compares the concentration of PSA in the serum to the volume of the prostate. The term PSA index or PSA ratio is more accurate. The mean PSA density for patients with prostate cancer in Benson's study was 0.581, whereas that for BPH was 0.044. Thirty-three of 34 patients with a PSA density greater than 0.1 had prostate cancer, leading these authors to conclude that PSA density is superior to serum PSA determination alone in predicting the presence or absence of prostate cancer. In conflict with these studies, however, are the data of Andriole and colleagues[52] that failed to support the concept that PSA density was superior to serum PSA alone as a means of detecting prostate cancer. Vesey and coworkers[53] found a significant correlation between the serum PSA level and the weight of prostatic tissue re-

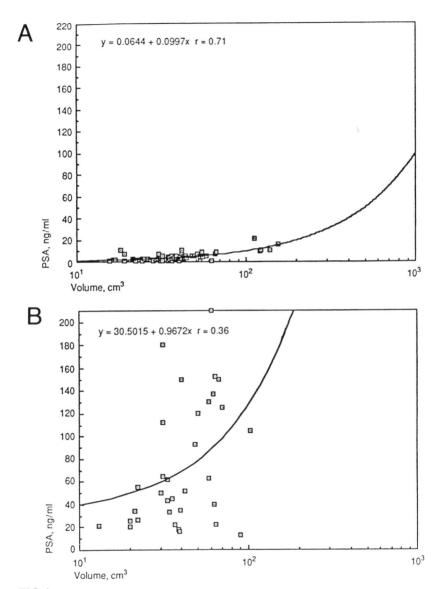

FIG 1.
A, simple linear correlation between serum prostate-specific antigen *(PSA)* and prostate volume in patients with benign prostatic disease (fibroadenomas and prostatitis). **B,** simple linear correlation between PSA and prostatic volume in patients with prostatic carcinoma. (From Veneziano S, Pavlica P, Querze R, et al: *Eur Urol* 1990; 18:112. Used by permission.)

sected at transurethral resection of the prostate in 58 men with BPH. By dividing the serum PSA by the prostatic weight, an index-corrected PSA in relation to prostatic size was devised. This same index in patients with prostate cancer was significantly higher than in patients with BPH. Further studies are needed to determine whether volume-related serum PSA values can be established to distinguish accurately between patients with BPH and those with prostate cancer.

Use of Serum Prostate-Specific Antigen Values in the Early Detection of Prostate Cancer

Despite early optimism, the available data clearly show that serum PSA values *alone* at a single point in time are not sufficiently specific to distinguish an individual patient with prostate cancer from one with BPH or other benign disorders of the prostate.[31, 34, 54, 55] Before the establishment of the currently accepted reference intervals for the different PSA assays, both Kuriyama and associates[54] and Bhatti and colleagues[55] reported that they were able to distinguish patients with advanced prostate cancer from those with BPH using serum PSA values. However, in neither of these studies could patients with early stage disease be distinguished from patients with BPH. Stamey and coworkers,[25] using the Pros-check PSA assay with an upper limit of 2.5 ng/mL, found that 86% of patients with histologically confirmed BPH had elevated serum PSA values as compared to 96% of those with prostate cancer. More recently, Oesterling[56] compared serum PSA values for patients with BPH with those with *organ-confined* prostate cancer using the data from three independent studies (Table 3). He found that 43% of men with organ-confined prostate cancer had PSA values in the normal range, whereas 32% of men with BPH had elevated PSA levels using the reference interval 0 to 4 ng/mL (Tandem R). The diagnostic accuracy of PSA as a screening test was evaluated using 4 ng/mL and 10 ng/mL as the upper limits of normal. The diagnostic accuracy for each of these levels was 64% and 70%, respectively. Although serum PSA values were able to distinguish whole patient populations with prostate cancer from populations with BPH, a single serum PSA value was not useful in predicting prostate cancer in an individual patient.

The use of serum PSA as a screening tool for prostate cancer has been viewed differently in a recent article by Catalona and colleagues.[57] In this study, it was suggested that, because a serum PSA value involves only a simple blood test, is more objective, and is relatively inexpensive, this test may be accepted more readily by patients than a DRE. In this study of 1,653 volunteers aged 50 years and over, only 10% had a PSA value greater than 4 ng/mL (Tandem R). Of the patients with an elevated PSA value between 4 and 10 ng/mL, 22% were found to have prostate cancer. Sixty-seven percent of patients whose PSA values were greater than 10 ng/mL were found to have prostate cancer. Additionally, 59% of the patients diagnosed with prostate cancer whose PSA levels were between 4

TABLE 3.
Prostate-Specific Antigen (PSA) Values for Benign Prostatic Hypertrophy (BPH) vs. Organ-Confined Prostate Cancer*

| | Number of Patients | | Percent of Patients With PSA Values in Specified Range (no./total) | | | | | | | |
| | | | 0.0–4.0 ng/mL† | | 4.1–10.0 ng/mL† | | >10.1 ng/mL† | |
References	BPH	Organ-Confined Prostate Cancer	BPH	Organ-Confined Prostate Cancer	BPH	Organ-Confined Prostate Cancer	BPH	Organ-Confined Prostate Cancer
Partin et al.[41]	72	185	47 (34/72)	45 (83/185)	46 (33/72)	44 (82/185)	7 (5/72)	11 (20/185)
Lange et al.[77]	357	31	79 (282/357)	45 (14/31)	18 (64/357)	32 (10/32)	3 (11/357)	23 (7/31)
Hudson et al.[34]	168	103	79 (133/168)	38 (39/103)	19 (32/168)	26 (27/103)	2 (3/168)	36 (37/103)
Totals	597	319	75 (449/597)	43 (136/319)	22 (129/597)	37 (119/319)	3 (19/597)	20 (64/319)

*Both diseases were confined histologically. $P < .0001$ for all PSA values.
†Tandem R PSA assay.

and 10 ng/mL were found to have organ-confined prostate cancer compared to only 13% of those with a PSA value greater than 10 ng/mL (Table 4). These findings were confirmed by Brawer and associates[58] in a similar study of 1,240 men who underwent initial screening for prostate cancer with a serum PSA value. Twenty-seven of 79 men in this study who underwent biopsy were found to have prostate cancer. Forty-four percent of those with prostate cancer were judged to have a normal or only asymmetric gland by DRE. Thus, it appears that serum PSA values may initiate a diagnostic work-up of some patients with prostate cancer in whom the condition otherwise would not have been detected by DRE alone.

Another potential use of serum PSA values in the early detection of prostate cancer is the serial monitoring of PSA values in an individual over time. Carter and coworkers[59] retrospectively reviewed banked frozen serum samples in men participating in a study on aging. Men were divided into three groups: those in whom no prostatic disease developed, those who underwent simple prostatectomy and had histologic confirmation of BPH, and those who developed prostate cancer confirmed histologically. Significant differences were noted in the slopes of the lines plotting serial PSA values in men who developed prostate cancer, in comparison to those with either BPH or no prostatic disease. They concluded that the percentage change in serum PSA per year may yield more information in detecting prostate cancer than any absolute PSA value (Fig 2). However, a short-term, prospective study by Catalona and associates of the rate of change of serum PSA values in men who underwent prostatic biopsies for a PSA greater than 4.0 ng/mL and benign findings on DRE or TRUS, measurement of rate of change of PSA levels or percent change of PSA levels over the 12- to 37-month interval before the biopsy failed to distinguish between men with positive biopsies and those with negative biopsies (Catalona R, unpublished data, 1992). Longer follow-up in a prospective study is needed to determine if measurement of the interval change in serum PSA values is useful to predict the development of prostate cancer in men who have normal levels initially.

Use of Serum Prostate-Specific Antigen in Conjunction With Digital Rectal Examination and Transrectal Ultrasound for the Detection of Prostate Cancer

As first suggested by Cooner and coworkers,[60] the value of serum PSA levels in detecting prostate cancer is greater when they are used in conjunction with other modalities, most commonly DRE and TRUS. Cooner and colleagues evaluated 1,807 men from a general urologic practice using serum PSA, DRE, and TRUS. The overall cancer detection rate in this series was 14.6%. The positive predictive value (PPV) with an abnormality on all three tests was 77%. Lee and associates[61] also confirmed a PPV of 71% for the detection of prostate cancer when all three tests were abnormal. Results from Prostate Cancer Awareness Week 1989 compared the

TABLE 4.
Serum Prostate-Specific Antigen (PSA) Concentrations and the Incidence of Cancer as a Function of Age in 1,653 Men in the Study Group and 235 Men in the Comparison Group*

Group/Age (yr)	Number of Men (% of total)	Serum PSA Level (µg/L)					
		<4.0		4.0–9.9†		≥10.0	
		No. (%)	No. (%) With Cancer‡	No. (%)	No. With Cancer/No. With Biopsy (%)§	No. (%)	No. With Cancer/No. With Biopsy (%)§
Study group							
50–59	629 (38)	613 (97)	—	12 (2)	2/11 (18)	4 (1)	1/3 (33)
60–69	737 (45)	669 (91)	—	53 (7)	8/40 (20)	15 (2)	12/15 (80)
70–79	264 (16)	215 (81)	—	39 (15)	9/32 (28)	10 (4)	4/8 (50)
80–89	23 (1)	19 (83)	—	3 (13)	0/2 (0)	1 (4)	1/1 (100)
All	1,653	1,516 (92)	—	107 (6)	19/85 (22)	30 (2)	18/27 (67)

Comparison group

Age							
50–59	46 (20)	27 (59)	0 (0)	13 (28)	0 (0)	6 (13)	4 (67)
60–69	93 (40)	51 (55)	6 (12)	37 (40)	12 (32)	5 (5)	3 (60)
70–79	80 (34)	37 (46)	7 (19)	21 (26)	5 (24)	22 (28)	13 (59)
80–89	16 (7)	1 (6)	0 (0)	3 (19)	2 (67)	12 (75)	9 (75)
All	235	116 (49)	13 (11)	74 (32)	19 (26)	45 (19)	29 (64)

*Serum PSA determinations were not performed in 65 patients in the comparison group.

†In addition to the numbers shown, 31 men in the study group with initial serum PSA values of 4.0 to 9.9 µg/L (most were 4.0 µg/L or just above) had values below 4.0 µg/L on repeated measurements and therefore did not undergo rectal examination or ultrasonography. We reanalyzed both samples in all 31 men. All but three of the results were within the limits of interassay variation, but in 2 men, a high value in the first assay could not be confirmed, and in 1, a lower value in the second assay could not be confirmed. For all 3, values less than 4.0 µg/L were detected in the second blood sample.

‡Dashes are shown for the study group because men with serum PSA levels below 4.0 µg/L were not evaluated with rectal examination, ultrasonography, or biopsy (see text). Three of 4 men who had further evaluation despite an initially normal serum PSA level were found to have prostate cancer; 3 of 8 men with serum PSA levels that were normal at first but elevated 6 months later had cancer; none of 6 men with serum PSA levels ≥4.0 µg/L and negative biopsies at first with a higher PSA value after 6 months had prostate cancer; one of 7 men with serum PSA levels ≥4.0 µg/L and negative biopsies initially and no change in serum PSA level 6 months later was found to have cancer on repeated biopsy.

§Numbers shown for the comparison group in this column are the number of men with cancer, followed in parentheses by the percentage created by dividing this number by the number of men shown in the preceding column.

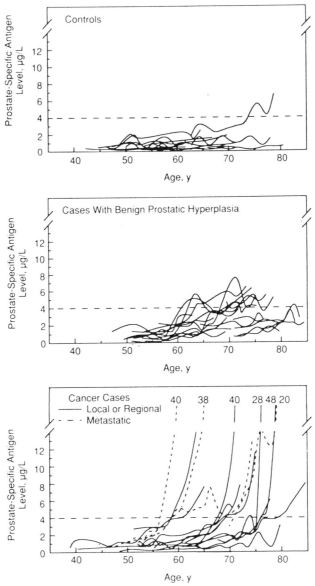

FIG 2.
Observed data on prostate-specific antigen levels (μg/L) plotted as a function of age for each individual in the three diagnostic groups *(solid lines).* The *broken horizontal line* marks the single PSA criterion of 4.0 μg/L. The PSA values at the visit closest to diagnosis are indicated for individuals who progress beyond a PSA value of 14 μg/L. (From Carter HB, Andres R, Metter J, et al: Longitudinal evaluation of prostate-specific antigen levels in men with and without prostate disease. *JAMA* 1992; 267:2215-2220. Used by permission.)

sensitivity, specificity, and predictive values of DRE and serum PSA values in detecting prostate cancer.[62] In this study of 196 biopsies performed, 41 cases of prostate cancer were detected; the sensitivity, specificity, PPV, and negative predictive value (NPV) of PSA vs. DRE are shown in Table 5. In all areas, PSA showed a significant advantage over DRE in detecting prostate cancer during screening. Babaian and colleagues[63] reviewed the use of DRE, TRUS, and serum PSA in 124 consecutive patients who underwent prostate biopsy because of an abnormality on either DRE or TRUS. These authors found that the cancer detection rate increased from 17.5% if the PSA values were less than 4 ng/mL to 68.7% if the values were greater than 4 ng/mL, and up to 83.3% for values greater than 20 ng/mL. They concluded that serum PSA levels were the most important of the diagnostic triad, and that patients with a PSA level greater than 10 ng/mL require biopsy regardless of their other findings because of the high likelihood of finding cancer. The data presented by Catalona and colleagues,[57] however, suggest that a PSA level greater than 4 ng/mL is a more appropriate point at which to initiate prostatic biopsy, because such a low percentage of patients with a PSA value greater than 10 ng/mL are found to have pathologically organ-confined prostate cancer. In another screening study performed at six different institutions (unpublished data, 1991), 183 prostate cancers were detected using DRE, TRUS, and serum PSA. The majority (70%) were detected by an abnormality on two or more of these

TABLE 5.
Results of Prostate Cancer
Awareness Week 1989*†

Parameter	PSA	DRE
Sensitivity	94	63
Specificity	49	17
PPV	46	12
NPV	95	64

*From Stone NN, Lazan D, Clejan S, et al: Comparison of digital rectal exam (DRE) and prostate-specific antigen (PSA) biopsy results from Prostate Cancer Awareness Week 1989. Presented at the annual meeting of the American Urological Association, Toronto, Canada, June 1991. Used by permission.
†One hundred and ninety-six patients with either an abnormal DRE, PSA, or both underwent prostate biopsy; 41 cases of prostate cancer were detected. PSA = prostate-specific antigen; DRE = digital rectal examination; PPV = positive predictive value; NPV = negative predictive value. All values are given as percentages.

screening tests. However, 13% were detected by PSA alone, 8% were found by DRE alone, and 9% were noted by TRUS alone, suggesting that serum PSA as a single screening modality is capable of detecting the largest number of cancers. The PPV for PSA in this study was 45%, compared to 22% for DRE and 18% for TRUS. Although neither Mettlin and colleagues[64] nor Lee and coworkers[65] used serum PSA as an initial screening modality for the detection of prostate cancer, both have reported cases of prostate cancer suspected solely on the basis of an elevated serum PSA value that were missed by both DRE and TRUS. In the Mettlin study,[64] the likelihood of an abnormality on DRE and TRUS proving to be prostate cancer increased from 14.6% to 68% when the PSA value was elevated. Thus, serum PSA in conjunction with DRE and TRUS appears to increase the cancer detection rate over any single modality used alone.

Serum Prostate-Specific Antigen in the Clinical Staging of Prostate Cancer

Preoperative serum PSA levels have been shown to increase with advancing clinical stage of prostate cancer. Using the Pros-check assay, Stamey and Kabalin[66] reported that serum PSA values can be used to distinguish among all clinical stages of prostate cancer, except between stages B2 and B3, and between stages A2 and B1. Although our own experience at Washington University also has shown that mean serum PSA values increase with advancing clinical stage, there is considerable overlap among all clinical stages (Fig 3). This has been substantiated in the studies by Chan and associates,[67] and by Myrtle.[39]

Use of Serum Prostate-Specific Antigen in Pathologic Staging of Prostate Cancer

Our early experience at Washington University,[34] along with that of numerous other investigators,[41, 54, 55, 62] mirrored the experience with preoperative serum PSA values for predicting the clinical stage of prostate cancer. Again, a direct correlation was noted between an increasing preoperative serum PSA value and advancing pathologic stage and tumor volume. The majority of studies have demonstrated a substantial overlap between patients with pathologically confirmed organ-confined disease and those with extracapsular tumor extension.

The time interval between procurement of the pretreatment serum PSA level and performance of the prostatic biopsy diagnosing the prostate cancer varied in these early studies. As mentioned previously, prostatic biopsy usually causes a transient marked elevation in serum PSA values that persists for several weeks after biopsy.[26] If, in some patients, the pretreatment PSA values were obtained shortly after a prostatic biopsy, then they may be elevated falsely over the true baseline value. A more recent study by

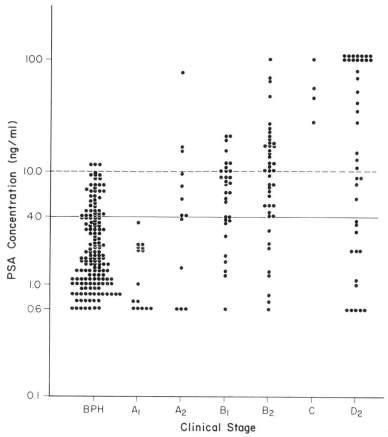

FIG 3.
Preoperative prostate-specific antigen *(PSA)* values in patients with benign prostatic hyperplasia, clinically localized prostate cancer, or metastatic prostate cancer. (From Hudson MA, Bahnson RR, Catalona WJ: *J Urol* 1989; 142:1011. Used by permission.)

Catalona and coworkers[68] found that, if the serum PSA value drawn prior to the diagnostic biopsy is greater than 10 ng/mL (Tandem R), then the radical prostatectomy specimen often will show extracapsular extension, positive surgical margins, or a persistently detectable PSA level.

More recent studies not only have focused on the correlation between serum PSA levels and pathologic stage, but also have sought to correlate serum PSA levels with either tumor grade or Gleason score, and with DNA ploidy. Babaian and colleagues[69] reported a significant correlation between PSA levels and progressive Gleason's scores 2 to 4, 5 to 7, and 8 to 10. These authors found that a PSA value greater than 20 ng/mL (Tandem R) was present more often in patients with extracapsular disease (57%) than in those with organ-confined disease (11%). In addition, 81%

of all patients with a serum PSA value greater than 50 ng/mL had metastatic disease, whereas only 28% of patients whose serum PSA value was below 50 ng/mL had metastases. Despite the statistically significant association between the serum PSA level and tumor grade and stage, this level was not recommended by these authors for use in differentiating reliably between organ-confined and extracapsular disease in an individual patient.

Badalament and associates[70] also studied 112 patients undergoing radical prostatectomy for clinically localized disease. Serum PSA values greater than 10 ng/mL (Tandem R) were associated with extraprostatic disease and a Gleason score of 6 to 10. Mean PSA values also were higher in patients with aneuploid tumors. The accuracy of a serum PSA value greater than 20 ng/mL in predicting regional lymph node metastases (D1 disease) was 80.6%, and the PPV and NPV for the identification of extracapsular disease were 84.2% and 74.0%, respectively. In distinguishing organ-confined prostate cancer and extracapsular disease, Winter and associates[71] used a preoperative serum PSA value of 10 ng/mL (Tandem R) as a cutoff value, and found that the sensitivity was 68%, the specificity was 66%, the PPV was 46%, and the NPV was 83%. Although a trend was noted of increasing serum PSA values with higher pathologic grade or stage, there was no preoperative serum PSA level that would serve as a useful cut-off in determining pathologic grade or stage in an individual patient. Partin and coworkers[41] found that, although mean PSA levels increased with advancing pathologic tumor stage, the usefulness of PSA to predict pathologic stage for an individual patient was limited for two reasons: (1) the unpredictable contribution from the BPH component of the gland, and (2) the decreasing production of PSA by higher-grade lesions as tumor volume increases. Lange[72] suggested the use of a table (Table 6) listing the preoperative serum PSA levels as a function of the relative likelihood of there being capsular perforation, seminal vesicle invasion, or lymph node metastases. These probabilities then could be taken into consideration with the patient's general health, age, tumor grade, and clinical staging information to arrive at an optimal treatment plan. Thus, serum PSA may provide some useful information in predicting the pathologic stage and likelihood of ultimate cure in patients undergoing radical prostatectomy.

Use of Prostate-Specific Antigen in Predicting the Need for Routine Radionuclide Bone Scan

Prostate cancer frequently has been shown to metastasize to the skeleton. Therefore, radionuclide bone scans have been performed routinely in the staging of prostate cancer. Chybowski and associates[73] retrospectively reviewed 521 cases of prostate cancer and correlated the bone scan findings with the pretreatment serum PSA values. In this study, only 1 of 306 men with a serum PSA value of less than 20 ng/mL had findings on a bone scan suggestive of metastatic prostate cancer. The NPV of a PSA value less than 20 ng/mL was 99.7%. The authors suggested that routine staging ra-

TABLE 6.
Distribution by Pathologic Stage of Serum Prostate-Specific Antigen (PSA) Levels in Men After Radical Prostatectomy*

PSA Level†	Number of Men	Number (%) With OC	Number (%) With CP	Number With +SV/+LN (%)
0–2.8	102	84 (82)	16 (16)	2 (2)
0–4	49	34 (69)	13 (27)	2 (4)
2.8–10	159	81 (51)	52 (33)	26 (16)
4–10	41	15 (37)	18 (44)	8 (20)
>4	40	23 (26)	26 (29)	47 (45)
>10	142	29 (20)	30 (21)	83 (59)
10–20	76	15 (20)	21 (28)	40 (52)
>20	62	14 (23)	7 (12)	41 (66)
20–50	43	11 (26)	4 (9)	28 (65)
>50	20	2 (10)	2 (10)	16 (80)
50–100	13	1 (8)	1 (8)	11 (84)
>100	6	0	0	6 (100)

*OC = organ-confined disease; CP = capsular perforation with or without positive margins; +SV = positive seminal vesicles; +LN = positive lymph nodes.
†Tandem-R assay.

dionuclide bone scanning is unnecessary if the serum PSA level is less than 20 ng/mL. Terris and colleagues[74] retrospectively reviewed follow-up bone scans in 118 men with clinically localized prostate cancer who previously had undergone radical prostatectomy. These authors found that serial serum PSA values more clearly represented the clinical situation than did routine bone scans. Routine bone scans provided little additional information when PSA levels were normal. These authors concluded that follow-up bone scans were indicated primarily if the postoperative serum PSA level became detectable or the patient became symptomatic. Freitas and coworkers[75] also confirmed these findings. In their review of 107 patients with prostate cancer who were treated with either definitive radiation therapy or radical prostatectomy, they used a serum PSA value of 8 ng/mL (Tandem R) to exclude bone metastases, with an NPV of 98.5%. Only on rare occasions have patients with untreated prostate cancer and a serum PSA value of less than 10 ng/mL been documented to have bone metastases.[76]

Use of Serum Prostate-Specific Antigen After Radical Prostatectomy

The greatest usefulness and most extensive application of serum PSA values has been for the follow-up of patients who have undergone radical prostatectomy for clinically localized prostate cancer. In theory, if all prostatic tissue is removed during the radical prostatectomy procedure, the serum PSA values should fall to an undetectable level. The presence of a persistently detectable or rising serum PSA level after radical prostatectomy is pathognomonic for the presence of residual prostatic tissue. Most commonly, residual carcinoma occurs in the pelvis or as occult metastases, although residual benign apical tissue also may be left inadvertently by the surgeon. Lange and coworkers[77] reported on 51 patients whose serum PSA values were measured 3 to 6 months after radical prostatectomy. Using a value of 0.4 ng/mL (Tandem R) as the lower limit of detectability, only 11% of men whose serum PSA was less than 0.2 ng/mL postoperatively demonstrated a recurrence within 6 to 50 months of follow-up. In contrast, 100% of those whose postoperative serum PSA was 0.4 ng/mL or higher demonstrated a recurrence during follow-up of 7 to 75 months. Ninety-five percent of those with a postoperative PSA value of 0.4 ng/mL or higher had positive surgical margins, seminal vesicles, or lymph nodes. These findings have been substantiated by Oesterling and colleagues[56] and by Stein and associates,[78] who noted that the frequency of an elevated PSA level following radical prostatectomy was higher with advancing pathologic stage and was similar to the progression rate for each stage at 5 to 10 years of follow-up. These authors also confirmed that all patients with a documented recurrence of prostate cancer after radical prostatectomy had an elevated postoperative serum PSA value. Killian and coworkers[79] similarly found serum PSA values to be elevated in 92% of patients who developed recurrence after definitive treatment with either radical prostatectomy or radiation therapy, with a lead time of up to 12 months before the recurrence was clinically apparent. In our experience at Washington University, we have found that only rarely has a patient with a documented tumor recurrence had an undetectable PSA value.[34]

Treatment of Patients With a Detectable Prostate-Specific Antigen Value Following Radical Prostatectomy

The question remains as to the optimal form of therapy for patients with a detectable PSA value following radical prostatectomy. A metabolic half-life of 2 to 3 days has been calculated on the rate of clearance of PSA from the circulation after this procedure.[25, 31] For patients with a persistently detectable or rising PSA postoperatively, its source may be either persistent disease in the pelvis, occult distant metastases, or both. A study by Lightner and colleagues[80] revealed a surprising number of patients with a local recurrence found by blind biopsy of the vesicourethral anastomotic site. Stein and associates[78] also found that, in patients with a detectable PSA level following radical prostatectomy, but no other sign of recurrence, an ultrasound-guided biopsy of the anastomosis confirmed local tumor recurrence in four of ten patients.

Adjuvant radiation therapy to the pelvis has been used to treat patients who have a detectable serum PSA level following radical prostatectomy. Our series[81] and that of Lightner and associates[82] have shown that serum PSA values fall to an undetectable level in about 40% of patients so treated. With further follow-up, however, 11 of 13 patients (84%) with persistently detectable PSA values despite adjuvant radiation therapy developed clinical evidence of recurrence. Adjuvant radiation therapy after radical prostatectomy for patients with tumor extension into the periprostatic fat or with seminal vesicle invasion also has been studied by Morgan and coworkers.[83] In this study, 94% of patients treated surgically and then with radiation had a PSA value of 0.2 ng/mL (Tandem R) compared to only 64% of those with tumors of the same pathologic stage who did not receive adjuvant radiation therapy at 1 year of follow-up. However, this effect of adjuvant radiation therapy on PSA levels was only temporary in the patients with longer follow-up. Thus, adjuvant radiation therapy for a detectable PSA level following radical prostatectomy appears to induce a long-term remission in only a minority of patients.

Use of Serum Prostate-Specific Antigen After Definitive Radiation Therapy

Several studies have addressed the role of serum PSA values used to follow patients with localized prostate cancer treated with definitive radiation therapy. The intent of radiation therapy is to eradicate the cancer cells, but it is not expected to eliminate the normal epithelium of the prostate gland. In contrast to patients who have undergone radical prostatectomy, serum PSA levels following radiation therapy are not expected to fall to undetectable levels. Chodak and colleagues[84] reported on 20 patients who underwent pelvic radiation for nonmetastatic prostate cancer. These authors found that 8 of 15 patients had a serum PSA value within the reference interval (Pros-check) by 7 months after the completion of therapy. A prostatic biopsy was positive for cancer in 4 of 5 patients with an abnormal PSA value, whereas all 3 patients with normal PSA values had negative biopsies more than 23 months after radiation was completed. Stamey and associates[85] reported on 183 men treated with either external beam radiation or radioactive iodine seeds for stages B and C prostate cancer and found that serum PSA values were decreasing in 82% of them 1 year after therapy. Of 80 patients followed for more than 1 year after the completion of therapy, 51% were noted to have rising PSA values (Pros-check). All men who had serum PSA values obtained prior to progression to clinical D2 disease demonstrated a rising serum PSA level before the progression was clinically evident. These authors also noted that, whereas serum PSA values were above the reference interval for the assay in men with progression after radiotherapy, they were not nearly as high as those seen in patients with untreated stage D2 disease. Meek and coworkers[86] reported on a series of patients receiving external beam radiotherapy for prostate cancer who underwent serial measurement of serum PSA levels (Tandem R) during treatment. A half-life of 43 ± 11 days for PSA clearance was calculated from this study. The authors also suggested that a prolonged PSA half-life may represent untreated or radiation-resistant disease in patients receiving radiation therapy for prostate cancer. An early study by Dundas and colleagues[87] reported on a mixed group of patients receiving external beam radiation therapy alone or in combination with either brachytherapy or hormonal therapy. Nine of 110 patients developed local and/or distant recurrences, and all 9 failed to have the PSA level return to normal after therapy. In contrast, 74 of 101 of the remaining patients (73%) demonstrated a PSA value within the reference interval (Tandem R). The greatest decrease in mean PSA values was noted in those patients treated with the combination of external beam radiation and hormonal therapy.

Another series of patients with localized prostate cancer treated with external beam radiation therapy is that of Zagars and associates.[88] In this series of 133 patients, 98% demonstrated a significant decrease in PSA values by the third month of follow-up. Overall, 85% of patients had their PSA value return to within the normal range (Tandem R) and none had a PSA level greater than 10 ng/mL by the sixth month after radiation therapy. During radiation therapy, PSA levels were noted to rise transiently to about a 1.15-fold increase over baseline in their study. The mechanism for this increase is unknown.

Use of Serum Prostate-Specific Antigen Values in Patients Treated With Hormonal Therapy

Our experience at Washington University[34] with serum PSA values in patients with untreated stage D2 prostate cancer reflects the experience of most authors. A pretreatment PSA value of greater than 50 ng/mL (Tandem R) is seen frequently in patients with metatastic prostate cancer. A marked decline in serum PSA values to below 10 ng/mL usually is noted following the institution of hormonal therapy in those who achieve clinically inactive disease. The majority of those with clinically progressive disease demonstrate rising or fluctuating PSA levels despite hormonal therapy. Stamey and colleagues[89] found that the level of serum PSA (Proscheck) 6 months after instituting hormonal therapy could distinguish patients who could expect a prolonged clinical remission from those in whom disease would progress more rapidly. Miller and coworkers,[90] measuring serum PSA values after hormonal therapy, found a significantly longer remission in those with a nadir PSA value below 4 ng/mL (Tandem R) than in those whose nadir PSA value remained elevated (median, 42 vs. 10 months). Killian[91] also demonstrated that elevations in serum PSA levels may precede evidence of clinical recurrence by a maximum of 6 months — the higher the initial serum PSA value, the greater the likelihood of disease progression and the shorter the interval to progression. Kuriyama and associates[92] also reported that serum PSA levels were inversely proportional to survival time. Leo and associates[93] recently compared serum PSA values in patients with untreated stage D2 disease with those in patients with stage D3 disease (recurrence after prior hormonal therapy). Median serum PSA values were significantly lower in patients who had undergone prior hormonal manipulation.

Serum Prostate-Specific Antigen Values in Patients With Hormone-Refractory Prostate Cancer Treated With Chemotherapy

Because the measurement of serum PSA levels has proven useful in monitoring the response in previously untreated patients with prostate cancer, it also has been proposed that those levels be used as an objective measure of response to chemotherapy in patients with hormone-refractory prostate cancer. Gerber and Chodak[94] assessed serial PSA levels in 15 patients with hormone-refractory prostate cancer treated with ketoconazole and prednisone. They found that 12 men with continually rising PSA levels before chemotherapy had a decrease in PSA levels with a median duration of response of 3 months. Three patients had prolonged responses to therapy as determined by continually decreasing PSA values and subjective improvement in bone pain. Scher and coworkers[95] recently reported on 31 patients with bidimensionally measurable hormone-refractory prostatic cancer who received trimetrexate. Serial PSA levels varied widely in these patients. A 50% increase from the patients' minimum PSA values on two successive determinations correlated with progression in 90% of these cases. Seidman and associates[96] studied the combination of estramustine and vinblastine in patients with hormone-refractory prostate cancer. Of the 24 patients with an elevated PSA level at the start of therapy, 54% had a greater than 50% reduction in the measured PSA values after treatment, 2 of 5 patients (40%) with bidimensionally measurable disease showed partial responses, and 6 of 9 patients (66%) reported subjective improvement in pain. Although the early data suggest that serum PSA values may reflect disease status in the patient with hormone-refractory prostate cancer, it also is possible, as suggested by Seidman and associates,[96] that PSA production or secretion may be decreased by chemotherapeutic agents without an effect on cell proliferation. Moreover, serum PSA levels did not reflect disease activity uniformly, and they must be used cautiously as an index of drug efficacy in clinical trials.

In conclusion, serum PSA values have proven useful to the clinician in several diagnostic and therapeutic situations. PSA has proven to be extremely specific to prostatic disease. When used in conjunction with other tests, serum PSA levels are helpful in the early detection of prostate cancer. Serum PSA values also appear to have a role in helping to distinguish between organ-confined prostate cancer and advanced disease. Serial PSA values can be used to help predict long-term response to therapy, to determine the need for additional testing (as with bone scans), and to determine the need for further adjuvant therapy.

References

1. Wang MC, Valenzuela LA, Murphy GP, et al: Purification of a human prostate specific antigen. Invest Urol 1979; 17:159.
2. Hara M, Norre T, Fukuyama T: Some physiochemical characteristics of gamma-seminoprotein, an antigenic component for human seminal plasma. Jpn J Legal Med 1971; 25:322.
3. Li TS, Beling CG: Isolation and characterization of two specific antigens of human seminal plasma. Fertil Steril 1973; 24:134.
4. Sensabaugh GF: Isolation and characterization of a semen-specific protein from human seminal plasma: A potential new marker for semen identification. J Forensic Sci 1978; 23:106.
5. Deguchi T, Kuriyama M, Shinoda I, et al: Immunological comparison between prostate specific antigen and gamma-seminoprotein. Urol Res 1991; 19:25.
6. Graves HC, Kamarei M, Stamey TA: Identity of a prostate specific antigen and the semen protein p30 purified by a rapid chromatography technique. J Urol 1990; 144:1510.
7. Papsidero LD, Wang MD, Valenzuela LA, et al: A prostate antigen in the sera of prostatic cancer patients. Cancer Res 1980; 40:24.
8. Wang MC, Kuriyama M, Papsidero LD, et al: Prostate antigen of human cancer patients, in Busch H, Yeoman LC (eds): Methods in Cancer Research XIX. New York, Academic Press, 1982, pp 179–197.
9. Bilhartz DL, Tindall DJ, Oesterling JE: Prostate-specific antigen and prostatic acid phosphatase: Bimolecular and physiologic characteristics. Urology 1991; 38:95.
10. Young CM, Montgomery BT, Andrews PE, et al: Hormonal regulation of prostate specific antigen messenger RNA in human prostatic adenocarcinoma cell line LN CaP. Cancer Res 1991; 51:3748.
11. Levine AC, Kirschenbaum A, Droller M, et al: Effect of the addition of estrogen to medical castration on prostatic size, symptoms, histology, and serum prostate specific antigen in 4 men with benign prostatic hypertrophy. J Urol 1991; 146:790.
12. Henttu P, Lukkarinen O, Vihko P: Expression of the gene coding for human prostate-specific antigen and related HGK-1 in benign and malignant tumor of the human prostate. Int J Cancer 1990; 45:654.
13. Killian CS, Chu TM: Prostate-specific antigen: Questions frequently asked. Cancer Invest 1990; 8:27.
14. Christenssen A, Laurell CB, Lilja H: Enzymatic activity of prostate-specific antigen and its reactions with extracellular serine proteinase inhibitors. Eur J Biochem 1990; 194:755.
15. Stenman UH, Leinonen J, Alfthan H, et al: A complex between prostate specific antigen in serum of patients with prostatic cancer: Assay of the complex improves clinical sensitivity for cancer. Cancer Res 1991; 51:222.
16. Papsidero LD, Kuriyama M, Wang MC, et al: Prostate antigen: A marker for human prostate epithelial cells. J Natl Cancer Inst 1981; 66:37.
17. Nadji M, Tabei SZ, Castro A, et al: Prostate-specific antigen: An immunohistochemical marker for prostatic neoplasms. Cancer 1981; 48:1229.
18. Kuriyama M, Wang MC, Papsidero LD, et al: Quantification of prostate-specific antigen in serum by a sensitive enzyme immunoassay. Cancer Res 1980; 40:4658.
19. Bruce, Chloe: Tumor markers in prostatic disease, in Bruce AW, Trachtenberg

J (eds): *Adenocarcinoma of the Prostate.* New York, Springer-Verlag, 1987, pp 196–219.

20. Qui SD, Young CY, Bilhartz DL, et al: In situ hybridization of prostate-specific antigen mRNA in human prostate. *J Urol* 1990; 144:1550.

21. Ersev A, Ersev D, Turkeri L, et al: The relation of prostatic acid phosphatase and prostate-specific antigen with tumor grade in prostatic adenocarcinoma: An immunohistochemical study. *Prog Clin Biol Res* 1990; 357:129.

22. Gallee MP, Visser-de-Jong JE, van der Korput JA, et al: Variation of prostate-specific antigen expression in different tumor growth patterns present in prostatectomy specimens. *Urol Res* 1990; 18:181.

23. Stege R, Lundh B, Tribukait B, et al: Deoxyribonucleic acid ploidy and the direct assay of prostatic acid phosphatase and prostate-specific antigen in fine needle aspiration biopsies as diagnostic methods in prostatic carcinoma. *J Urol* 1990; 144:299.

24. Stowell LI, Sharman LE, Hamel K: An enzyme-linked immunosorbent assay (ELISA) for prostate-specific antigen. *Forensic Sci Int* 1991; 50:125.

25. Stamey TA, Yang N, Hay AR, et al: Prostate-specific antigen as a serum marker for adenocarcinoma of the prostate. *N Engl J Med* 1987; 317:909.

26. Yuan JJJ, Coplen DE, Petros JA, et al: Effects of digital rectal examination, prostate massage, ultrasonography and needle biopsy on serum prostate specific antigen levels. *J Urol* 1992; 147:810.

27. Brawn PN, Speights VO, Kuhl D, et al: Prostate-specific antigen levels from completely sectioned clinically benign whole prostate. *Cancer* 1991; 68:1592.

28. Hughes HR, Penney MD, Ryan PG, et al: Serum prostatic-specific antigen: In vitro stability and the effect of ultrasound rectal examination in vivo. *Ann Clin Biochem* 1987; 24(suppl):206.

29. Brawer MK, Schifman RB, Ahmann FR, et al: The effect of digital rectal examination on serum levels of prostate specific antigen. *Arch Pathol Lab Med* 1988; 112:1110.

30. el-Shirbiny AM, Nilson T, Pawar HN: Serum prostate-specific antigen: Hourly change/24 hours compared with prostatic acid phosphatase. *Urology* 1990; 35:88.

31. Oesterling JE, Chan DW, Epstein JI, et al: Prostate-specific antigen in the preoperative and postoperative evaluation of localized prostate cancer treated with radical prostatectomy. *J Urol* 1988; 139:766.

32. Hortin GL, Bahnson RR, Daft M, et al: Differences in values obtained with 2 assays of prostate-specific antigen. *J Urol* 1988; 139:762.

33. Vaidya HC, Wolf BA, Garrett N, et al: Extremely high values of prostate-specific antigen in patients with adenocarcinoma of the prostate; demonstration of the "hook effect." *Clin Chem* 1988; 34:2175.

34. Hudson MA, Bahnson RR, Catalona WJ: Clinical use of prostate-specific antigen in patients with prostate cancer. *J Urol* 1989; 142:1011.

35. Turkes A, Nott JP, Griffiths K: Prostate specific antigen: Problems in analysis. *Eur J Cancer* 1991; 27:650.

36. Dnistrian AM, Schwartz MK, Smith CA, et al: Evaluation of the Abbott IMx assay for prostate specific antigen in serum. Presented at the Annual Meeting of the American Urologic Association, Washington, DC, May 1992.

37. Stamey TA, Wehner N, Graves HCB, et al: Usefulness of a new ultrasensitive assay in follow-up of patients after radical prostatectomy. Presented at the Annual Meeting of the American Urological Association, Washington, DC, May 1992.

38. Villers A, Boccon-Gilbod L, Meaulemens A, et al: Hypersensitive PSA test for

detection of PSA below 0.1 ng/ml: Results of serum and urine PSA in prostatectomy and cystoprostatectomy patients. Presented at the Annual Meeting of the American Urological Association, Washington, DC, May 1992.

39. Myrtle JF, Klimey PG, Ivor LP, et al: Clinical utility of prostate specific antigen (PSA) in the management of prostate cancer, in *Adv Cancer Diagnostics.* Hybritech, 1986, p 1.

40. Ercole CJ, Lange PH, Mathisen M, et al: Prostatic-specific antigen and prostatic acid phosphatase in the monitoring and staging of patients with prostatic cancer. *J Urol* 1987; 138:1181.

41. Partin AW, Carter HB, Chan DW, et al: Prostate-specific antigen in the staging of localized prostate cancer: Influence of tumor differentiation, tumor volume and benign hyperplasia. *J Urol* 1990; 143:747.

42. Lindstedt G, Jacobsson A, Lundberg PA, et al: Determination of prostate-specific antigen in serum by immunoradiometric assay. *Clin Chem* 1990; 36:53.

43. Cooner WH, Mosley BR, Rutherford CL Jr, et al: Clinical application of transrectal ultrasonography and prostate specific antigen in search for prostate cancer. *J Urol* 1988; 139:758.

44. Yang N: PSA values in BPH and stage A1 prostate cancer, in Catalona WJ, Coffey DS, Karr JP (eds): *Clinical Aspects of Prostate Cancer.* New York, Elsevier, 1989, pp 197–200.

45. Brawer MK: Prostate specific antigen: A review. *Acta Oncol* 1991; 30:161.

46. McNeal J: Pathology of benign prostatic hyperplasia. *Urol Clin North Am* 1990; 17:477.

47. Weber JP, Oesterling JE, Peters CA, et al: The influence of reversible androgen deprivation on serum prostate-specific antigen levels in men with benign prostatic hyperplasia. *J Urol* 1989; 141:987.

48. Littrup PJ, Kane RA, Williams CR, et al: Determination of prostate volume with transrectal US for cancer screening. Part. Comparison with prostate specific antigen assays. *Radiology* 1991; 178:537.

49. Babaian RJ, Fritsche HA, Evans RB: Prostate specific antigen and prostate gland volume: Correlation and clinical application. *J Clin Lab Anal* 1990; 4:135.

50. Veneziano S, Pavlica P, Querze R, et al: Correlation between prostate-specific antigen and prostate volume evaluated by transrectal ultrasonography: Usefulness in diagnosis of prostate cancer. *Eur Urol* 1990; 18:112.

51. Benson MC, Whang S, Pantuck A, et al: Prostate-specific antigen density: A means of distinguishing BPH and prostate cancer. *J Urol* 1992; 147:815.

52. Andriole GL, Coplen DE, Catalona WJ: PSA "density": Does it enhance detection of prostate cancer in men with symptoms of BPH and/or digital rectal exam (DRE) findings of prostatic enlargement? Presented at the annual meeting of the American Urologic Association, Toronto, Canada, June 1991.

53. Vesey SG, Goble M, Ferro MA, et al: Quantification of prostatic cancer metastatic disease using prostate-specific antigen. *Urology* 1990; 35:483.

54. Kuriyama M, Loor R, Wang MC, et al: Prostatic acid phosphatase and prostate-specific antigen in prostate cancer. *Int Adv Surg Oncol* 1982; 5:29.

55. Bhatti PG, Ray P, Guinan P: An evaluation of prostate-specific antigen in prostatic cancer. *J Urol* 1987; 137:686.

56. Oesterling JE: Prostate-specific antigen: A critical assessment of the most useful tumor marker for adenocarcinoma of the prostate. *J Urol* 1991; 145:907.

57. Catalona WJ, Smith DS, Ratliff TL, et al: Measurement of prostate-specific an-

tigen in serum as a screening tool for prostate cancer. *N Engl J Med* 1991; 324:1156.

58. Brawer MK, Chetner MP, Beatie J, et al: Prostate-specific antigen and early detection of prostatic carcinoma. Presented at the annual meeting of the American Urological Association, Toronto, Canada, June 1991.

59. Carter HB, Andres R, Metter J, et al: Longitudinal evaluation of prostate-specific antigen levels in men with and without prostate disease. *JAMA* 1992; 267:2215-2220.

60. Cooner WH, Mosley BR, Rutherford CL Jr, et al: Prostate cancer detection in a clinical urological practice by ultrasonography, digital rectal examination and prostate-specific antigen. *J Urol* 1990; 143:1146.

61. Lee F, Littrup PJ, Torp-Pedersen ST, et al: Prostate cancer: Comparison of transrectal US and digital rectal examination for screening. *Radiology* 1988; 168:389.

62. Stone NN, Lazan D, Clejan S, et al: Comparison of digital rectal exam (DRE) and prostate-specific antigen (PSA) biopsy results from Prostate Cancer Awareness Week 1989. Presented at the annual meeting of the American Urological Association, Toronto, Canada, June 1991.

63. Babaian RJ, Camps JL: The role of prostate-specific anitgen as part of the diagnostic triad and as a guide when to perform a biopsy. *Cancer* 1991; 68:2060.

64. Mettlin C, Lee F, and the investigators of the American Cancer Society National Prostate Cancer Detection Project: The American Cancer Society National Prostate Cancer Detection Project: Findings on the detection of early prostate cancer in 2425 men. *Cancer* 1991; 67:2940.

65. Lee F, McHugh TA, Solomon MH, et al: Transrectal ultrasound, digital rectal examination, and prostate-specific antigen: Preliminary results of an early detection program for prostate cancer. *Scand J Urol Nephrol Suppl* 1991; 137:101.

66. Stamey TA, Kabalin JN: Prostate-specific antigen in the diagnosis and treatment of adenocarcinoma of the prostate I. Untreated patients. *J Urol* 1989; 141:1070.

67. Chan DW, Bruzek DJ, Oesterling JE, et al: Prostate-specific antigen as a marker for prostatic cancer: A monoclonal and polyclonal immunoassay compared. *Clin Chem* 1987; 33:1916.

68. Catalona WJ, Ratliff TL, Yuan JJJ: Serum prostate-specific antigen as a first-line screening test for prostate cancer (abstract). *J Urol* 1990; 143:313A.

69. Babaian RJ, Camps JL, Frangos DN, et al: Monoclonal prostate-specific antigen in untreated prostate cancer. Relationship to clinical stage and grade. *Cancer* 1991; 67:2200.

70. Badalament RA, O'Toole RV, Young DC: DNA ploidy and prostate-specific antigen as prognostic factors in clinically resectable prostate cancer. *Cancer* 1991; 67:3014.

71. Winter HI, Bretton PR, Herr HW: Preoperative prostate-specific antigen in predicting pathologic stage and grade after radical prostatectomy. *Urology* 1991; 38:202.

72. Lange PH: Prostate-specific antigen for staging prior to surgery and for early detection of recurrence after surgery. *Urol Clin North Am* 1990; 17:813.

73. Chybowski FM, Larson-Keller JJ, Bergstrahl EJ, et al: Predicting radionuclide bone scan findings in patients with newly diagnosed untreated prostate cancer:

Prostate-specific antigen is superior to all other clinical parameters. *J Urol* 1991; 145:313.

74. Terris MK, Klonecke AS, McDougall IR, et al: Utilization of bone scans in conjunction with prostate-specific antigen levels in the surveillance for recurrence of adenocarcinoma after radical prostatectomy. *J Nucl Med* 1991; 32:1713.

75. Freitas JE, Gilvydas R, Fetty JD, et al: The clinical utility of prostate-specific antigen and bone scintigraphy in prostate cancer follow-up. *J Nucl Med* 1991; 32:1387.

76. Andriole GL, Catalona WJ, Becich M: Letter to editor. *J Urol* 1992; 147:474.

77. Lange PH, Ercole CJ, Lightner DJ, et al: The value of serum prostate-specific antigen determination before and after radical prostatectomy. *J Urol* 1989; 141:873.

78. Stein A, de Kernion JB, Smith RB, et al: Prostate-specific antigen levels after radical prostatectomy in patients with organ-confined and locally extensive prostate cancer. *J Urol* 1992; 147:942.

79. Killian CS, Yang N, Emich LJ, et al: Prognostic importance of prostate specific antigen for monitoring patients with stages B2 to D1 prostate cancer. *Cancer Res* 1985; 45:886.

80. Lightner DJ, Lange PH, Reddy PK, et al: Prostate-specific antigen and local recurrence after radical prostatectomy. *J Urol* 1990; 144:921.

81. Hudson MA, Catalona WJ: Effect of adjuvant radiation therapy on prostate-specific antigen following radical prostatectomy. *J Urol* 1990 143:1174.

82. Lightner DJ, Reddy PK, Lange PH: PSA response to radiation therapy (RT) after radical prostatectomy (RP). *J Urol* 1989; 141:183A.

83. Morgan WR, Zincke H, Rainwater LM, et al: Prostate-specific antigen values after radical prostatectomy for adenocarcinoma of the prostate: Impact of adjuvant treatment (hormonal and radiation). *J Urol* 1991; 145:319.

84. Chodak GW, Neumann J, Blix Sutton H, et al: Effect of external beam radiation therapy on serum prostate-specific antigen. *Urology* 1990; 35:288.

85. Stamey TA, Kabalin JN, Ferrari M: Prostate-specific antigen in the diagnosis and treatment of adenocarcinoma of the prostate III. Radiation treated patients. *J Urol* 1989; 141:1084.

86. Meek AG, Park TL, Oberman E, et al: A prospective study of prostate-specific antigen levels in patients receiving radiotherapy for localized carcinoma of the prostate. *Int J Radiat Oncol Biol Phys* 1990; 19:733.

87. Dundas GS, Porter AT, Venner PM: Prostate-specific antigen: Monitoring the response of carcinoma of the prostate to radiotherapy with a new tumor marker. *Cancer* 1991; 66:45.

88. Zagars GK, Sherman NE, Babaian RJ: Prostate-specific antigen and external beam radiation therapy in prostate cancer. *Cancer* 1991; 67:412.

89. Stamey TA, Kabalin JN, Ferrari M, et al: Prostate-specific antigen in the diagnosis and treatment of adenocarcinoma of the prostate IV. Anti-androgen treated patients. *J Urol* 1989; 141:1088.

90. Miller JI, Ahmann FR, Drach GW, et al: The clinical usefulness of serum prostate specific antigen after hormonal therapy of metastatic prostate cancer. *J Urol* 1992; 147:956.

91. Killian CS, Yang N, Emich LJ, et al: Relative reliability of five serially measured markers for prognosis of progression in prostate cancer. *J Natl Cancer Inst* 1986; 76:176.

92. Kuriyama M, Wang ME, Lee CL, et al: Use of human prostate-specific antigen in monitoring prostate cancer. *Cancer Res* 1981; 41:3874.

93. Leo ME, Bilhartz DL, Bergstrahl EJ, et al: Prostate-specific antigen in hormonally-treated stage D2 prostate cancer: Is it always an accurate indicator of disease status? *J Urol* 1991; 145:802.
94. Gerber GS, Chodak GW: Prostate-specific antigen for assessing response to ketoconazole and prednisone in patients with hormone refractory metastatic prostate cancer. *J Urol* 1990; 144:1177.
95. Scher H, Curley T, Geller N, et al: Trimetrexate in prostatic cancer. Preliminary observations in the use of prostate-specific antigen and acid phosphatase as a marker in measurable hormone-refractory disease. *J Clin Oncol* 1990; 8:1830.
96. Seidman AD, Scher HI, Petrylak D, et al: Estramustine and vinblastine: Use of prostate-specific antigen as a clinical trial endpoint for hormone refractory prostatic cancer. *J Urol* 1992; 147:931.

Expectant Management of Carcinoma of the Prostate*

Ian M. Thompson, M.D.

Chief, Urology Service, Brooke Army Medical Center, San Antonio, Texas

Samuel J. Peretsman, M.D.

Vice-Chairman, Department of Urology, Wilford Hall United States Air Force
Medical Center, San Antonio, Texas

Carcinoma of the prostate is the most common tumor in U.S. men, surpassing lung cancer in the number of cases in 1989.[1] It is estimated by the American Cancer Society that in 1992 there will be 132,000 new cases and 34,000 deaths from prostate cancer.[2] In 1985, Seidman and colleagues estimated that white and black males born in 1985 had 8.7% and 9.4% risks, respectively, of developing prostate cancer, and that these same two groups had 2.6% and 4.3% risks, respectively, of dying of the disease.[3] Although data from the early 1980s suggested that the age-specific mortality curve was flat, more recent evidence finds the age-specific mortality rate to be increasing.[4] The United States is on the threshold of a demographic period in which a large number of men will be at an age associated with a high risk for having prostate cancer. The life expectancy of the U.S. population has increased from 66.6 years in 1960 to 72.1 years in 1990.[5] This has resulted in an estimated 31.6 million men over the age of 65 years in 1990. This number will increase to 34.9 million in the year 2000 and to 39.4 million in 2010.[5] With the dramatic age-dependent prevalence of prostate cancer, we can anticipate a similarly dramatic increase in the number of cases diagnosed and a corresponding increase in the prostate cancer death rate, assuming that no major change occurs in either diagnostic or therapeutic efforts.

With this bleak assessment of the current impact of prostate cancer, and anticipating a worsening of the situation, it seems almost antithetical to the practice of medicine to discuss the option of expectant management of this disease. The purpose of this chapter is to present aspects of the enigma that is prostate cancer and reasons why expectant management may be a reasonable option for some patients. Prognostic factors for individual pa-

---

*The opinions contained herein are those of the authors and do not necessarily reflect those of the Departments of the Air Force, Army, or Defense.

Advances in Urology®, vol 6
© 1993, Mosby–Year Book, Inc.

tients are discussed in an attempt to provide practical guidance for the implementation of an expectant management strategy.

The Basis of Expectant Management of Prostate Cancer

The Whitmore Concept

Dr. Willet Whitmore has defined best the crucial issue in the treatment of prostate cancer: for treatment of this disease to be justified, cure of the disease must be both *necessary* and *possible*.[6] Although this statement seems to be self-evident, as it provides the foundation for the subsequent discussion, it is worth proving. The "necessary" concept is based upon the natural history of the disease. If prostate cancer proved to cause morbidity or lead to death rarely if ever (i.e., a so-called "toothless lion"), treatment would be unnecessary. On the other hand, if prostate cancer progressed inexorably to metastatic disease and death regardless of attempts to arrest its growth, cure could be regarded as impossible. It is only for patients in whom treatment for cure is both necessary and possible that such efforts are appropriate.

Contention One: Treatment for a Significant Number of Patients With Prostate Cancer Is Unnecessary

There are patients with prostate cancer in whom the treatment for cure is not necessary. Figure 1 demonstrates this concept in an idealized fashion. The figure presumes a relationship among tumor volume, biologic behavior, tumor stage, and time. The concept has been supported by the work of McNeal.[7] In general, as the volume of a tumor increases, so does its propensity to spread and metastasize. As tumor volume continues to increase, a level is reached at which death of the host occurs. The appearance of symptoms occurs variably (rarely before extraprostatic disease has developed), but can occur at almost any time from the development of a small tumor volume to the occurrence of distant metastases.[8] A threshold for tumor detection has been placed arbitrarily at the point at which a tumor nodule is present. On the x-axis are arrows corresponding to repetitive examinations over time to detect prostate cancer.

Figure 1 displays the clinical course of two patients who develop prostate cancer. Patient A develops a prostatic tumor at a comparatively early age, but, due to the relatively slow tumor growth rate, it never reaches a detectable size. The patient dies at an older age of other causes. Patient B develops a prostate tumor at a slightly older age, but this tumor, having a more aggressive biologic behavior, is clinically evident at a later age. Without treatment, the patient develops symptoms (e.g., bladder outlet obstructive symptoms) during the last year of his life and dies of other causes shortly thereafter.

These two theoretical patients both had prostate cancer. In neither was the cancer treated, and neither developed serious consequences from its

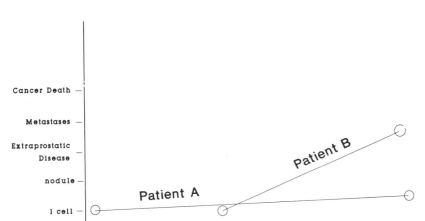

FIG 1.
Natural history of prostate cancer in two hypothetical patients. *Arrows* on the x-axis represent repeated examinations to detect prostate cancer, which can be detected only at the "nodule" stage. The y-axis represents increasing volume of disease, with increased risk of metastases and death associated with increasing volume. Both patients A and B expire of causes other than prostate cancer.

presence. In both patients, treatment for prostate cancer was unnecessary. Let us now examine the evidence demonstrating that, for a number of men with prostate cancer, treatment is unnecessary.

Most Men With Prostate Cancer Do Not Develop Clinical Disease.—Perhaps the most confounding aspect of the natural history of prostate cancer is that many men in the second half of their lives have the disease, but never become aware of it. Rich and Moore each reported in 1935 on the incidence of prostate cancer in consecutive autopsy series. In Rich's series, only a single section was obtained through the prostate;[9] nevertheless, a considerable incidence of prostate cancer was detected, ranging from 5.6% at 50 to 55 years of age and 11.4% at 56 to 60 years of age to 37.5% at 76 to 80 years of age. Overall, 14% of all autopsied men were found to have prostate cancer. Examining more sections from the prostate, yet still able to detect only lesions larger than 4 mm, Moore noted 52 incidental cases of prostate cancer in 364 autopsies (14%).[10] As many as 29% of the prostates (in the men aged 81 to 90 years) were found to have unsuspected prostate cancer. Reporting in 1954, Hudson and associates attempted to determine the incidence of prostate cancer in unselected patients.[11] Performing open perineal biopsies in 300 men whose average age was 62 years, and obtaining a 1-cm specimen for analysis, 39 cases (13%) of unsuspected disease were detected.

Recognizing that many prostate tumors were small enough to be missed by obtaining single sections or seeking only large tumors, Scott and coworkers examined the results of autopsy evaluations of the prostate using step sectioning of the gland.[12] The authors found that the detection rate almost doubled with this technique, with 36% of men aged 70 to 80 years and 44% of those aged over 80 years having unsuspected prostate cancer.

These and two additional series[13, 14] can be combined to approximate the rate of histologically evident prostate cancer in the U.S. population. The average as well as the high and low estimates by age are shown in Figure 2. As can be seen, a significant proportion of men have prostate cancer. Using data from 1988, when 28,000 deaths due to prostate cancer occurred, a total of 1,125,540 deaths were recorded in men.[15, 16] Fewer than 2.5% of deaths in U.S. men are due to prostate cancer, yet more than 30% of all men over 50 years of age have histologic evidence of the disease; therefore, only about 1 man in 12 with histologic evidence of prostate cancer will die of his disease. Returning to our premise, in only 1 man in 12 with prostate cancer is cure necessary to prevent death from the disease.

Many Men With Clinical Prostate Cancer Do Not Experience Morbidity or Mortality From the Disease.—At a time (1940) when prostate cancer was thought to be a condition rarely leading to patient morbidity, Young suggested that frequent digital rectal examination (DRE) may allow for early diagnosis and more frequent cure of the disease, thereby preventing its ravages.[17] Authors in the early half of the 20th century lent credence to the suggestion that prostate cancer could be a virulent disease. The first such report was presented by Bumpus in 1926.[18] Among 485 patients who were treated for prostate cancer, he reported 2-

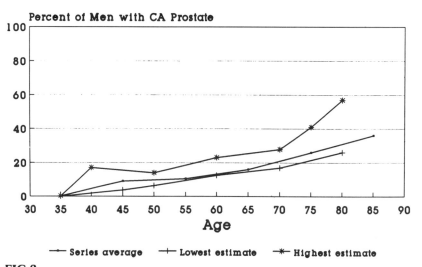

FIG 2.
Incidence of prostate cancer autopsy data. Prevalence of prostate cancer *(CA)* in the U.S. population. Based upon six series using autopsy or arbitrary perineal biopsy.[9–14]

and 5-year survival rates of 30% and 12%, respectively. Nesbit and Plumb, reporting on the experience of 477 patients without metastases at diagnosis at the University of Michigan in Ann Arbor, found that the mean survival from diagnosis was only 23.6 months.[19] Half of the patients were dead within 12.8 months. Hanash in 1972 also reported on patients from the preendocrine era.[20] He found 5-, 10- and 15-year survival rates of 60 patients with stage B disease to be 19%, 4%, and 1%, respectively, dramatically lower than the expected survival rates of 71%, 45%, and 25%.

These earliest series confirmed the notion that prostate cancer was indeed a malignant disease resulting in the death of up to half of all patients within 3 to 5 years of diagnosis. This concept, however, meshes poorly with our increasing awareness of the significant pool of men who have disease that never becomes clinically apparent. Such divergent concepts led to a series of reports over the past 2 decades of the experience with untreated, localized prostate cancer—the so-called "natural history" studies.

Cook and Watson surveyed the experience at the Ellis Fischel Cancer Center in Columbia, Missouri and found 20 patients with localized nodules of cancer who were not treated for cure.[21] Five patients died of prostate cancer within 10 years of diagnosis, but 1 remained alive and 14 had died of other causes, and the 10-year cancer-specific survival rate was 53%. Barnes and colleagues similarly reviewed 115 patients with clinical stage B prostate cancer who received only treatment for symptoms (i.e., transurethral resection of the prostate) or hormonal therapy.[22] Survival rates at 5, 10, and 15 years for this group were 71%, 58%, and 28%—remarkably better than those reported in series from 30 years earlier.

Moskovitz and associates presented an experience with 101 patients with T0b, T1-3N0m0 prostate cancer who were followed for a mean of 58 months.[23] The only treatment rendered in these patients was nonradical prostatectomy (transurethral prostatic resection or simple retropubic prostatectomy) for obstructive symptoms. Although 29 patients (28.7%) died of prostate cancer, another 22.8% died of other causes, and 48.5% were alive at the time of the report. A larger, randomized experience was reported by Madsen and coworkers.[24] These authors provided 15-year follow-up on the Veterans Administration Cooperative Urologic Research Group (VACURG) studies of the 1960s and 1970s. Fifty patients with stage B prostate cancer were randomized to receive either placebo or placebo plus radical prostatectomy. Staging of these patients was accomplished primarily with DRE and determination of serum acid phosphatase levels. Bone scans were not required. Despite seemingly disparate treatment programs, no survival difference was detected between the treatment groups. (Indeed, an average 12% advantage in survival was found for placebo over that provided by radical prostatectomy.)

Although widely recognized as acceptable treatment in the United Kingdom,[25, 26] the principal report of conservative treatment for prostate cancer in Britain was published by George in 1988.[27] Of 120 evaluable patients in whom bone scans were normal during a 7-year study period, 13 (11%) developed metastases and 5 (4%) died of prostate cancer. This compares to 48 patients (40%) who died of unrelated causes (other malignancies or cardiovascular disease).

Between 1989 and 1991, two series of untreated patients with prostate cancer were reported from Scandinavia. Johansson and associates, in a population-based study, described 223 patients with T0I (stage A1) to T4NXM0 tumors staged with DRE and bone scanning who received no definitive treatment for cure.[28] Eighty-three patients died during follow-up, 16 of prostate cancer and 67 of other causes. The 5-year survival rate for all patients was 68.6% and, using the expected survival of an age-matched male Swedish population, the authors calculated that the 5-year corrected survival rate of these untreated patients was 93.8% (95% confidence interval = 90% to 97.6%).

The second Swedish series from Stockholm included 61 patients with prostate cancer, all of whom were under 70 years of age and received no treatment for cure.[29] The median patient age was 63 years and the mean follow-up period was 96 months. Local progression (to T3 disease) was detected in 69% of patients and extraprostatic tumor extension occurred in 61%. By 10 years, the risk of local disease progression was 72%. Metastatic disease developed in 9 patients (15%), all but 1 of whom had T2 tumors at diagnosis. Eight patient deaths occurred during follow-up, 4 caused by prostate cancer and 4 by other causes. At 5 and 10 years, the probability of dying of prostate cancer was 2% and 8%, respectively.

The series with perhaps the longest follow-up of the natural history of prostate cancer is from Memorial Sloan-Kettering Cancer Center (New York). Whitmore and colleagues collected 75 patients with clinical stage B1, B2, or B3 tumors (T1 to T3) diagnosed between 1949 and 1986 who received no treatment at the time of diagnosis for cure of their disease.[30] Mean follow-up periods for B1, B2, and B3 tumors were 133, 130, and 108 months, respectively. As expected, progression occurred in a high proportion of patients. The median time to progression for patients with B1, B2, and B3 tumors was 63, 78, and 175 months, respectively. In almost all patients, local progression preceded the development of distant metastatic disease. The median time to the development of distant metastases was 138 months in patients with B2 disease, but with follow-up periods as reported previously, the median time to metastasis for B1 and B3 tumors had not been reached yet. Only 11 of the 75 patients with follow-up in excess of 10 years died of prostate cancer.

These recent series describing the natural history of prostate cancer suggest several characteristic behaviors. First, with close attention to the DRE and with sufficient follow-up, virtually all tumors will progress, and such progression almost always occurs before the development of distant metastases. The median time to progression is between 5 and 7 years. Less likely is the risk of the development of metastatic disease, and even more rare is the risk of death due to prostate cancer, as many patients in these series died of other causes. It is possible to combine the results of these series to attempt to quantify the behavior of prostate cancer. Although admittedly biased and inexact, Figure 3 combines these series, weighted for

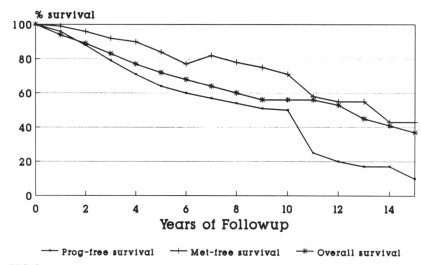

% survival

Years of Followup

—●— Prog-free survival   —+— Met-free survival   —*— Overall survival

FIG 3.
Summary of series of survival criteria comparisons. Experience with untreated prostate cancer.[21-24, 27-30] *Prog* = progression; *met* = metastasis.

the number of patients in each one. It is readily apparent that the contention of this section is well supported: *many (if not the majority) of men with clinical prostate cancer will not experience morbidity or mortality from the disease.*

Summary.—Referring back to Figure 1, the scenario of patient A represents a significant proportion of men with histologic prostate cancer, as evidenced by the six autopsy series cited. These men not only do not develop morbidity from the disease, but they live without any knowledge of its presence. Patient B also seems to be represented frequently, as demonstrated by the number of patients in the series of those with untreated prostate cancer in whom morbidity and mortality did not occur. Certainly, for all of these patients with prostate cancer, treatment for cure is not necessary.

Contention Two: Treatment for Cure for a Significant Number of Patients With Prostate Cancer Is Not Possible

The basis for the concept that treatment for cure is not always possible in prostate cancer is that there exists a population of patients with biologically aggressive tumors that progress to extraprostatic and metastatic disease so quickly that, with the standard frequency of tests for prostate cancer detection (e.g., annually), by the time the tumor is detected, cure is no longer possible. Using the same type of graph as used in our first contention, Figure 4 demonstrates two examples of this concept. Patient A has a tumor with such a rapid growth rate that it progresses from a microscopic focus to metastatic disease between screening evaluations. Patient B, a more theoretical case, has a longer microscopic interval, but proceeds rapidly from a

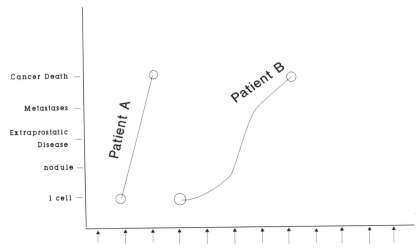

FIG 4.
Natural history of two patients in whom prostate cancer cannot be cured despite repetitive examinations for the disease. In both patients, growth rate of the disease is so rapid between the detectable stage and a stage at which metastatic disease occurs, that detection is missed despite frequent examinations.

detectable size to metastatic disease before the periodic examination is performed. For both of these patients, the interval between examinations may be too infrequent or the examination itself not sensitive enough to detect the tumor within the window of curability.

Although the curves in Figure 4 are theoretical, there is some evidence to corroborate these concepts. Chodak and Thompson combined the results of two long-term experiences with serial screening for prostate cancer using DRE.[31] The proportion with clinically localized disease was similar in patients with disease diagnosed through the first DRE and those with a history of normal prior annual DREs in whom a subsequent DRE was abnormal and prostate cancer was detected. Overall, 62% of all patients had tumors diagnosed at a clinically localized stage (stage B). Although overall survival was similar in patients with prostate cancer diagnosed on initial and subsequent examinations, the 5-year disease-specific mortality rates of these two groups were 97% and 81%, respectively—a dramatic difference.

One would expect a patient who had a normal DRE 1 year prior to the diagnosis of prostate cancer to do better than one who never previously had undergone DRE, but Chodak and Thompson's data suggest the reverse to be true. The explanation can be found in the concept of length-time bias. This supports the concept shown in Figure 4. Figure 5 has combined two theoretical patients from Figures 1 and 4. As can be seen readily, the repeat screening examinations are more likely to detect patient A, who has a tumor with a slow growth rate that will never pose a threat to

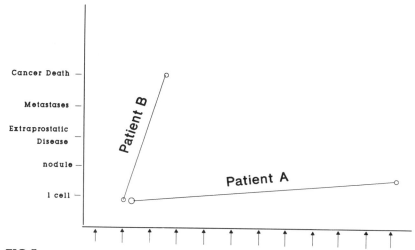

FIG 5.
Two hypothetical patients in whom treatment for cure either is not necessary or is not possible. In patient A, cure is not necessary. In patient B, detection occurs after metastatic disease has occurred and, therefore, cure is not possible.

his survival. On the other hand, patient B, who will die of his disease, has a tumor with such a rapid growth rate that, despite frequent screening examinations, it cannot be detected in time to be curable. Thus, the bias occurs. Repetitive screening tests have a bias toward the detection and cure of patients with indolent, slow-growing tumors and may not detect those whose tumors pose the most serious threat to survival.

A second area of support for the contention that cure is not possible in a proportion of patients with newly diagnosed prostate cancer derives from known problems with our tests for tumor detection. If these tests cannot detect the disease early enough to guarantee cure, then detection and treatment may be of no avail. The two most commonly employed tests are DRE and prostate-specific antigen (PSA). The former has some serious drawbacks. We and others have found that a significant number of patients with cancer diagnosed through DRE alone who are thought to have localized disease based on clinical staging are found to have extraprostatic disease on surgical staging.[32] In a unique study of 96 men who died of prostate cancer, we found that 25% had a normal DRE at the time of diagnosis.[33] Thus, reliance on DRE alone could not have prevented 25% of the cancer deaths within this group of men from a population-based study.

It is unfortunate that a similar experience has been noted with PSA. Catalona's series from 1991 is illustrative.[34] Of 1,653 men screened for prostate cancer, half of all those with cancer who had an elevated PSA had a serum level of 4.0 to 9.9 ng/mL, and half had a value greater than 10.0 ng/mL. Of these two groups, 41% and 87%, respectively, had extraprostatic disease when surgically staged. The prognostic importance of surgical staging has been emphasized by many authors, all of whom have demonstrated a significant increase in disease-specific mortality due to the high risk of local and distant metastases.[35]

Thus, even though we are able to detect prostate cancer in a large number of men, we frequently are unable to do so before the disease has spread beyond the confines of the prostate and is beyond our ability to cure. Both this concept and the concept of length-time bias inherent to detection efforts support the contention that cure may not be possible in a significant number of patients with prostate cancer and, thus, expectant management may not be an unreasonable option.

Contention Three: There May be Drawbacks to the Treatment of Patients in Whom Treatment Is Both Necessary and Possible

We have discussed evidence supporting the concept that there are two groups of patients for whom treatment for cure of prostate cancer is neither necessary nor possible. The exact proportion of patients these represent is unknown. To calculate this, it would be necessary to randomize patients with prostate cancer to receive either observation or treatment for cure. With the exception of the VACURG series, this has not been done. One can use a liberal statistical license, however, to compare series of patients who are not treated for prostate cancer to those who are treated. In Figure 6, we have taken this liberty. The figure displays survival curves for three groups of patients. Combining the series of untreated patients from Figure 3 yields the expected survival associated with a policy of expectant management. Two survival curves have been added representing the results of

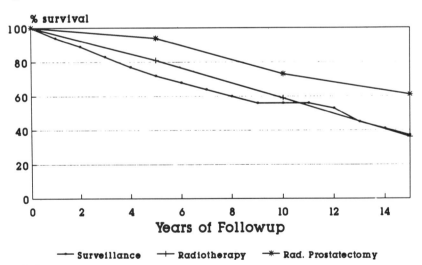

FIG 6.
Survival comparisons: surveillance vs. radiotherapy vs. radical (rad.) prostatectomy.[21–24, 27–30, 36, 37]

treatment. One represents the Stanford experience of radiotherapy for patients in whom disease was limited to the prostate.[36] The second illustrates a series of patients from the Virginia Mason Clinic (Seattle) with extended follow-up following treatment with radical prostatectomy.[37] As is readily apparent, the marginal improvement in survival seen at 10 years does not seem to be excessively large for radical prostatectomy, and the curves for expectant management and radiotherapy are virtually the same. Although such a comparison is fraught with considerable bias, it does illustrate that the number of patients who truly benefit from treatment may be small.

Despite the nihilistic tone of this discussion, there are certainly great numbers of patients who will receive significant survival benefit from treatment of their prostate cancer. Figure 7 demonstrates such a characteristic patient. If his prostate cancer is left undiagnosed and untreated, the patient will die of this disease before he would die otherwise of other causes. Interval "A" in the figure refers to this prolongation of life. Additionally, the patient would be free from symptoms of his disease for an even longer period of time; this is represented by interval "B." These two periods of time

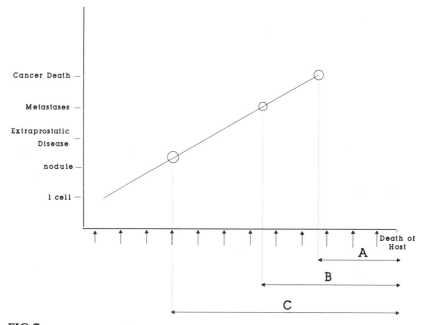

FIG 7.

Example of a patient in whom cure of prostate cancer is both necessary and possible. If untreated, patient would die "A" years before an otherwise "natural" death. Interval "B" represents the duration of symptoms from metastatic disease that does not occur, which benefit the patient gains by treatment. Interval "C" represents the time between tumor detection and death of other causes. It is during this interval that the patient may experience side effects of treatment for the disease.

are concrete benefits to this patient as a result of early detection and treatment.

Despite his improved survival, there are two ways in which treatment may prove to be deleterious to this patient. The first is portrayed graphically in interval "C." This represents the period of time following treatment during which the patient may suffer from treatment-related morbidity. Although, for many patients, this may represent only the pain and recuperation from radical prostatectomy or the nuisance-level symptoms of radiotherapy, for some, it may be lifelong symptoms, including impotence, incontinence, urethral stricture, and voiding dysfunction. To what degree this longer period of time decreases the value of interval "A" must be evaluated within the context of the patient's own sense of priorities.

A more bothersome drawback to treatment for cure of prostate cancer lies in the extension of life well into old age, which is a period of increasing disability for the U.S. male. It first must be established what period of time interval "A" represents. Horm and Sondik have calculated the total number of years of life lost annually to various neoplasms as well as the average number of years of life lost to prostate cancer.[38] Although prostate cancer was the fifth most common cause of cancer death and the eighth most common cause of person-years of life lost, among 21 different neoplasms, it led to the least number of years of life lost due to the disease. The authors calculated that an average patient who died of prostate cancer lost an average of 9.0 years of life expectancy due to the disease.

Gerontologists remind us of the multiplicity of problems associated with old age that occur during the additional years of life expectancy that are gained by treatment for prostate cancer. Schneider and Guralnik reported that 10% of men aged 65 to 74 years either live in a nursing home or live at home and need the assistance of another person to accomplish their everyday activities.[39] By the age of 85 years, this number increases to 46%. Rogers and colleagues have calculated the relative increase in the dependent population based on age.[40] Figure 8 demonstrates that, at the age of 70 years, the dependent population is only 10% of the independent population, but that this increases to about 50% at the age of 80 years, and the curves cross in the middle of the ninth decade. Brody and Miles, referring to the work of Guralnik and Fitzsimmons, have crystallized this concern, stating, "At present, our best data indicate that for each year of life expectancy gained, we incur almost four years of compromised health." [41, 42] Finally, in 1985, Fries calculated the ideal average life span and found it to be 85 years.[43] Using demographic data from the past century, incorporating trends of health care and public health, he concluded that, "Clearly, the medical and social task of eliminating premature death is largely accomplished."

There is no doubt that the previous discussion is bothersome, both medically and ethically. However, it would be naive to expect that decisions regarding health care should be made without concern for the patient's quality of life. Referring again to Figure 7, the absolute gain in life expectancy (interval "A") requires several trade-offs: (1) a period of variable treatment-related morbidity (interval "C"); (2) an increasing risk of an in-

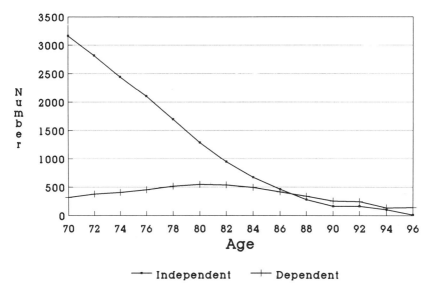

FIG 8.
Number of dependent and independent persons in the United States, by age.[40]

active and dependent (possibly institutionalized) life-style during some portion of interval "A"; and (3) an increasing risk of many other disease processes associated with aging, including abnormal carbohydrate metabolism, osteoporosis, dementia, arthritis, incontinence, and depression. The relative value of these two choices (a shorter life with less aging-related morbidity vs. a longer life with more aging-related morbidity) must be judged by the individual patient. It must be conceded, however, that for some patients, this trade-off may not warrant treatment for cure.

Summary of Expectant Management

The three contentions just presented above have suggested that, for a proportion of patients who develop prostate cancer, diagnosis and treatment are not warranted, as cure of the disease is either not possible or not necessary. The relative number of patients in each of these three groups (treatment unnecessary, treatment impossible, and treatment possible and necessary) is unknown. The task of the clinician is to attempt to discern which patient needs treatment. Identification of the patient who requires therapy may be assisted by the use of several prognostic factors. Each is discussed in detail following.

Predictors of Progression

The previously described hypothetical cases reveal that the crux of the problem in treating prostate cancer is how to predict the future of an individual patient. How can we separate one patient from the multitudes with prostate cancer and accurately predict the outcome if he is left untreated? Clearly, if we had a biologic crystal ball that could reveal a patient's outcome, then expectant management could be applied selectively and safely.

Our knowledge of the natural history of prostate cancer has increased in recent decades, but, with few exceptions, was acquired by retrospective review of the results of patients already treated. As noted earlier, application of these results to present and future patients may introduce biases. However, the retrospective analyses have allowed us to improve our general understanding of the disease process and to develop new techniques and instrumentation for analysis.

The future behavior of a malignancy may be fixed from its onset or may change over time. With the exception of certain neuroblastomas, spontaneous differentiation of a tumor from a malignant to a benign phenotype cannot be expected. Much more commonly, transformation of a localized tumor will occur, exhibiting the biochemical ability to invade beyond the organ of origin or metastasize to distant sites. A fundamental requirement to enable us to treat a patient expectantly is the ability to predict whether transformation will occur or already has occurred. A patient with a tumor that is still organ-confined, but has demonstrated transformation to a more malignant phenotype, is an individual in whom treatment probably is both necessary and possible.

Many tumor characteristics have been described that provide prognostic information (Table 1). Macroscopic features such as distant or local tumor spread, or tumor size were analyzed earliest. Microscopic analyses led to characterization of tumor architecture (e.g., Gleason's grade) or qualitative nuclear grading. With the advent of newer techniques, more quantitative features have been described, such as DNA ploidy, nuclear roundness, and labeling index. Finally, the genetic code, or nucleic acid sequencing, is being unraveled in tumors and ultimately may become predictive of a tumor's future behavior.

TABLE 1.
Characteristics of Tumors Used to Access Their Biologic Potential Past, Present, and Future

Tumor Features	Detection Techniques
Stage	DNA ploidy
Volume	Nuclear morphometry
Grade	DNA synthesis
	oncogenes

Stage

Early efforts to categorize patients in order to assess outcome were based on the clinician's assessment of tumor extent. Tumors that were clinically occult and found incidentally were designated stage A. Tumors noted on DRE that were confined to the prostate were called stage B. Stage C tumors included those with evidence of direct extension outside the prostate gland. Tumors that had metastasized to lymph nodes, bone, or other distant sites were designated stage D. Long ago, urologists noted that the prognosis was poorer in the more advanced tumor stages, and the risk of developing metastases also was related to the local stage.[44] In addition, clinicians observed that not all tumors progressed over time, and that not all patients with tumors of similar stage had similar outcomes.[45, 46]

Stage was demonstrated to be predictive of outcome in the first VA-CURG study (Table 2).[47] When the tumor was localized clinically, the patient's 5-year survival rate was 69% to 79%. However, a patient with distant metastases and an elevated acid phosphatase level had only a 14% 5-year survival rate.

The inherent limitation of clinical stage as a predictor of cancer progression lies in the fact that advancement in clinical stage defines progression itself. Thus, tumor stage serves as a marker along the time line of progression, but does not determine independently that further progression will occur. As noted by Whitmore, stage A prostate cancer is the source of all

---

TABLE 2.
Relationship of 5-Year Survival to Tumor Stage*

Stage	5-Year Survival, %
Stage I: clinical occult	69
Stage II: palpable tumor, organ-confined	79
Stage III: local extension	52
Stage IV: distant metastases or elevated serum acid phosphatase level;	25
distant metastases and elevated serum acid phosphatase level	14

*Adapted from Whitmore WF: *Cancer* 1973; 5:1104–1112.

---

clinically evident tumors, although most stage A tumors never become clinically manifest.[47] The passage of time allows the occult tumor to advance in stage by continued local growth or transformation into an altered phenotype that advances in stage at a different rate (Figure 9). A stage A or B tumor may be an early nontransformed lesion that needs no therapy or an early transformed lesion that will progress and requires treatment. Tumors may become stage C by slow local growth without transformation and still be amenable to treatment. Other stage C tumors may be late transformed malignancies associated with progression to metastatic disease and are not curable by any local therapy. Metastatic tumors (stage D) represent the late outcome of transformed stage A, B, or C tumors.

Expectant therapy for low-stage tumors is reasonable if the time required for tumor progression to a lethal burden is predictable and exceeds the life expectancy of the host. Unfortunately, the time to tumor progression for any given patient is not predictable. The clinician's ability to determine whether transformation has occurred is important in deciding if expectant therapy is reasonable. The key to understanding the future behavior of localized prostate tumors lies in finding the transforming factors or biologic predictors of progression.

Tumor Volume

In 1962, McNeal reported that prostate cancer became less differentiated as the size of the tumor increased. He noted that lesions greater than 1 cm in diameter usually were of high grade.[48] His work laid the foundation for establishing the relationship between tumor volume and tumor grade.

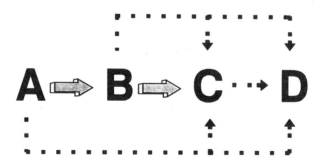

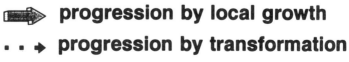

FIG 9.
Stage progression can occur by local growth in an orderly sequence or by transformation of tumor cell lines, allowing advancement to late stages without passage through all clinical stages.

Subsequent work showed that the distinction between stage A and B disease is less important than the difference in tumor volume, particularly since tumors of both stages spanned the same volume range.[49] Tumor volume correlated with tumor differentiation, local invasion, and metastasis. Stamey reported on retrospective studies showing that patients having cancers with volumes greater than 3 cc (based on pathologic examination) did poorly. The high volume of tumor correlated with invasion of the seminal vesicles, pelvic lymph node metastases, and early postoperative progression to bone metastases.[50] In his series, no patient with a pathologically determined tumor volume of 3cc or less had positive lymph nodes at surgery or progressed to bone metastases.

Tumor Grade

Fifty years ago, Evans and others described a correlation between the microscopic appearance of a tumor and the patient's clinical outcome.[51] During the 1960s, it rapidly became apparent that histologic differentiation, or grade, correlated with the clinical course of the disease and with patient survival.[52–55]

Multiple grading systems have been developed, but the system described by Gleason has become preeminent because of its simplicity, reproducibility, and prognostic significance.[56, 57] Using only 40 to 100× magnification, he described a grading system based upon the overall pattern of tumor growth, and not on the assessment of cytologic details at higher magnification. Gleason considered both the predominant and the lesser histologic pattern of the tumor. Each pattern is assigned a grade on a scale of 1 through 5, with the highest value representing loss of any pattern of organization.[57] He and others combined the clinical stage with the cumulative Gleason's score to arrive at a category score.[57] The range of category scores from 3 through 15 was obtained by adding the primary and secondary Gleason's grade (1 to 5 each) to the VACURG tumor stages, which were assigned numeric equivalents (I=1, II=2, III=3, IV=5). The investigators noted that cancer deaths per patient-year of follow-up were the same for a given category score and were independent of stage alone (Table 3). They also noted that cancer-specific deaths were the same for each tumor grade regardless of which was the primary and which was the secondary pattern (i.e., 4+2 = 2+4). Only 8 of 302 patients with scores of 8 or less died of prostate cancer, and there were no cancer-specific deaths among the 68 patients with category scores of less than 7. Of 18 patients with the highest category score (15 = highest grade and highest stage), 10 died of cancer and 6 died of other causes (including DES-related cardiovascular deaths). The VACURG report also noted that patients with low-grade stage III and IV tumors treated with hormonal therapy fared as well as did those with stage I and II tumors treated with radical prostatectomy.

More contemporary studies relating tumor grade to cancer progression or patient outcome include patients treated with surgical or medical therapy, not expectantly. Some of these studies, however, provide pathologic

TABLE 3.
Cancer Deaths Per Patient-Year of Follow-up*

Stage	Combined Stage and Grade Category						
	4–6	7–8	9	10	11–12	13–14	15
Stage I and II (N=148)	0.0	≤0.01	0.02	0.05	†	†	†
Stage III and IV (N=884)	0.0	≤0.01	0.02	0.05	0.10	0.172	0.30

*Adapted from Gleason DF, Mellinger GT, the Veterans Administration Cooperative Urological Research Group: *J Urol* 1974; 111:58–64.
†No patients in this group.

staging information that further illuminates the relationship between tumor grade and patient outcome. Pathologic staging information also highlights the obstacles inherent in expectant therapy, such as understaging and undergrading.

Regional lymph node metastases occur most commonly in patients with poorly differentiated tumors; well-differentiated tumors are associated with nodal metastases only rarely.[58, 59] Zincke and associates reported that no patient had metastases to the pelvic lymph nodes if the primary tumor was Mayo grade 1 or 2, pathologic stage B1, or Mayo grade 1 and stage B2 or C.[60] Also, a "Mayo sum" was derived by adding the Mayo grade of 1 through 4 to the Mayo stage of 1 through 6. The authors reported a significant difference between tumors with a Mayo sum of 5 and those with a Mayo sum of 6. No patients with tumors having a Mayo sum of 5 or less had positive lymph nodes, whereas eight patients with tumors having a Mayo sum of 6 had positive nodes. They concluded that the Mayo sum could identify patients who already had nodal metastases.

Fowler described the relationship between Gleason's grade and pathologic tumor extent in a series of 75 patients with clinically organ-confined prostate cancer treated with radical prostatectomy.[61] He demonstrated that the clinical stage and Gleason grade correlated with the presence of local extension beyond the surgical specimen (pathologic stage C). Surgical margins were always negative in patients with stage A2 tumors and a Gleason score of 7 or below, whereas all 3 patients with tumors having a score of 8 or above had positive margins. Of the patients with clinical stage B tumors, positive surgical margins were found in 2 of 10 (20%) with Gleason grade 5 or below in 13 of 37 (35%) with grade 7 or below, and in 7 of 11 (64%) with grade 8 or above. Patients with clinical stage B2 tumors had such a high incidence of positive margins by stage alone that grade had no additive effect. The highest predictive value for surgical upstaging to stage C was a Gleason score of 8 or above. Only 5% of the surgically organ-confined tumors were high-grade (Gleason 8 or above), again emphasizing the relationship between tumor grade and tumor extent/local progression. Fowler also found that no patient with a low-volume tumor (cancers histologically confined to one lobe or involving 33% or less of the transurethral prostatic specimen) had a Gleason score of 8 or above. Finally, he noted that postoperative progression to distant metastases was related to tumor grade. All patients with a grade of 6 or below remained disease-free, but 31% of those with a grade of 8 or above had progression.

The studies discussed previously add to our understanding of the influence of tumor grade on cancer progression; however, the patients were treated with surgery or androgen deprivation. The question remains, can tumor grade be used to help select patients who can be treated expectantly?

Two early reports, by Byar (VACURG) in 1972 and Cantrell in 1981, showed that incidentally found microscopic cancer of the prostate (stage I or A), particularly if it was low-grade, had low progression rates when managed expectantly.[62, 63] Cantrell presented 117 patients with stage A tumors, 84 of whom had been followed for at least 4 years and 24 of whom had been followed for 10 or more years. Patients with tumor volumes of less than 5% of the resected specimen and a Gleason grade of 4 or below were classified as having stage A1 disease and were observed. No patient with a low-grade tumor progressed with expectant management during the initial study; however, subsequent follow-up revealed an increase in progression with time.[64]

Two studies published in the late 1980s related the initial tumor grade to treatment outcome when patients were treated expectantly. Johansson reported 223 patients with clinically localized prostate cancer who were treated expectantly and found that 28.2% progressed and 6.2% died of prostate cancer during a 5-year follow-up period.[28] Table 4 shows the relationship of tumor grade to progression and death. Grade 1 tumors (World Health Organization classification) progressed in only 19% of cases, usually only locally to stage T3 (or C) disease. Grade III tumors progressed in 66% of cases, and five of six progressions were to distant metastases. Progression-free survival for grade I, II, and III tumors was 82.9%, 50.3%, and 26.7%, respectively. Moderately differentiated tumors had a risk of progression 2.9-fold higher than that of well-differentiated tumors. Poorly differentiated tumors had a risk of progression 18.7-fold higher than that of well-differentiated tumors.

In 1988, Adolfsson reported 91 patients with prostate cancer diagnosed by transrectal fine needle aspiration biopsy. The patients were treated by observation alone. Their outcome was dramatically dependent on tumor grade.[65] Fifty-seven of the patients were considered to have clinically localized cancer (i.e., normal prostatic acid phosphatase levels and bone scans). Using Willems' system of cytologic diagnosis and grading, only 1 of 23 well-differentiated tumors, but 18 of 19 poorly differentiated tumors, had

TABLE 4.
Relationship of Grade to Progression and Survival in 223 Patients With Newly Diagnosed Prostate Cancer That Was Nonmetastatic and Managed Expectantly*

Grade	Patient Number (Percent of Total)	Local Progression	Distant Metastases	Total Progression (%)	Deaths Due to Prostate Cancer	Deaths Due to Unrelated Causes
I	148 (66)	20	8	28 (19)	4	48
II	66 (30)	24	7	31 (47)	7	16
III	9 (4)	1	5	6 (66)	5	3

*Adapted from Johansson JE, Adami HO, Andersson SO, et al: *Lancet* 1989; 1:799–803.

distant metastases at the time of diagnosis.[66] There was no significant difference in frequency of local progression, development of metastases, or death from prostate cancer between well- and moderately well-differentiated tumors (Table 5).

These reports suggest that the initial tumor grade may be a good predictor of prostate cancer progression. Occasional low-grade tumors do progress, however, revealing the limitations of the initial tumor grade alone as a prognostic indicator. The explanations for progression include the following possibilities: (1) certain truly low-grade tumors have the capacity to invade and metastasize, (2) there is an element of undergrading of expectantly treated tumors due to sampling error, and (3) the phenotype of these progressing tumors may have changed over time to a higher-grade subline.

As an extension to analysis by tumor grade, Lowe and Listrom combined tumor grade and tumor volume in 232 patients with stage A lesions and calculated the risks of progression in multiple subsets.[67, 68] Group 1 consisted of two patient sets. The first set included 143 patients with tumor volumes of 5% or less and the second set included 34 patients with tumor volumes of greater than 5%. Patients were treated with radical prostatectomy or radiation therapy. Group 2 consisted of 55 patients with tumor volumes greater than 5% who were treated expectantly. Progression was defined as symptomatic local recurrence or distant metastases. There was a high mortality rate from intercurrent disease; therefore, survival was not used as an endpoint. The study population had the following distribution of Gleason tumor grades: 2 or 3 (32%), 4 (36%), 5 or 6 (23%), and 7 through 9 (9%). Gleason grade and tumor volume correlated with the risk of disease progression (Table 6). Progression rates ranged from 0% with Gleason grade 2 tumors to 57% with Gleason grade 7 to 9 tumors. Tumor volume also was related to progression. Focal tumors (less than 1% by volume) rarely progressed, but tumors with volumes greater than 5% progressed in over half the cases. After eliminating the patients in group 1 who

---

TABLE 5.
Relationship of Cytologic Grade to Outcome in 57 Patients With Clinically Localized Prostate Cancers That Were Managed Expectantly*

Tumor Grade	Patient Number	Local Progression (%)	Metastases (%)	Died of Prostate Cancer (%)	Died of Unrelated Cause (%)
1	22	8 (36)	6 (27)	3 (14)	6 (27)
2	34	16 (47)	12 (35)	6 (18)	4 (12)
3	1	1	0	0	1

*Adapted from Adolfsson J, Farhaus B: *J Urol* 1988; 140:1452–1454.

TABLE 6.
Relationship of Tumor Grade and Tumor Volume to Subsequent Tumor Progression *

Tumor Grade (Gleason Sum)	Percent Progression	Tumor Volume (Percent of Specimen Involved)	Percent Progression
2	0	Less than 1	6
3	7		
4	27	1–5	12
5–6	38		
7–9	57	Greater than 5	53

*Adapted from Lowe BA, Listrom MB: *J Urol* 1988; 140:1340–1344.

received treatment, the authors analyzed the remaining 188 expectantly managed patients to determine the probability of progression based on tumor grade and volume. All patients were found to be at risk for progression except for the rare patient with Gleason grade 2 cancer. The probability of a 60-year-old man with a tumor volume of less than 1% and a Gleason grade 2 or 3 lesion developing progressive disease was 0.03 at 5 years and 0.06 at 10 years. At the other extreme, a 70-year-old man with a tumor volume of greater than 5% and a Gleason grade 7, 8, or 9 lesion had a probability of progression of 80% at 5 years and one of 95% at 10 years. Unfortunately, the more frequently encountered patients with moderately differentiated tumors had an equal chance of progressing or not progressing. For example, a 70-year-old man with a tumor volume of 1% to 5% and a Gleason grade 5 or 6 lesion would have a 0.051 probability of progression. A 60-year-old man with a tumor volume of greater than 5% and a Gleason grade 4 tumor would have a 0.051 probability of progression. Lowe and Listrom recommended that treatment should be offered to patients with at least a 5-year life expectancy and a 10% chance of progression based on their analysis of age, grade, and tumor volume.[68] As the investigators themselves acknowledge, choosing any single level of probability as a determinant of therapy is arbitrary. Their calculations provide a broad range of risk probabilities that can be used as a guide to weigh the benefits and risks of expectant management. As revealed by the aforementioned studies, limitations exist in using tumor grade to predict the outcome of expectant therapy. Tumor grade predicts progression best at the extremes of the grading scales. Patients with well-differentiated cancers fare well and those with poorly differentiated cancers fare poorly, but grade alone is of limited use in predicting progression in the majority of patients who have moderately differentiated tumors. Perhaps tumor grade, similar to tumor stage, is not a predictor of progression. Decreasing tumor differentiation may indicate that progression or transformation already has occurred, at least at the cellular level. Consequently, to help differentiate the course of moderately differentiated cancers, investigators may need to analyze more closely intracellular abnormalities that are more fundamental than the histologic appearance.

Nuclear Features as Predictors of Behavior

The ultimate behavior of a malignancy, including its ability to invade locally or spread to distant sites, is regulated by its nuclear content. Analyses of nuclear shape or contour, DNA or RNA content, karyotype, nuclear synthesis, and oncogenes may provide investigators with insights into a tumor's future behavior. Stenkvist and colleagues reported the use of computerized nuclear morphometry to characterize human cancer cell populations in 1978.[69] Since then, different approaches to analyzing tumor cell nuclei and their nucleic acid content have been developed and continue to be refined. The clinical utility of these techniques remains in its infancy.

DNA Ploidy

Flow cytometry of prostatic carcinoma tissue can determine ploidy status, which can be related to tumor progression and patient survival. Flow cytometry determines ploidy by comparing the position of the G1 peak of the tumor cell population to that of normal diploid cells and defining the proportions of cells distributed throughout the cell cycle. Diploid nuclei have a normal complement of DNA (2C) and a single G1 peak that deviates less than 10% from normal reference nuclei. Cells with twice the normal complement (4C) are tetraploid and may be considered aneuploid if the peak deviates greatly from the G2M peak of normal cells. Aneuploid nuclei have a second peak more than 10% from the internal standard or, less commonly, a single peak deviating more than 10% from standard nuclei. Retrospective studies have reported the ploidy status of stage B, C, or D prostate cancers that already had been treated.[70-74] Two studies analyzed tumor ploidy in incidental or expectantly managed cancers.[75, 76]

Montgomery and associates reported the Mayo Clinic analysis of DNA ploidy in organ-confined prostate cancer.[73] Two hundred and sixty-one patients had pathologic stage B disease and adequate histograms by flow cytometry. The overall progression rate was 20%, with a mean follow-up period of 9.4 years. Local recurrence occurred in 22 patients, and metastases developed in 23. Eight patients suffered both local and distant tumor progression. Of the tumors that progressed, 51% were diploid and 49% were nondiploid (tetraploid and aneuploid). In this retrospective analysis, 100% of aneuploid tumors progressed. Only 15% of diploid tumors progressed, and 31% of nondiploid tumors (nearly all tetraploid) progressed. Survival, both crude and cause-specific, was diminished in aneuploid tumors (Table 7). The authors' multivariate analysis demonstrated that only

TABLE 7.
Survival Probabilities (Crude and Cause-Specific) for Patients With Pathologic Stage B Prostate Cancer Treated by Radical Prostatectomy*

| Ploidy | Patient Number | Crude/Cause-Specific Survival Rates (%) | |
		10 Years	15 Years
Diploid	177	75/96	65/90
Tetraploid	74	78/95	75/92
Aneuploid	10	58/58	58/58

*Adapted from Montgomery BT, Nativ O, Blute ML, et al: *Arch Surg* 1990; 125:327–331.

aneuploidy was predictive of progression and cause-specific survival. After adjusting for aneuploidy, only a Gleason grade of 6 to 10 had significant predictive value for progression.

Mayo Clinic investigators also have reported DNA ploidy analysis of pathologic stage C prostate cancers. The study was performed on archival specimens from 143 patients treated with radical prostatectomy and pelvic lymphadenectomy.[71] The median time to progression (defined as local recurrence or metastases) was not reached in the diploid groups, as only 23% had progressed after 18 years of follow-up. However, the median time to progression was only 7 years for aneuploid tumors and 7.8 years for tetraploid tumors. High-grade tumors had a poor prognosis regardless of ploidy status. Patients with low-grade tumors had a 92% progression-free survival rate if the tumor was diploid, but only a 57% progression-free survival rate if the tumor was tetraploid or aneuploid. Importantly, ploidy was found not to vary with tumor volume (Table 8). Ploidy was comparable in tumors with volumes of less than 3 cc and those with volumes more than 10 cc. In this study, multivariate analysis revealed that tumor grade was the most important predictor of progression.

Lee and coworkers reported on a series of 80 patients treated with radical prostatectomy and followed for progression.[77] Tumor extension into the seminal vesicles was present in two thirds of patients, which decreased the probability of them remaining disease-free at 5 years from 87% to 28%. Flow cytometry was performed on the deparaffinized specimens. Aneuploidy (tetraploid aneuploid and aneuploid) resulted in only a 9% probability of being disease-free at 5 years, but diploidy was associated with an 85% chance of remaining disease-free. None of the 18 patients with seminal vesicle invasion and a diploid tumor had tumor recurrence. The probability of tumor progression was 92% if the seminal vesicles were involved and the tumor was aneuploid. Interestingly, patients with diploid tumors

TABLE 8.
Relationship of Tumor Volume to Ploidy in 146 Patients With Pathologic Stage C Prostate Cancer Treated by Radical Prostatectomy and Pelvic Lymphadenectomy*

Tumor Volume (cc)	Patient Number	DNA Ploidy (Percent of Patient Number)		
		Diploid	Tetraploid	Aneuploid
Less than 3	63	51	43	6
3 to 10	62	42	50	8
Greater than 10	21	43	48	9

*Adapted from Nativ O, Winkler HA, Raz Y, et al: *Mayo Clin Proc* 1989; 64:911–919.

with seminal vesicle extension, had a greater than 70% chance of remaining disease-free for 5 years. Those with aneuploid tumors without seminal vesicle invasion fared worse.

Tumor ploidy also has been useful in predicting patient survival in men with metastatic disease. Miller and colleagues stratified patients with stage D2 disease into those with poor outcome (dead of disease within 12 months) and those with good outcome (alive for 5 years or more).[78] DNA ploidy analysis of the primary tumor was a significant independent indicator of outcome ($P<.001$). Forty-six of 52 patients (88%) with nondiploid (tetraploid and aneuploid) tumors had poor outcomes, but only 16 of 45 (36%) patients with diploid tumors did poorly. Tumor grade also was an independent predictor of outcome.

Although these studies demonstrate a relationship between ploidy and progression, others have not confirmed ploidy as an independent predictor of patient outcome. Detjer reported 69 patients with pathologic stage B, C, and D1 prostate cancer and clinical stage D2 disease.[79]Table 9 shows the relationship of Gleason grade and pathologic stage to tumor ploidy. Table 10 demonstrates that the frequency of aneuploidy increases as tumor grade or stage increases. Ploidy status approaches its extremes as the Gleason score or stage approaches the extremes of the respective scales. Aneuploidy was found in only 5.8% of tumors with a Gleason score of 2 to 4, but was present in 62.5% of high-grade tumors (Gleason score 8 to 10). Aneuploidy was a feature of 2.7% of pathologic stage B tumors and 72.2% of stage D2 tumors. Unfortunately, even the extreme cases of ploidy and grade were not completely predictive. Of diploid clinical stage B tumors that were Gleason grade 6 or less, 13.9% still had extracapsular tumor extension or metastatic disease. Of clinical stage B aneuploid tumors with Gleason scores of 7 to 10, one of six patients still had organ-confined disease at the time of surgery. Most importantly, the authors noted that,

TABLE 9.
Relationship of Gleason Score and Pathologic Stage to Ploidy Status in 69 Patients With Prostate Cancer*

Stage	Number of Diploid Tumors	Number of Aneuploid Tumors	Frequency of Aneuploidy, %
Gleason stage			
2–4	16	1	5.8
5–7	25	3	10.7
8–10	9	15	62.5
Pathologic stage			
B	36	1	2.7
C	9	5	35.7
D	5	13	72.2

*Adapted from Detjer SW Jr, Cunningham RE, Noguchi PD, et al: *Urology* 1989; 33:361–366.

after adjusting for stage, there was no significant difference in survival between patients with aneuploid and diploid tumors.

Using flow cytometry, McIntire evaluated the ploidy status of 39 stage A prostate cancers (Table 11).[75] Stage A2 disease (tumor volume greater than 5% of the specimen) was identified in 25 of the 39 specimens. Three patients in each stage had histograms inadequate for analysis. None of the stage A1 nonaneuploid tumors progressed, whereas 67% of the stage A2 aneuploid tumors progressed (see Table 11). This supports the notion that

TABLE 10.
Relationship Between Ploidy, Grade, and Pathologic Stage for 51 Patients With Clinically Localized Prostate Cancer*

DNA Ploidy	Gleason Score	Pathologic Stage B (%)	Pathologic Stage C and D1 (%)	Total Patients
Diploid	2–6	31 (86.1)	5 (13.9)	36
Diploid	7–10	5 (55.6)	4 (44.4)	9
Aneuploid	2–6	0	0	0
Aneuploid	7–10	1 (16.7)	5 (83.3)	6

*Adapted from Detjer SW Jr, Cunningham RE, Noguchi PD, et al: *Urology* 1989; 33:361–366.

TABLE 11.
Patterns of Progression in Stage A1 and A2 Tumors in Relation to NA Ploidy Status*

Stage and Ploidy Status (Number of Patients)	Number That Progressed (%)	Number That Did Not Progress (%)
Stage A1 (11)	1 (9)	10 (91)
Aneuploid (1)	1 (100)	0
Nonaneuploid (10)	0	10 (100)
Stage A2 (22)	8 (36)	14 (64)
Aneuploid (9)	6 (67)	3 (33)
Nonaneuploid (13)	2 (15)	11 (85)

*Adapted from McIntire TL, Murphy WM, Coon JS, et al: *Am J Clin Pathol* 1988; 89:370–373.

stage A1 nonaneuploid tumors should be treated expectantly. The authors, however, defined tumor progression only as documented metastases or death from prostate cancer, and only tumor registry records were used as the source of follow-up and documentation. Patients alive with localized disease only were not considered to have progressed. The authors did not comment on whether any of the localized tumors were enlarging, advancing from stage A to stage B or C disease. Finally, it was not specified whether the patients were managed expectantly or received therapy. These omissions diminish the value of the results.

Tribukait presented a series of patients with newly diagnosed prostate cancer managed by observation alone.[76] The diagnosis of cancer was made by fine-needle aspiration and the specimens were assigned a cytologic grade and analyzed by flow cytometry. Only 7% of diploid tumors had distant metastases at diagnosis. Metastatic disease was more common in tetraploid tumors (17%), aneuploid tumors (25%), and tumors with multiple aneuploid cell lines (52%). Table 12 shows the relationship between cytologic grade and ploidy status. Regretfully, the moderate-grade tumors, for which the most help is needed in predicting progression, were diploid in 29% of cases and nondiploid in the remaining 71% of cases (including 6% with multiple aneuploid cell lines). The relationship between ploidy and tumor stage was not surprising. Diploid cancers accounted for 80% of T1 tumors, 34% of T2 tumors, and only 2% of T4 tumors. Survival was related to ploidy, but progression was not addressed specifically. Interestingly, ploidy status for the study was assessed at the time of initial diagnosis; however, 124 patients underwent repeat biopsy during a mean follow-up period of 20 months. Advancement in ploidy occurred at an annual rate of 9%. Adolfsson and Tribukait later reported this progression in

TABLE 12.
Relationship Between Cytologic Findings on Fine-Needle Aspiration of the Prostate and DNA Ploidy of the Same Biopsy Specimen*

Cytologic Findings	Diploid, %	Aneuploid		
		Multiple Tetraploid Lines (%)	Nontetraploid (%)	Cell (%)
Benign	91	7	2	0
Malignant				
Well-differentiated	58	32	7	3
Moderately differentiated	29	37	28	6
Poorly differentiated	10	23	41	26

*Adapted from Tribukait B: Rapid-flow cytometry of prostatic fine-needle aspiration biopsies, in Karr JP, Coffey DS, Gardner W Jr (eds): *Prognostic Cytometry and Cytopathology of Prostate Cancer.* New York, Elsevier Science Publishing, 1989, p 236.

ploidy and cytologic grade in patients with at least 2 years of repeated tumor sampling.[80] They found increased ploidy in 17 of 72 patients (23%) samples. In a 3-year period, one patient's cancer progressed from diploid to tetraploid to aneuploid. He developed local tumor progression to T3 disease at the time tetraploidy was noted and a positive bone scan when aneuploidy was found.

Flow cytometry studies enhance our understanding of prostate cancer, but add little predictive value when considering the future behavior of untreated tumors. Patients with aneuploid tumors frequently have a poor outcome, even if clinically localized and treated. The preponderance of untreated but still treatable tumors are diploid. We remain unable to predict reliably which individual, within a cohort of those with low-stage diploid cancers, will experience tumor progression if left untreated. In a low-stage, moderate-grade tumor that is aneuploid, ploidy status may determine the need for intervention to prevent progression. The demonstration that tumor ploidy can advance over time is disturbing to those planning expectant therapy based on a single sampling at the time of diagnosis. The alteration from diploid to nondiploid cell lines over time represents a form of progression itself and must be a consequence of a more fundamental change in the nuclear content of the cancerous cells.

Nuclear Morphometry

Nuclear morphometry objectively measures the size, shape, and contour of cancer cell nuclei. Recent improvements in computer hardware and software have made this analysis possible for large populations of cells. Complex statistical analyses of the data are feasible now, given the advances made in software programming. Initially, these tests were very time-consuming and the necessary equipment was expensive. However, continued modifications have made these analyses more practical and affordable. The technical aspects of these studies are beyond the scope of this chapter. The interested reader is referred to the methods sections of the references cited.

Computerized image analysis of nuclear shape was reported as a prognostic factor in prostate cancer in 1982. Diamond then showed how relative nuclear roundness could identify tumors that had metastatic potential.[81, 82] Nuclear roundness factor was reported to discriminate perfectly between patients who were disease-free for at least 14 years and those who developed metastases within 9 years following radical prostatectomy for stage B disease. Nuclear roundness also was shown to be predictive of prognosis in patients with untreated stage A2 disease.[83] Paulson and associates studied the clinical outcome of 105 patients with clinically localized prostate cancer.[84] They found no correlation between treatment failure and nuclear roundness and no correlation between Gleason grade and nuclear roundness.[84] Mohler noted that differences in equipment and a lack of standardized methods for acquiring and reporting data contributed to discrepancies in results between these investigators.[85, 86] Mohler and others, by standardizing equipment with standard objects, have achieved an accuracy of at least 95% while holding intraobserver and interobserver variation to less than 5%.[85] Partin discredited the idea of using only average nuclear roundness to assess an individual cancer because it negates the importance of the variability of the malignant cell population, which may influence the tumor's ultimate behavior.[87] He reported a series of 18 patients with stage A2 prostate cancer (5% or more of the transurethral prostatic specimen involved by tumor or a Gleason score of 7 to 10). Patients were treated expectantly until local progression or distant metastases occurred. Using the Johns Hopkins morphometry system software, they analyzed 15 different shape descriptors of tumor nuclei and subjected them to 17 different statistical analyses, thus creating 255 test pairs. Since the outcomes of the patients were known, the test pairs were assessed retrospectively for the ability to discriminate between tumors with good and those with poor outcomes. The Gleason grade was only a moderate discriminator; 177 of 255 test pairs provided better prediction of outcome. Average nuclear roundness provided good separation by prognosis, but the best shape descriptor was an ellipticity factor that correctly predicted 17 of the 18 outcomes. Nuclear morphometry continues to show promise as an avenue of investigation.

DNA Synthesis

Another approach to assessing the biologic potential of a tumor is to examine the synthesis of nuclear material. Nuclear proliferative activity has been shown to be prognostic in tumors such as breast cancer.[88]

An advantage of this technique is the fact that the labeling can be done on the biopsy specimen, thereby also permitting histologic examination. Tritiated thymidine often is impractical to use in the study of human tumors. Bromodeoxyuridine (BrDU) is a halopyrimidine, like thymidine, that is incorporated into cellular nuclei at the time of DNA synthesis for mitosis (S phase of the cell cycle). The development of a monoclonal antibody to BrDU has allowed rapid determination of BrDU uptake, avoidance of autoradiography, and better visibility of nuclear detail.

Scrivner and coworkers reported cell kinetics by BrDU labeling and DNA ploidy in prostate cancer needle biopsies.[89] The labeling indices were a mean of 1.6%, a median of 0.87%, and a range of 0.1% to 29%. The extreme case (i.e., 29%) occurred in a patient with stage D2 disease, a Gleason score of 10, and multiple aneuploid cell lines. The authors found no relationship between labeling index and age, clinical stage, or tumor size by ultrasound. They noted that the highest labeling indices occurred in association with high Gleason scores or aneuploidy, but the overlap was extensive. The 75th percentile of the labeling index was defined as the lower limit of a "high" labeling index. Only with this cutoff did the relationship between high labeling index and Gleason score become statistically significant. The finding that labeling index was independent of tumor stage may allow investigators to use the labeling index in predicting outcomes in intermediate-grade tumors. Data regarding patient outcome are not available yet.

Nemto reported the results of BrDU uptake in 15 patients with prostate cancer.[90] Only 5 patients had nonmetastatic disease. He found that the higher the tumor grade, the higher the labeling index. Grade 1 tumors were labeled in 1.36% of cells, and grade 3 tumors were labeled in 4.37%. Thus, even poorly differentiated tumors had a low growth rate. In this study, samples from different parts of the tumor exhibited different growth rates. BrDU labeling has not been used yet in a cohort of patients with clinically localized disease who have been managed expectantly.

Ki-67 is a mouse monoclonal antibody that recognizes a proliferation-associated nuclear antigen expressed in the G1, S, G2, and M phases of all cycling human cells, but is absent in G0 and early G1 cells. Oomens and colleagues used Ki-67 to assess the proliferative cell fraction in 50 human prostate cancers.[91] The Ki-67 index was significantly higher in cancer specimens than in benign prostatic hypertrophy specimens. The Ki-67 index also decreased with therapeutic intervention—either radiotherapy or endocrine deprivation (Table 13). The prognostic relevance or predictive capability of Ki-67 currently is under investigation.

Oncogenes

Recently, considerable interest has been directed at investigating gene patterns in prostate cancer. To date, no specific alteration in oncogenes or tumor suppressor genes has been identified consistently. Although some investigators have reported altered *ras* and *myc* expression, others have

TABLE 13.
Ki-67 Response to Therapy Aspiration Biopsy*

Months Following Initiation of Therapy†	Patient Number	Mean Ki-67 Index	Mean Percentage of Initial Ki-67 Index
0	9	5.0	100
1	8	1.9	58.2
2	6	1.0	27.3
3	6	0.4	6.6

*Adapted from Oomens EHGM, Van Steenbrugge GJ, Van Der Kwast THH, et al: *J Urol* 1991; 145:81–85.
†Tissue stained for KI-67 before (0), and at 1, 2, and 3 months following the initiation of therapy.

found no correlation between increased levels of their expression and tumor progression or prognosis.[92] Overexpression of the *neu* oncogene has been associated with higher histologic tumor grade, increased nuclear synthesis, and aneuploid cell lines.[93] Future progress in the field of oncogenes, tumor suppressor genes, and chromosome analysis may improve our ability to predict the natural history of a tumor based on its genetic features.

Summary

Patients with localized prostate cancer who are managed expectantly may do well, but some will manifest progression of their disease. If we could foresee which patients would not experience clinically significant progression during their lifetime, we could better advise them concerning therapy. If patients at substantial risk for progression could be identified accurately, we could recommend appropriate therapy confidently. Unfortunately, there is no single aspect of the tumor's phenotype that can identify accurately the individual patient who is at risk. Tumor stage and grade fail to be predictive for the individual patient. Grade may be helpful in making therapeutic decisions if it is high or low, but the majority of cancers are moderately differentiated, and their prognosis is uncertain. Generally, DNA ploidy has the same limitations as tumor grade. Nuclear morphometry and nuclear kinetics have not been employed widely to assess their true value. The ultimate predictor(s) of prostate cancer progression remains unknown. Expectant management of prostate cancer should be based on the clinician's best judgment, using the available modalities, recognizing that no one as yet has a "biologic crystal ball."

References

1. Silverberg E, Lubera JA: Cancer statistics, 1989. *Cancer* 1989; 39:3–20.
2. Boring CC, Squires TS, Tong T: Cancer statistics, 1992. *Cancer* 1992; 42:19–38.
3. Seidman H, Mushinski MH, Gelb SK, et al: Probabilities of eventually developing or dying of cancer—United States, 1985. *Cancer* 1985; 35:36–56.
4. Byar DP: Incidence, mortality and survival statistics for prostatic cancer, in Coffey DS (ed): *Current Concepts and Approaches to the Study of Prostate Cancer.* New York, Alan R Liss, 1987, pp 785–796.
5. US Department of Commerce: *Vital Statistics of the U.S., 1990.* Washington DC, Bureau of the Census.
6. Whitmore WF: Natural history of low-stage prostatic cancer: The impact of early detection. *Urol Clin North Am* 1990; 17:689–697.
7. McNeal JE, Kindrachuk RA, Freiha FS, et al: Patterns of progression in prostate cancer. *Lancet* 1986; 1:60–63.
8. Kimbrough JC: Carcinoma of the prostate: Five-year followup of patients treated by radical surgery. *J Urol* 1956; 76:287–291.
9. Rich ARR: On the frequency of occurrence of occult carcinoma of the prostate. *J Urol* 1935; 33:215–220.
10. Moore RA: The morphology of small prostatic carcinoma. *J Urol* 1935; 33:224–234.
11. Hudson PB, Finkle AL, Hopkins JA, et al: Prostatic cancer XI. Early prostatic cancer diagnosed by arbitrary open perineal biopsy among 300 unselected patients. *Cancer* 1954; 7:690–703.
12. Scott R, Mutchnik DL, Laskowski TZ, et al: Carcinoma of the prostate in elderly men: Incidence, growth characteristics, and clinical significance. *J Urol* 1969; 101:602–607.
13. Hirst AE, Bergman RT: Carcinoma of the prostate in men 80 or more years old. *Cancer* 1954; 7:136–141.
14. Halpert B, Sheehan EE, Schmalhorst WR, et al: Carcinoma of the prostate: A survey of 5,000 autopsies. *Cancer* 1963; 16:737–742.
15. Silverberg E, Luberg JA: Cancer statistics, 1988. *Cancer* 1988; 38:5.
16. US Public Health Service: *Vital Statistics of the United States, 1988.* Washington DC, US Department of Health and Human Services, 1988.
17. Young HH: *A Surgeon's Autobiography.* New York, Harcourt Brace & Co, 1940.
18. Bumpus HC: Carcinoma of the prostate: A clinical study of 1,000 cases. *Surg Gynecol Obstet* 1926; 43:150–155.
19. Nesbit RM, Plumb RT: Prostatic carcinoma. A followup on 795 patients treated prior to the endocrine era and a comparison of survival rates between these and patients treated by endocrine therapy. *Surgery* 1946; 20:263–272.
20. Hanash KA, Utz DC, Cook EN, et al: Carcinoma of the prostate: A fifteen year followup. *J Urol* 1972; 107:450–453.
21. Cook GB, Watson FR: Twenty single nodules of prostate cancer not treated by total prostatectomy. *J Urol* 1968; 100:672–674.
22. Barnes R, Hirst A, Rosenquist R: Early carcinoma of the prostate: Comparison of stages A and B. *J Urol* 1976; 115:404–405.
23. Moskovitz B, Nitecki S, Levin DR: Cancer of the prostate: Is there a need for aggressive treatment? *Urol Int* 1987; 42:49–52.
24. Madsen PO, Graversen PH, Gasser TC, et al: Treatment of localized prostatic

cancer. Radical prostatectomy versus placebo: A 15-year followup. *Scand J Urol Nephrol* 1988; 110(suppl):95–100.

25. Newling DWW, Hall RR, Richards B, et al: The normal history of prostatic carcinoma: The argument for a no-treatment policy, in Pavone-Macaluso M, Smith PH, Bagshaw MA (eds): *Testicular Cancer and Other Tumors of the Genitourinary Tract,* vol 18. New York, Plenum Press, 1983, pp 443–448.

26. Parker MC, Cook A, Riddle PR, et al: Is delayed treatment justified in carcinoma of the prostate? *Br J Urol* 1985; 57:724–728.

27. George NJR: Natural history of localized prostatic cancer managed by conservative therapy alone. *Lancet* 1988; 1:494–496.

28. Johansson JE, Adami HO, Andersson SO, et al: Natural history of localized prostatic cancer: A population-based study in 223 untreated patients. *Lancet* 1989; 1:799–803.

29. Adolfsson J, Carstensen J: Natural course of clinically-localized prostatic adenocarcinoma in men less than 70 years old. *J Urol* 1991; 146:96–98.

30. Whitmore WF, Warner JA, Thompson IM: Expectant management of localized prostatic cancer. *Cancer* 1991; 67:1091–1096.

31. Chodak GW, Thompson IM, Gerber GS, et al: Results from two prostate cancer screening programs. *J Urol* 1991; 145:251A.

32. Thompson IM, Ernst JJ, Gangai MP, et al: Adenocarcinoma of the prostate: Results of routine urological screening. *J Urol* 1984; 132:690–692.

33. Thompson IM, Zeidman EJ: Presentation and clinical course of patients ultimately succumbing to carcinoma of the prostate. *Scand J Urol Nephrol* 1991; 25:111–114.

34. Catalona WJ, Smith DS, Ratliff TL, et al: Measurement of prostate-specific antigen as a screening test for prostate cancer. *N Engl J Med* 1991; 324:1156–1161.

35. Paulson DF, Moul JW, Walther PJ: Radical prostatectomy for clinical stage T1-2NOMO prostatic adenocarcinoma: Long-term results. *J Urol* 1990; 144:1180–1184.

36. Bagshaw MA: Potential for radiotherapy alone in prostatic cancer. *Cancer* 1985; 55:2079–2085.

37. Gibbons RP, Correa RJ, Brannen GE, et al: Total prostatectomy for clinically-localized prostatic cancer: Long-term results. *J Urol* 1989; 141:564–566.

38. Horm JW, Sondik EJ: Person-years of life lost due to cancer in the United States: 1970 and 1984. *Am J Public Health* 1989; 79:1490–1493.

39. Schneider EL, Guralnik JM: The aging of America. *JAMA* 1990; 263:2335–2340.

40. Rogers A, Rogers RG, Berlanger A: Longer life but worse health? Measurement and dynamics. *Gerontologist* 1990; 30:640–649.

41. Brody JA, Miles TP: Mortality postponed and the unmasking of age-dependent non-fatal conditions. *Aging* 1990; 2:283–289.

42. Guralnik JM, Fitzsimmons SC: Aging in America: A demographic perspective. *Geriatr Cardiol* 1986; 4:175–183.

43. Fries JF: Aging, natural death, and the compression of morbidity. *N Engl J Med* 1980; 303:130–135.

44. Flocks RH: Clinical cancer of the prostate. *JAMA* 1965; 193:559–562.

45. Franks LM, Durh MB: Latency and progression in tumors, the natural history of prostatic cancer. *Lancet* 1958; 1:1037.

46. Franks LM, Fergusson JD, Murnaghan GF: An assessment of factors influencing survival in prostatic cancer: The absence of reliable prognostic features. *Br J Cancer* 1958; 12:321.

47. Whitmore WF: The natural history of prostatic cancer. *Cancer* 1973; 5: 1104–1112.
48. McNeal JE: Regional morphology and pathology of the prostate. *Am J Clin Pathol* 1968; 49:374–357.
49. McNeal JE, Price HM, Redwine EA, et al: Stage A versus stage B adenocarcinoma of the prostate: Morphological comparison and biological significance. *J Urol* 1988; 139:61–65.
50. Stamey TA: Prostate cancer: Some basic clinical and morphometric observations. *Monogr Urol* 1989; 10:79.
51. Evans N, Barnes RW, Brown AF: Carcinoma of the prostate—correlation between the histological observations and the clinical course. *Arch Pathol* 1942; 34:473–483.
52. Wiederanders RE, Stuber RV, Mota C, et al: Prognostic value of grading prostatic carcinoma. *J Urol* 1963; 89:881–888.
53. Bailer JC III, Mellinger GT, Gleason DF: Survival rates of patients with prostatic cancer, tumor stage, and differentiation—preliminary report. *Cancer Chemother Rep* 1966; 50:129–136.
54. Mobley TL, Frank IN: Influence of tumor grade on survival and on serum acid phosphatase levels in metastatic carcinoma of the prostate. *J Urol* 1968; 99:321–323.
55. Schirmer HKA, Murphy GP, Scott WW: Hormonal therapy of prostatic cancer—a correlation between histological differentiation of prostatic cancer and the clinical course of the disease. *Urology Digest* 1965; 3:15.
56. Gleason DF: Classification of prostatic carcinomas. *Cancer Chemother Rep* 1966; 50:125–128.
57. Gleason DF, Mellinger GT, the Veterans Administration Cooperative Urological Research Group: Prediction of prognosis for prostatic adenocarcinoma by combined histological grading and clinical staging. *J Urol* 1974; 111:58–64.
58. Wilson JWL, Morales A, Bruce AW: The prognostic significance of histological grading and pathological staging in carcinoma of the prostate. *J Urol* 1983; 130:481–483.
59. Kramer SA, Spahr J, Brendler CB, et al: Experience with Gleason's histopathological grading in prostate cancer. *J Urol* 1980; 124:223–225.
60. Zincke H, Farrow GM, Myers RP, et al: Relationship between grade and stage of adenocarcinoma of the prostate and pelvic lymph node metastases. *J Urol* 1982; 128:498–501.
61. Fowler JE Jr, Mills SE: Operable prostatic carcinoma: Correlations among clinical stage, pathological stage, Gleason histological score, and early disease-free survival. *J Urol* 1985; 133:49–52.
62. Byar DP, the Veterans Administration Cooperative Urological Research Group: Survival of patients with incidentally found microscopic cancer of the prostate: Results of a clinical trial of conservative treatment. *J Urol* 1972; 108:908–913.
63. Cantrell BB, DeKlerk DP, Eggleston JC, et al: Pathological factors that influence prognosis in stage A prostatic cancer: The influence of extent versus grade. *J Urol* 1981; 125:516–520.
64. Epstein JI, Paull G, Eggleston JC, et al: Prognosis of untreated stage A1 prostatic carcinoma: A study of 94 cases with extended followup. *J Urol* 1986; 136:837–839.
65. Adolfsson J, Fårhaeus B: The natural course of prostatic carcinoma in relation to initial cytological grade. *J Urol* 1988; 140:1452–1454.
66. Willems J-S, Lowhagen T: Transrectal fine-needle aspiration biopsy for cytologic diagnosis and grading of prostatic carcinoma. *Prostate* 1981; 2:381–395.

67. Lowe BA, Listrom MB: Incidental carcinoma of the prostate: An analysis of the predictors of progression. *J Urol* 1988; 140:1340–1344.

68. Lowe BA, Listrom BM: Management of stage A prostate cancer with a high probability of progression. *J Urol* 1988; 140:1345–1347.

69. Stenkvist B, Westman-Naeser S, Holmquist J, et al: Computerized nuclear morphometry as an objective method for characterizing human cancer cell populations. *Cancer Res* 1978; 38:4688–4695.

70. Winkler HZ, Rainwater LM, Myers RP, et al: Stage D1 prostatic adenocarcinoma: Significance of nuclear DNA ploidy patterns studied by flow cytometry. *Mayo Clin Proc* 1988; 63:103–112.

71. Nativ O, Winkler HZ, Raz Y, et al: Stage C prostatic adenocarcinoma: Flow cytometric nuclear DNA ploidy analysis. *Mayo Clin Proc* 1989; 64:911–919.

72. Lee SE, Currin SM, Paulson DF, et al: Flow cytometric determination of ploidy in prostatic adenocarcinoma: A comparison with seminal vesicle involvement and histopathological grading as a predictor of clinical recurrence. *J Urol* 1988; 140:769–774.

73. Montgomery BT, Nativ O, Blute ML, et al: Stage B prostate adenocarcinoma: Flow cytometric nuclear DNA ploidy analysis. *Arch Surg* 1990; 125:327–331.

74. Blute ML, Nativ O, Zincke H, et al: Pattern of failure after radical retropubic prostatectomy for clinically and pathologically localized adenocarcinoma of the prostate: Influence of tumor deoxyribonucleic acid ploidy. *J Urol* 1989; 142:1262–1265.

75. McIntire TL, Murphy WM, Coon JS, et al: The prognostic value of DNA ploidy combined with histologic substaging for incidental carcinoma of the prostate gland. *Am J Clin Pathol* 1988; 89:370–373.

76. Tribukait B: Rapid-flow cytometry of prostatic fine needle aspiration biopsies, in Karr JP, Coffey DS, Gardner W Jr (eds): *Prognostic Cytometry and Cytopathology of Prostate Cancer.* New York, Elsevier Science Publishing, 1989, p 236.

77. Lee SE, Currin SM, Paulson DF, et al: Flow cytometric determination of ploidy in prostatic adenocarcinoma: A comparison with seminal vesicle involvement and histopathological grading as a predictor of clinical recurrence. *J Urol* 1988; 140:769–774.

78. Miller J, Horsfall DJ, Marshall VR, et al: The prognostic value of deoxyribonucleic acid flow cytometric analysis in stage D2 prostatic carcinoma. *J Urol* 1991; 145:1192–1196.

79. Detjer SW Jr, Cunningham RE, Noguchi PD, et al: Prognostic significance of DNA ploidy in carcinoma of the prostate. *Urology* 1989; 33:361–366.

80. Adolfsson J, Tribukait B: Evaluation of tumor progression by repeated fine needle biopsies in prostate adenocarcinoma: Modal deoxyribonucleic acid value and cytological differentiation. *J Urol* 1990; 144:1408–1410.

81. Diamond DA, Berry SJ, Umbricht C, et al: Computerized image analysis of nuclear shape as a prognostic factor for prostatic cancer. *Prostate* 1982; 3:321–332.

82. Diamond DA, Berry SJ, Jewett HJ, et al: A new method to assess metastatic potential of human prostate cancer: Relative nuclear roundness. *J Urol* 1982; 128:729–734.

83. Epstein JI, Berry SJ, Eggleston JC: Nuclear roundness factor: A predictor of prognosis in untreated stage A2 prostate cancer. *Cancer* 1984; 54:1666–1671.

84. Paulson DF, Stone AR, Walther PJ, et al: Radical prostatectomy: Anatomical predictors of success or failure. *J Urol* 1986; 136:1041–1043.

85. Mohler JL, Partin AW, Lohr WD, et al: Nuclear roundness factor measurement

for assessment of prognosis of patients with prostatic adenocarcinoma. I. Testing of a digitization system. *J Urol* 1988; 139:1080–1084.

86. Mohler JL, Partin AW, Epstein JI, et al: Nuclear roundness factor measurement for assessment of prognosis of patients with prostatic carcinoma. II. Standardization of methodology for histologic sections. *J Urol* 1988; 139:1085–1090.

87. Partin AW, Walsh AC, Pitcock RV, et al: A comparison of nuclear morphometry and Gleason grade as a predictor of prognosis in stage A2 prostate cancer: A critical analysis. *J Urol* 1989; 142:1254–1258.

88. Meyer JS, Province M: Proliferative index of breast carcinoma by thymidine labeling: Prognostic power independent of stage, estrogen, and progesterone receptors. *Breast Cancer Res Treat* 1988; 12:191–204.

89. Scrivner DL, Meyer JS, Rujanavech N, et al: Cell kinetics by bromodeoxyuridine labelling and deoxyribonucleic acid ploidy in prostatic carcinoma needle biopsies. *J Urol* 1991; 146:1034–1039.

90. Nemto R, Uchida K, Shimazui T, et al: Immunocytochemical demonstration of S phase cells by anti-bromodeoxyuridine monoclonal antibody in human prostate adenocarcinoma. *J Urol* 1989; 141:337–340.

91. Oomens EHGM, Van Steenbrugge GJ, Van Der Kwast THH, et al: Application of the monoclonal antibody Ki-67 on prostate biopsies to assess the proliferative cell fraction of human prostatic carcinoma. *J Urol* 1991;145:81–85.

92. Schalken JA, Bussemakers MJG, DeBruyne FMJ: Oncogene expression in prostate cancer. *Oncogene* 1990; 7:97–105.

93. Sadasivan R, Morgan R, Jennings S, et al: Overexpression of Her-2/neu may be an indicator of poor prognosis in prostate cancer. *Proc Am Assoc Cancer Res* 1991; 32:A992.

Hormonal Therapy in Prostate Cancer

David F. Paulson, M.D.

Professor and Chief, Division of Urologic Surgery, Duke University Medical Center, Durham, North Carolina

The observation that adult prostatic epithelium atrophies when the sustaining physiologic effect of androgenic hormones is removed led to the therapeutic application of androgen ablation or suppression in the management of prostatic adenocarcinoma.[1-4] The biologic effect of androgens on prostatic epithelium seems dependent on the ability of testosterone to be converted to dihydrotestosterone, the principal intracellular androgen.[5-9]

Circulating testosterone enters the prostatic cell, where it is converted by the enzyme 5α-reductase to dihydrotestosterone, which then is bound to a specific intracellular macromolecular receptor protein. The resulting dihydrotestosterone-receptor complex, after penetrating the cytoplasm undergoes a conformational change that permits the intranuclear translocation of this complex[10] (Fig 1). Once within the nucleus, chromatin binding occurs with initiation of transcription and subsequent messenger RNA formation. The binding site within the nucleus is unknown. Whether the steroid receptors bind to the nuclear matrix or to specific sequences of DNA,[11, 12] it is felt that specific nucleotide sequences are bound and genes activated. Androgens are necessary for prostate growth and androgen ablation will produce marked involution of the prostate. In the intact animal, androgen withdrawal disrupts this orderly growth and results in marked atrophy of the prostatic epithelium.

Testosterone production in the adult male is dependent on an intact hypothalamic-pituitary-testicular axis[13] (Fig 2). Decreased levels of circulating testosterone initiate the hypothalamic release of luteinizing hormone releasing hormone (LHRH). This in turn initiates the pituitary release of luteinizing hormone, which subsequently prompts testosterone synthesis by the Leydig cells of the testis. The Leydig cells of the testis are the major source of testicular androgen. Stimulated by the luteinizing hormone to synthesize testosterone from acetate and cholesterol, the Leydig cells release testosterone into the testicular venous drainage. The testes produce 6 to 7 mg of testosterone per day, usually in a peripheral venous serum testosterone of approximately 600 ng/dL. The resultant enhanced levels of circulating testosterone produce feedback inhibition of LHRH at the hypothalamic level. In response to Leydig cell stimulation, the testis produces 95% of the circulating androgens.[14] The remaining androgens, andro-

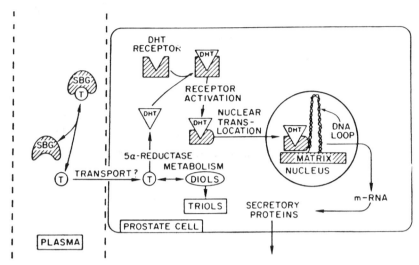

FIG 1.
A schematic of the effects of testosterone growth in an epithelial cell. In the plasma, testosterone is bound to serum-binding globulins *(SBG)*, such as testosterone-binding globulin and albumin. Unbound testosterone *(T)* is transported by diffusion into the prostate, where it is converted enzymatically to dihydrotestosterone *(DHT)* through the action of 5α-reductase, metabolized further to diols (3α or 3β, and metabolized irreversibly into the inactive triols (6α or 7α). DHT binds to a cytoplasmic receptor (which actually may be nuclear), which then is activated and translocated to the nucleus. There, the DHT receptors interact with the acceptors on the nuclear matrix and with DNA. This nuclear binding of the receptor stimulates specific messenger RNA *(m - RNA)* synthesis that is translated at the ribosomes in the cytoplasm to form secretory proteins. (From Coffey DS: The biochemistry and physiology of the prostate and seminal vesicles, in Walsh PC, Gitter RF, Perlmotter AD, et al (eds): *Campbell's Urology,* 5th ed. Philadelphia, Saunders, 1986, p 243. Used by permission.)

stenedione and dehydroepiandrosterone, are of adrenal origin. Ninety-five percent of the circulating androgens either are bound specifically to steroid-binding globulin or are bound nonspecifically to albumin. The unbound androgens are believed to be responsible for the cellular response.[15, 16] Plasma testosterone concentration in adult males averages approximately 600 ng/dL, a level that stays remarkably stable between the ages of 25 and 70 years. Episodic and diurnal variations of the production rate of testosterone occur, with plasma concentrations varying widely within any 24-hour period. Longer cycles averaging 21 days have been observed, superimposed on the daily variation (Table 1).[17] A decrease in testosterone levels has been observed as men age, being seen in the seventh, eighth, and ninth decades of life (Fig 3). Controversy exists as to whether this decreased testicular function occurs through aging or reflects the associated illnesses seen in aged men. Both pituitary and testicular abnormalities have been identified. However, supporting evidence for a pitu-

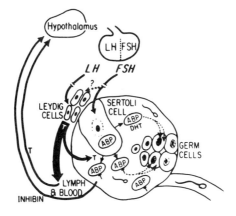

FIG 2.
In response to circulating levels of serum testosterone *(T)* and the degree to which hypothalamic sex steroid receptors are occupied, the hypothalamus releases luteinizing hormone releasing hormone. This prompts release of luteinizing hormone *(LH)* from the anterior pituitary. LH then is carried through the systemic circulation, where it prompts synthesis of T by the Leydig cells. The T is released to body fluids, picked up by the vascular system, and returned, where it establishes a systemic level of serum T. The T in the serum then occupies sex steroid receptors within the hypothalamus. *FSH* = follicle-stimulating hormone; *DHT* = dihydrotestosterone.

itary defect is based on the observations that, while testosterone levels are below normal, the testes can respond following the administration of exogenous gonadotropins. Whether this specific observation accounts for the decreased response of prostatic malignancies in older men to androgen deprivation is as yet undetermined.

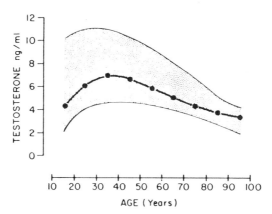

FIG 3.
Decline with age of total testosterone. The *shaded area* represents the range of individual values. (From Coffey DS: The biochemistry and physiology of the prostate and seminal vesicles, in Walsh PC, Gitter RF, Perlmotter AD, et al (eds): *Campbell's Urology,* 5th ed. Philadelphia, Saunders, 1986, p 194. Used by permission.)

TABLE 1.
Plasma Levels of Steroids in Healthy Human Males*

Common Name	Chemical Name	Plasma Concentration			Blood Production Rate (mg/day)	Relative Androgenicity Rat V.P. Assay
		ng/dL	Molarity	Relative Molarity		
Testosterone	17β-hydroxy-4-androstene-3-one	611 ± 186	2.1×10^{-8}	100	6.6 ± 0.5	100
Dihydrotestosterone (DHT; Stanolone)	17β-hydroxy-5α-androstan-3-one	56 ± 20	1.9×10^{-9}	9	0.3 ± 0.06	181
5α-Androstane-3α,17β-diol (3α-androstanediol)	5α-androstan-3α,17β-diol	14 ± 4	4.8×10^{-10}	2	0.2 ± 0.03	126
5α-Androstane-3β,17β-diol (3β-androstanediol)	5α-androstan-3β,17β-diol	<2	$<7 \times 10^{-11}$	<0.3		18
Androstenediol	5-androstene-3β,17β-diol	161 ± 52	5.6×10^{-9}	26		0.21
Androsterone	3α-hydroxy-5α-androstan-17-one	54 ± 32	1.9×10^{-9}	9	0.28	53

Androstenedione	4-androstene-3,17 dione	150 ± 54	5.2×10^{-9}	25	1.4	39
Dehydroepiandrosterone (DHA)	3β-hydroxy-5-androstene-17-one	501 ± 98	1.7×10^{-8}	81	29	15
Dehydroepiandrosterone sulfate (DHAS)	17-oxo-5-androstene-3β-γl-sulfate	$135,925 \pm 48,000$	3.7×10^{-6}	17,619		<1
Progesterone	4-pregnene-3,20-dione	30	9.5×10^{-10}	4.5	0.75	
17β-Estradiol (E$_2$)	1,3,5(10)-estratriene-3,17β-diol	2.5 ± 0.8	9.2×10^{-11}	0.4	0.045	
Estrone	3-hydroxyl-1,3,5(10)-estratriene-17-one	4.6	1.7×10^{-10}	0.8		

*From Coffey DS: The biochemistry and physiology of the prostate and seminal vesicles, in Walsh PC, Gittes RF, Perlmatter AD, et al (eds): *Campbell's Urology*, 5th ed. Philadelphia, Saunders, 1986, p 250. Used by permission.

The hormonal treatment of prostatic adenocarcinoma is based on the assumption that malignant prostatic epithelium is androgen-dependent, as is nonmalignant prostatic tissue. However, most prostatic malignancies are of a heterogeneous population of cells differing in androgen requirements. Although some cells of the tumor mass require physiologic levels of androgen in order to survive, others not only survive, but even may thrive in the absence of androgen. Tumors composed primarily of androgen-dependent cells undergo involution, with the clinical indication of a good response to androgen deprivation therapy. Tumors that are composed primarily of androgen-independent cells do not respond well to the removal of androgen. Thus, the variation in clinical response is dependent upon the biologic androgen-dependent or -independent characteristics of the tumor, rather than upon the treatment itself.

Controversies in the Use of Androgen Deprivation

Is Immediate or Delayed Androgen Deprivation of Greater Benefit?

Physicians are faced with the dilemma as to whether they should initiate androgen deprivation at the time that metastatic disease is identified or

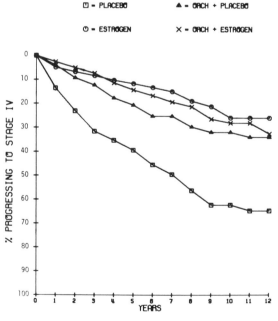

FIG 4.
Prostate I Study using diethylstilbestrol 5 mg/day, orchiectomy plus placebo, or orchiectomy plus diethylstilbestrol 5 mg/day demonstrated that these three active forms of androgen deprivation were more effective than placebo in preventing progression of disease.

whether they are permitted ethically to delay androgen deprivation until the patient experiences pain or other ravages of disease progression. The early Veterans Administration Cooperative Research Group examined the impact of active androgen deprivation using either orchiectomy, estrogen plus orchiectomy, or estrogen alone vs. a placebo in a population of patients with stage C prostatic adenocarcinoma (Figs 4 and 5). Their trial effectively demonstrated that active androgen deprivation using either orchiectomy, orchiectomy and diethylstilbestrol, or diethylstilbestrol alone, each was more effective (in that order) at slowing the progression of disease from stage C to stage D. When overall survival was examined, however, it was noted that the patients on the placebo arm survived as long as did those who received active androgen deprivation. Although initially interpreted as indicating that placebo was as effective as androgen deprivation, reexamination of the data showed that patients who received the placebo were treated with androgen deprivation when progression occurred. Thus, this large-volume randomized trial demonstrated that early and delayed androgen deprivation seemed to have equivalent effectiveness when survival alone was examined.

A nonrandomized trial from the Duke Medical Center used androgen deprivation in patients with minimal localized residual disease. In the early 1970s, patients with margin-positive residual disease after radical prostatectomy were subjected to either immediate androgen deprivation or no

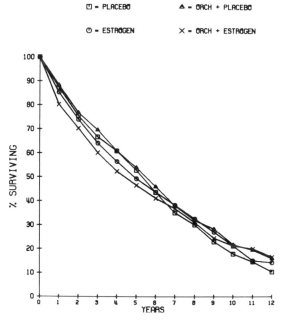

FIG 5.
Active androgen deprivation using diethylstilbestrol 5 mg/day, orchiectomy plus placebo, or orchiectomy plus diethylstilbestrol 5 mg/day were no more effective than placebo alone (or delayed androgen deprivation) in affecting survival.

androgen deprivation based upon the personal preference of both the physician and the patient. An analysis of this cohort of patients in the late 1980s demonstrated that, although immediate androgen deprivation at the time of radical prostatectomy produced a delay in the subsequent appearance of either local or distant recurrent disease, when survival was examined, this conferred no advantage (Fig 6). This leads to the conclusion that the physician has an ethical basis for delaying androgen deprivation in an asymptomatic patient if that is the decision reached by both physician and patient. The rationale for such occurrence is based on the premise that the doubling time of the tumor mass remains constant throughout the residual survival experience of the host, and upon the secondary assumption that the percentage of patients who are "androgen-dependent" remains constant throughout the lifetime of that tumor mass. Thus, a tumor mass of 10 billion cells that is 90% androgen-dependent would have a residually active population of 1 billion cells after androgen deprivation. Assuming a doubling time of 6 months, at the end of 2 years, this residual population of 1 billion cells would number 8 billion. If the original 10 billion cells experienced a similar doubling time, within 2 years, the 10 billion cells would become 80 billion cells. If androgen deprivation were initiated then, assuming 90% reduction, only 10% of the cells (8 billion) would be viable at the 24-month mark. Thus, in both instances, the host would be left with a similar number of active residual cancer cells. Although growth kinetics may alter somewhat depending upon the nutritional status of the host, the survival rate observed in patients treated with immediate vs. delayed androgen deprivation seems to support the above scenario.

What Is the Optimal Form of Single-Agent Androgen Deprivation?

Reduction of androgenic support of prostatic epithelium can be accomplished therapeutically by (1) removing the primary source of circulating androgens, (2) suppressing the reduced hypothalamic LHRH, (3) reducing the release of luteinizing hormone by the anterior pituitary, (4) inhibiting androgen synthesis directly at the cellular level, and (5) blocking androgens or their effect at the cellular level (Fig 7).

Removal of the Primary Androgen Source

Serum testosterone levels in the normal male range between 400 and 1,000 ng/dL. Bilateral orchiectomy will reduce plasma testosterone levels by 90%.[15, 16, 18-21] In the adult human male, there is no detectable increase in plasma testosterone levels from the activation of secondary androgen sources following orchiectomy. Patients treated by orchiectomy alone experience a median survival of 18 to 28 months, depending on the extent of disease at the initiation of therapy. The appearance of endocrine-unresponsive symptomatic disease after bilateral orchiectomy is not associated with demonstrable increases in the level of circulating plasma andro-

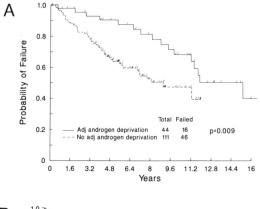

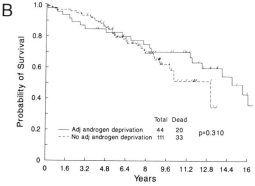

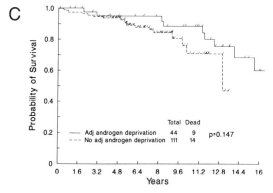

FIG 6.
Kaplan-Meier projections of failures **(A)**, death of any cause **(B)**, and death of prostatic cancer **(C)** as a function of immediate or no immediate adjunctive *(adj)* androgen deprivation. Four patients who underwent cystoprostatectomy for transitional cell tumors but who had incidental prostate carcinoma were excluded from analysis. Note that only probability of failure curve demonstrates a statistically significant difference in outcome.

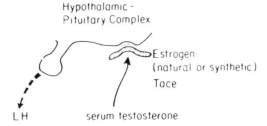

FIG 7.
Certain exogenously administered agents block hypothalamic receptors, sequentially suppressing both luteinizing hormone releasing hormone and luteinizing hormone *(LH)* secretion. The activity of chlorotrianisene *(Tace)* at this site is debated.

stenedione, dehydroepiandrosterone, or testosterone, indicating that symptomatic recurrence is not associated with an increase in circulating androgens or their metabolic end products.[14, 20, 22]

Bilateral orchiectomy appears to be the most cost-effective method of treatment for prostatic carcinoma. McClinton and coworkers from the Aberdeen Royal Infirmary examined the relative expense of bilateral orchiectomy vs. outpatient treatment with either cyproterone acetate or the LHRH analogue goserelin.[23] Orchiectomy was one tenth to one fifth the cost of treatment with either drug. In this study, all patients were admitted to the hospital for operation. It is current practice in the United States to perform orchiectomy either in the office or as an outpatient at the hospital. In these settings, bilateral orchiectomy appears to be the most cost-effective method of initiating androgen deprivation.

Manipulation of the Hypothalamic-Pituitary Axis With Exogenous Sex Steroids

Estrogens establish their major effect at the hypothalamic level by occupying the hypothalamic binding site of testosterone. Thus, they inhibit the release of LHRH, which produces subsequent suppression of luteinizing hormone release by the pituitary and a reduction in testosterone production by the testis. In the adult human male, no evidence exists that estrogens directly induce regression of prostatic epithelium. Studies in the intact dog have indicated that estrogens (stilbestrol) may influence directly the secretory ability of the prostate. In addition, in vitro studies have shown that stilbestrol in high levels can inhibit directly DNA polymerase and 5α-reductase.[24, 25] However, the level of estrogen required for in vitro enzyme inhibition is far greater than the pharmacologic levels that can be achieved in humans.[24, 26]

Plasma testosterone levels in males treated with 1 mg/day of stilbestrol or its equivalent show variation not only between individuals, but also with respect to serial values obtained during longitudinal observations in a single person. Serum testosterone levels may not reach anorchid levels.

TABLE 2.
Effect of Bilateral Orchiectomy or Treatment With Stilbestrol on Plasma Levels of Testosterone in Men With Carcinoma of the Prostate*

| | | | Mean Plasma Testosterone Levels (ng/dl ± SD) | | | | | |
| | | | | Stilbestrol (mg/day)† | | | | |
Authors	Reference	Pretreatment	Bilateral Orchiectomy	0.2	1.0	3.0	5.0
Young HH, Kent JR	21	560	<50				<50
Robinson MRG, Thomas BS	15	607 ± 235	30			<10a	
Mackler MA, et al.	20	620 ± 260	50 ± 50		80c	46 ± 19b	190d
Kent JR, et al.	22						
Stage C		620 ± 288		570 ± 335b	320 ± 220b		210 ± 246b
Stage D		640 ± 335		700 ± 276	410 ± 359		130 ± 110
Shearer RJ, et al.	16	280	47 ± 23		66–86 ± 58	45 ± 20e	47 ± 25

*From Walsh PC: Urol Clin North Am 1975; 2:132.
†Treatment key: a = <6 months; b = >6 months; c = 7 days; d = 2 days; e = 6 to 24 months.

Three milligrams per day of stilbestrol suppresses testosterone levels to the castrate range (Table 2).

Doses greater than 3 mg/day do not produce any additional androgen-suppressing effect and are accompanied by unacceptable cardiovascular risks. As identical goals can be achieved with both orchiectomy and exogenous sex steroids, there does not seem to be any evidence to support simultaneous treatment with both methods. Responses to diethylstilbestrol and orchiectomy appear equivalent (Table 3).

There is increasing evidence that diethylstilbestrol carries unacceptable cardiovascular hazard. One recently published study examined the cardiovascular toxicity of the agent vs. orchiectomy and found that approximately 25% of men receiving diethylstilbestrol experienced a cardiovascular event during the first 12 months of treatment. Risk of cardiovascular toxicity could not be predicted by screening for clinical evidence of atherosclerotic disease (Tables 4 and 5). Aro and colleagues from Finland have provided additional information on the adverse cardiovascular consequences of using exogenous estrogens to achieve androgen deprivation. Although their trial of 150 patients with locally advanced prostatic cancer (T3–4M0) originally was designed to examine the impact of orchiectomy, estrogens, or radiation therapy, their 4-year follow-up period was too brief for any significant difference in progression rates to be seen between the therapy groups. However, 13 of 50 patients who had been randomized to receive exogenous estrogens experienced thromboembolic or other cardiovascular complications. This high rate of cardiovascular problems argues strongly against the use of exogenous estrogens.[27] Henriksson and co-workers, in an attempt to predict cardiovascular complications in patients with prostatic cancer who were receiving exogenous estrogen, subjected patients to an exercise stress test, a physiologic evaluation of peripheral blood circulation, a blood value estimation, chest radiographs, and blood tests including determinations of hormone, lipoprotein, and antithrombin III levels. In their randomized trial, 25% of the patients treated with estrogen therapy had cardiovascular complications during the initial treatment

---

TABLE 3.
Initial Response Rate of Previously Untreated Patients With Advanced Prostatic Cancer*

Diethylstilbestrol or Orchiectomy	Number of Patients	Response Rate, %
Murphy et al.	83	80.7
Leuprolide Study Group	94	87

*Data from Murphy GP, et al: *Cancer* 1983; 51:1264 and Leuprolide Study Group: *N Engl J Med* 1984; 311:1281.

TABLE 4.
Cardiovascular Hazard of Estrogens vs. Orchiectomy*

Method of Treatment	Number of Patients (n = 91)	Major Cardiovascular Event in 12 Mo
Orchiectomy	44	0/44
Estrogens	47	13/47(25%)

*From Henriksson P, Edhag O, Eriksson A, et al: *Br J Urol* 1989; 63:186–190. Used by permission.

year. Their study permitted the identification of two discriminating variables for cardiovascular complications of estrogen therapy in patients without overt clinical cardiovascular disease: luteinizing hormone elevation and ST segment depression during exercise. They concluded that patients with ST segment depression during exercise testing or with a high luteinizing hormone concentration should not be treated with exogenous estrogens. No explanation for the link between luteinizing hormone levels and cardiovascular risk could be provided.[28] As cardiovascular toxicity cannot be predicted by screening for clinical evidence of atherosclerotic disease, and as the risk of an adverse cardiovascular event is so high using exogenous diethylstilbestrol, I believe that exogenous sex steroids should not be used.

TABLE 5.
Incidence of Major Cardiovascular Events in Estrogen Treatment Group in Relation to Prevalence of Minor Signs of Atherosclerosis at Entry to Study*

Patient Status	Minor Signs of Atherosclerosis (n = 10)	No Sign of Atherosclerosis (n = 43)
Number of patients who had a cardiovascular event	3 (30%)	10 (23%)
Number of patients who did not have a major cardiovascular event	7 (70%)	33 (77%)

*From Henriksson P, Edhag O, Eriksson A, et al: *Br J Urol* 1989; 63:186–190. Used by permission.

Many other available agents provide an equivalent effect without such high toxicity.

Patients who have received exogenous estrogens for an extended period occasionally may be removed from diethylstilbestrol without substituting orchiectomy. Tomic and colleagues withdrew diethylstilbestrol from a group of patients who had received it for 8 years or more. Serum testosterone levels remained at castrate levels in all patients (Fig 8). Patients removed from exogenous estrogen treatment due to an adverse cardiovascular event do not need to receive an alternative form of therapy immediately. It is totally appropriate to monitor the serum testosterone level on a longitudinal basis and to initiate another type of androgen deprivation only when levels begin to rise.

Radiation of Luteinizing Hormone Release by the Use of Luteinizing Hormone Releasing Hormone Analogues

The recent demonstration that LHRH analogues may function at a central level to suppress testosterone synthesis has prompted examination of this alternative method of achieving disease control. LHRH is a hypothalamic decapeptide that induces the release of luteinizing hormone and follicle-stimulating hormone from the pituitary. Native LHRH has a short-lived ef-

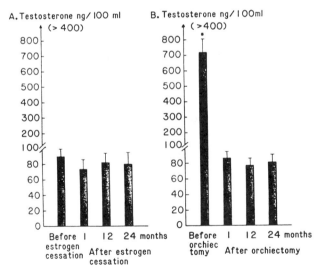

FIG 8.
Serum concentrations of testosterone both before and after withdrawal of estrogen treatment (**A**) in 14 patients treated for prostatic carcinoma for more than 4 years compared to age-matched patients treated with orchiectomy (**B**). (From Tomic, Bergman: J Urol 1987; 138:801. Used by permission.)

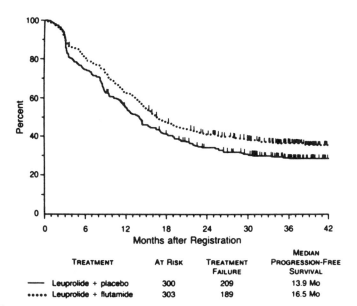

TREATMENT	AT RISK	TREATMENT FAILURE	MEDIAN PROGRESSION-FREE SURVIVAL
—— Leuprolide + placebo	300	209	13.9 Mo
•••• Leuprolide + flutamide	303	189	16.5 Mo

FIG 9.
Progression-free survival (*P* = .039). (From Crawford ED: *N Engl J Med* 1989; 321:419. Used by permission.)

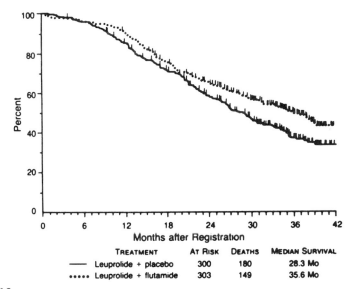

TREATMENT	AT RISK	DEATHS	MEDIAN SURVIVAL
—— Leuprolide + placebo	300	180	28.3 Mo
•••• Leuprolide + flutamide	303	149	35.6 Mo

FIG 10.
Overall survival (P = .035). (From Crawford ED: *N Engl J Med* 1989; 321:419. Used by permission.)

fect on gonadotropin secretion and, therefore, is not suitable for long-term therapy. By substituting other amino acids within the decapeptide chain, LHRH analogues have been synthesized that produce a marked and prolonged effect.

Randomized trial data indicate that the LHRH analogue leuprolide is as effective as diethylstilbestrol in affecting survival (Figs 9 and 10).[29, 30] A similar trial comparing goserelin acetate to orchiectomy also has demonstrated no specific benefit of either treatment (Fig 11). The mode of action of these agents is not understood fully. Current hypotheses include pituitary depletion of luteinizing hormone, pituitary desensitization to pituitary luteinizing hormone feedback, and direct extrapituitary action of the luteinizing hormone analogue on the testis. Following treatment with the LHRH analogues, there is an initial increase in serum testosterone production (Fig 12, A). This may be accompanied by a disease "failure" characterized by an increase in bone pain and elevation in serum prostate specific antigen (PSA) and prostate acid phosphatase (PAP) levels. However, after several days, serum androgens will decrease to the castrate level. Serum prolactin will not change significantly and serum estradiol will decrease. The accumulated evidence indicates that these agents are as effective as orchiectomy in managing previously untreated disease, but that they will not permit rescue of patients who have failed alternative forms of androgen deprivation therapy.

Both leuprolide and goserelin acetate are available in depo formulations. Randomized clinical trials have demonstrated that depo leuprolide is as effective as daily injection (see Fig 12,B).

Inhibitors of Androgen Synthesis at the Cellular Level

Selective inhibitors of androgen synthesis should produce pharmaceutical orchiectomy; however, although certain of these agents are available for

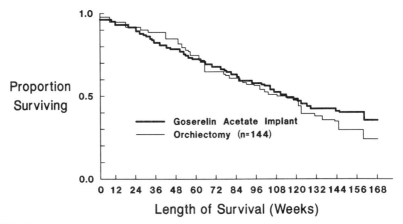

FIG 11.
Survival rates of patients receiving goserelin vs. orchiectomy. (From Peeling WB: *Urology* 1989; 33(suppl):45. Used by permission.)

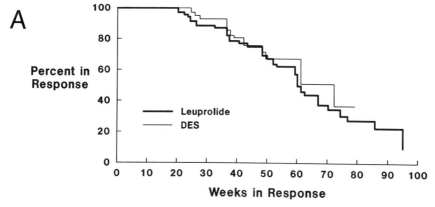

N Engl J Med 1984;311:1281-1286

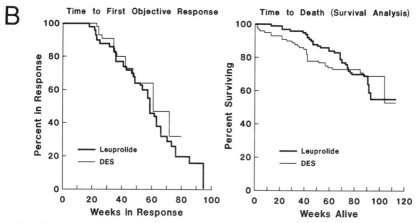

FIG 12.
Leuprolide compared to diethylstilbestrol *(DES).* **A,** time to first objective progression. **B,** time to death. (From Leuprolide Study Group: *N Engl J Med* 1984; 311:1281. Used by permission.)

clinical trials, none has been released yet with this specific indication. Aminoglutethimide blocks side-chain cleavage of cholesterol and subsequent hydroxylation, inhibiting the production of both cortisone and aldosterone (Fig 13).[15] Cyproterone acetate blocks 17,20-desmolase and, thus, interferes with androgen synthesis.[13, 31] Both agents have been evaluated in the treatment of endocrine-unresponsive, malignant prostatic disease, but neither has been found to be effective in reversing the clinical course of this patient population.[15, 16] Although Robinson and Thomas showed that aminoglutethimide suppressed plasma testosterone levels to below 10 ng/ dL, Shearer and associates failed to demonstrate any significant suppression in their study of 12 patients.

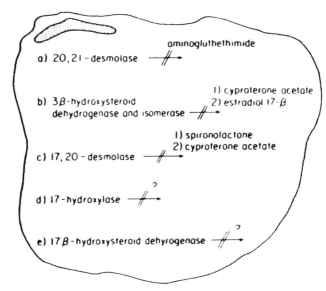

FIG 13.
Three of the five major enzymes involved in androgen synthesis may be selectively inhibited.

Worgul and associates, in a study of 25 previously castrated men with progressive stage D carcinoma who were treated with 1,000 mg of amino-glutethimide and 40 mg of hydrocortisone daily, demonstrated a complete response in 1 patient and a partial response in 4.[32] Significant suppression of both serum testosterone and dihydrotestosterone was noted after treatment. Although these observations are of interest, whether they imply that lowering serum testosterone below castrate levels will induce a further clinical response is unproved. Nonetheless, these results do prompt further clinical study.

Walsh and Siiteri, using spironolactone, found that plasma testosterone levels were suppressed by 90%, and that plasma androstenedione and dehydroepiandrosterone levels were suppressed by 40% to 60%.[13, 33, 34] Since it has not been demonstrated that the symptomatic reactivation of malignant prostatic disease is associated with residual androgen production either by the adrenal or by a residual testis, the theoretic lack of efficacy of these agents is unconfirmed in practice.

Ketoconazole is an orally administered synthetic imidazole dioxolan that has been used in the treatment of superficial and deep fungal infections. This drug has been demonstrated to reduce adrenal and testicular androgen production in both animals and humans. Ketoconazole is believed to exert its effect by interfering with cytochrome P-450–dependent 14-demethylation, thereby interfering with conversion of lanosterol to cholesterol. The predominant effect is inhibition of the formation of androstenedione, dehydroepiandrosterone, and testosterone. When ketoconazole is administered at a dosage of 400 mg every 12 hours, serum testosterone initially will decrease to castrate levels, and previously untreated patients will demonstrate a clinical response evidence by improvement in pain and decrease in serum prostatic acid phosphatase levels. Preliminary data indicate that, as an initial treatment, the drug is effective in the management of previously untreated patients, but again no advantage is achieved by combining this with alternative medication, nor will it rescue previously treated patients.[35-37]

Antiandrogens

The antiandrogens do not lower serum androgen levels, but do block the cellular uptake of androgens at the target organ by inhibiting the nuclear uptake of dihydrotestosterone.[38, 39] Antiandrogens come in two forms: steroidal and nonsteroidal. The steroidal androgens include megestrol acetate and cyproterone acetate. The nonsteroidal antiandrogens include flutamide and anandron.

Antiandrogens block the effectiveness of androgens at the target level by interfering with the intracellular events that mediate androgenic action. These agents are capable of inhibiting both endogenously secreted and exogenously administered androgens.[35, 40, 41] All effective compounds tested to date act through a common mechanism by inhibiting the formation of the receptor-dihydrotestosterone complex, interrupting the binding of a dihydrotestosterone-receptor complex to nuclear chromatin and thereby suppressing RNA formation and protein synthesis (Fig 14). Cyproterone acetate is the most potent of the steroidal antiandrogens. It is well absorbed locally, and not only produces target organ inhibition, but also interferes with gonadotropin release and inhibits steroidogenesis.

Cyproterone acetate is a derivative of 17-hydroxyprogesterone. It functions in a manner similar to the progestational agents in that the drug blocks gonadotropin release from the pituitary. Cyproterone acetate inhibits the formation of dihydrotestosterone-receptor complex in the prostatic nuclei while also inhibiting the C21–19-desmolase enzyme, which is responsible for the synthesis of adrenal androgens. The drug does not seem to be more effective than other monotherapies. It may be administered with low-dose diethylstilbestrol to prevent the escape phenomenon that has been observed with other progestational agents.

The peripheral antiandrogenic action of cyproterone acetate on the adult untreated male is accompanied by a decrease in total plasma testosterone concentration and suppression of the plasma follicle-stimulating hormone concentration.[33] Cyproterone acetate has been used as the initial form of therapy in a small series of previously untreated males with malignant prostatic disease. Plasma testosterone and luteinizing hormone concentrations were determined at varying levels during therapy. The plasma testosterone concentration showed a sharp decline from control levels within the first week of therapy and was maintained at greatly reduced levels for at

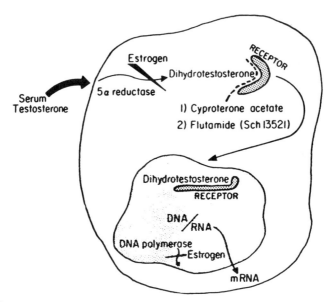

FIG 14.
The antiandrogens cyproterone acetate and flutamide block the formation of the dihydrotestosterone receptor complex. Estrogens in vitro will inhibit 5α-reductase and DNA polymerase activity. *mRNA* = messenger RNA.

least 16 weeks. The plasma follicle-stimulating hormone levels were suppressed significantly during the second and fourth weeks of therapy, whereas the plasma luteinizing hormone concentration was essentially unchanged during cyproterone acetate treatment. The findings suggest that the peripheral antiandrogenic action of cyproterone acetate may be augmented by a reduction in plasma testosterone concentration and suppression of pituitary gonadotropin secretion. No special benefit seems to be derived from the use of cyproterone acetate in the treatment of estrogen-unresponsive males.[34, 42]

Flutamide (Eulixin) is a nonsteroidal antiandrogen that does not reduce either gonadotropin or plasma testosterone levels.[40, 43, 44] Flutamide apparently inhibits the binding of testosterone and dihydrotestosterone to androgen receptors within the cell.[45] As the drug neither inhibits gonadotropin release nor suppresses testosterone synthesis, patients maintain normal or slightly elevated serum testosterone levels. The drug does not appear to be more effective than standard endocrine therapy when used as a single agent. Most patients will develop gynecomastia when the drug is used alone. Side effects include nausea, vomiting, and diarrhea. Serum testosterone levels do not drop, and many patients retain libido and potency. Anandron, another antiandrogen, functions in a manner similar to flutamide. It does produce visual disturbances in some patients. The antiestrogen tamoxifen has been used in both previously untreated and androgen-independent prostatic carcinoma. No significant response in either treatment group has been identified with tamoxifen, and it is felt that the accrued data do not support continued investigation of the agent in advanced prostatic malignancy.[46, 47]

Controversy: The Benefit of Relative Androgen Deprivation (Monotherapy) Vs. Complete Androgen Blockage (Combination Therapy)

Current discussions focus upon a comparison of the effectiveness of relative androgen blockade vs. total or complete androgen blockade. Relative androgen blockade refers to the use of therapies that produce anorchid levels of serum testosterone and that do not consider adrenal androgens to be of importance in the maintenance of malignant prostatic growth. Complete or total androgen blockade refers to those therapies designed to ablate the effect of adrenal and testicular androgen production. Those who promote total androgen blockade argue that up to 30% of patients with advanced prostatic cancer who relapse with disease progression after treatment with therapies designed to control only the influence of testicular androgens do respond to both surgical and medical adrenalectomy. However, careful review of the impact of medical or surgical adrenalectomy or hypophysectomy in patients whose condition has not responded to monotherapy reveals an overall response rate of only about 7%. Thus, those who emphasize this aspect of total androgen blockade interpret previous studies with excessive enthusiasm. It also must be recognized that these patients receive supplemental corticosteroids; it may be that their apparent clinical improvement is related not so much to disease control as to the feeling of well-being produced by the exogenous androgens. The administration of exogenous steroids has been reported to produce a marked decrease in pain and disease activity in patients who have been treated by relative androgen deprivation. Those who support total androgen deprivation have argued that these observations indicate that there is a continued low level of androgen dependence, and they conclude that low levels of adrenal androgens may contribute to the continued growth of prostatic malignancies. However, current data strongly indicate that this "exogenous androgen–induced flair" probably occurs through the activation of prolactin and estrogen receptors.

Several hypotheses have been developed to explain the phenomenon of clinical relapse in patients treated with relative androgen deprivation. One theory is that prostatic cancer cells are variably sensitive to androgens and that the relapse observed following an initial response results from inadequate suppression of androgenic impact. This hypothesis sustains enthusiasm for total androgen blockade, since this should produce complete reduction in the androgen-dependent clones and increase both time to progression and survival. The second hypothesis focuses on the heterogeneity of the malignant cells and proposes that this heterogeneity produces a differential growth requirement for androgens, with relapse resulting from the emergence of androgen-independent cell lines. If this hypothesis is correct, total androgen blockade should have little or no effect.[48]

Animal studies support both hypotheses. The androgen-sensitive Shionogi mouse mammary tumor model has been used both to support and to deny the value of total androgen blockade. Incubation of androgen-sensitive Shionogi mouse mammary cancer cells for 2 weeks in the absence of androgen produces androgen-independent cell growth. However, since cells are preincubated with flutamide in the presence of androgens, the cells remain androgen-sensitive. The study implies that the administration of androgens might delay the development of androgen insensitivity. Other investigators have used this same model to explain the variable sensitivity of prostatic cancer cells. Figure 15 indicates the percentage of cells surviving with increasing levels of dihydrotestosterone.[48] Some clones require higher levels of dihydrotestosterone to sustain cell growth than do others. The tumor mass is made of multiple clones, certain of which within this tumor mass are able to grow at reduced androgen levels. This model supports control strategies designed to reduce the impact of any circulating androgen.

Isaacs and coworkers examined the effect of partial vs. total androgen deprivation in rats bearing the Dunning 3327H (well-differentiated) and

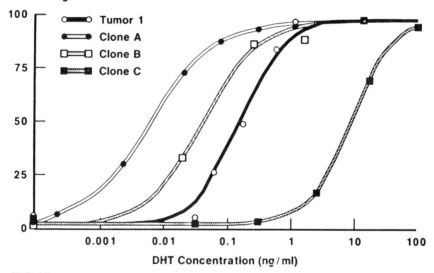

FIG 15.
The percent survival with increasing levels of dihydrotestosterone *(DHT)*. Clones of cells to the right require higher levels of DHT in the media to grow than do ones to the left. (From Crawford ED: Total androgen blockade, in Crawford ED, Lynch JH (eds): *Progress Report on the Clinical Treatment of Prostatic Cancer.* Colorado Springs, Colo, Tap Pharmaceuticals, 1990, p 73. Used by permission.)

3327R (poorly differentiated) prostatic malignancies. Appropriate control subjects were used. Tumor-bearing rats were treated either with orchiectomy alone or with orchiectomy and cyproterone acetate, a progestational antiandrogen. No difference in growth or survival could be observed in the two groups.

The U.S. Intergroup Study was designed to determine the potential benefit of total androgen blockade using leuprolide and flutamide. The study design was placebo-controlled, double-blinded, prospective, and randomized. Six hundred and three patients were eligible for evaluation; all of them had untreated, histologically confirmed, D2 prostatic carcinoma with bone or measurable soft-tissue metastases. Three hundred and three patients received leuprolide plus flutamide and 300 received leuprolide plus placebo. When both survival and progression were examined, an increase in time to progression from 13.9 to 16.5 months was noted in patients receiving the combination therapy and a statistically significant difference in survival of 35.6 months was observed with combination therapy as compared to 28.3 months in patients receiving leuprolide alone (Figs 16 and 17 and Tables 2 and 3).[49] The Canadian trial stratified patients to orchiectomy with or without Nilutamide. Patients treated with orchiectomy plus Nilutamide experienced both an increase in time to progression and a sur-

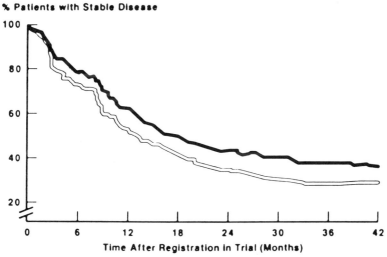

% Patients with Stable Disease

Treatment Regimen	No. at Risk	No. of Failures	Median Time to Progression
■■■ Leuprolide Acetate + Flutamide	303	189	16.5 Months
▭ Leuprolide Acetate + Placebo	300	209	13.9 Months

FIG 16.
Progression-free survival by treatment regimen. (From Crawford ED: Total androgen blockade, in Crawford ED, Lynch JH (eds): *Progress Report on the Clinical Treatment of Prostatic Cancer.* Colorado Springs, Colo, Tap Pharmaceuticals, 1990, p 74. Used by permission.)

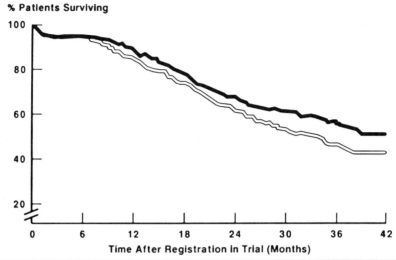

FIG 17.
Overall survival by treatment regimen. (From Crawford ED: Total androgen blockade, in Crawford ED, Lynch JH (eds): *Progress Report on the Clinical Treatment of Prostatic Cancer.* Colorado Springs, Colo, Tap Pharmaceuticals, 1990, p 75. Used by permission.)

vival advantage over those treated with orchiectomy alone (Fig 18). Patients receiving orchiectomy plus Nilutamide experienced a median survival of 24 months as compared to over 18 months in patients receiving orchiectomy alone.

A recent but as yet unpublished report of a multi-institutional, multinational trial comparing orchiectomy with or without the antiandrogen Nilutamide also demonstrated a 6-month survival advantage in patients treated with the combination of orchiectomy and antiandrogen administration. The median survival rates approximated those seen in the U.S. Intergroup Trial.

It must be concluded that total (or complete) androgen deprivation achieved by use of an antiandrogen plus any other therapy that ablates testicular androgen production provides a survival advantage over monotherapy alone. The combination therapies appear to add about 6 months to the median survival time. It seems appropriate to inform patients who are about to embark on a course of androgen deprivation of the relative benefit of combination therapy.

Androgen Deprivation in Stage C Cancer

Stage C (T3N0M0) prostatic carcinoma has presented difficulties in treatment selection. A randomized trial comparing radiation vs. observation

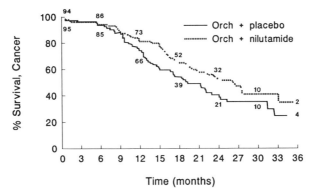

FIG 18.
Demonstrated median survival advantage in patients treated with orchiectomy *(orch)* plus nilutamide vs. orchiectomy plus placebo.

demonstrated no advantages of radiation, suggesting that the purported impact of radiation could be nothing more than an observation of the natural history of the disease. This has prompted others to explore alternative treatments such as androgen deprivation for stage C disease. Early androgen deprivation delays the appearance of extension, but does not enhance survival.[50–53] Some investigators have used androgen deprivation as an adjunct to other therapy to determine if any disease control benefit would emerge. Zagars and coworkers sought to determine whether adjunctive androgen deprivation achieved by the early administration of diethylstilbestrol would change the course of clinical stage C adenocarcinoma of the prostate. In their study, 78 patients with such disease were randomized prospectively to receive either radiation alone or radiation and adjunctive androgen deprivation using diethylstilbestrol. No patient had received any prior treatment. Patients who were not treated initially with androgen deprivation were provided with it when disease progression or failure was identified. Disease-free survival was enhanced by the use of androgen deprivation (Fig 19)[54]; when overall survival was examined, however, no advantage was accorded to the group that received early adjunctive androgen deprivation. These data strongly suggest that the dominant disease-control modality is androgen deprivation and not radiation. This trial also suggests that any disease-control trial that examines therapies other than androgen deprivation should not include androgen deprivation as an adjunctive treatment, since its impact probably will outweigh that of any other treatment modality.

The therapeutic dilemma posed by patients with stage C adenocarcinoma of the prostate combined with enthusiasm to establish a beneficial treatment prompted early investigators to determine if an initial course of androgen ablation would reduce a clinical T3 lesion enough in size to make it amenable to surgical extirpation. In 1969, Scott and Boyd reported their experience, which extended over 25 years.[55] It is interesting to examine the patient population that subsequently received radical surgery. All patients with obvious metastatic disease were excluded. Furthermore,

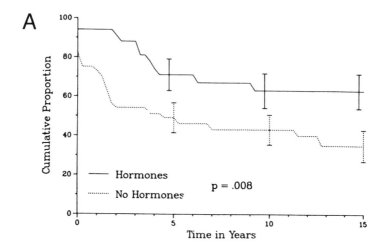

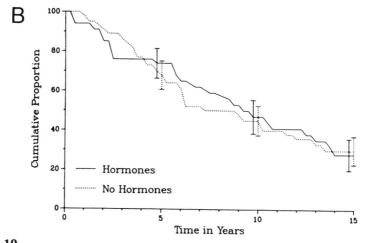

FIG 19.
A, actuarial survival curves according to treatment actually received. **B,** disease-free survival curves according to treatment actually received. *Vertical bars* are standard errors. (From Zagars GK, Johnson DE, von Eschenback AC, et al: *Int J Radiat Oncol Biol Phys* 1988; 14:1085–1091. Used by permission.)

only patients with tumor grades I and II were included in the treatment group, as it was the researchers' experience that those with grade III disease would not have survived sufficiently long to accept them for subsequent surgical therapy. No patient who maintained a persistent elevation of either alkaline or acid phosphatase level was included in the surgical group, and any patient with a markedly advanced local lesion was excluded from receiving the combined form of therapy.

All patients were treated with combined therapy, which consisted of orchiectomy and estrogens. Patients were treated for 6 months or more before they were considered for surgery. Only when maximum regression had occurred was surgical intervention initiated. Last, following radical perineal prostatectomy, all patients were urged to remain on the androgen deprivation protocol they had received previously.

In their 1969 article, Scott and Boyd reported on 44 patients who had been selected and treated as outlined above. Thirty-nine patients had been followed for 5 years or more and 24 (61%) had survived without evidence of cancer. Thirty-three patients were followed for 10 years or more and 17 (51%) were alive without obvious evidence of disease. Determining the impact of this study design is difficult, as there are two treatments to evaluate. Was the survival in this highly selected group of patients promoted by the androgen deprivation or by the surgery? As the patients all had demonstrated a good response to androgen deprivation, and a response that had lasted for at least 6 months, the primary impact of this combined therapy probably was afforded by androgen deprivation and not by subsequent surgical intervention.[55]

Nonetheless, based on these early observations, many investigators began again to explore the possibility of using preoperative androgen deprivation to downstage tumors and render them operable. The basic flaw in this thinking is the belief that androgen deprivation merely rolls or pushes all of the tumor cells back into the original tumor mass and confines them within its anatomic capsule. Preoperative androgen deprivation may reduce the size of the primary tumor mass and the thickness of the "tentacles" of tumor that extend along vascular spaces and fascial planes, but it does not roll these tumor cells back into the primary tumor mass as one would a window shade. The largest experience to date in using preoperative androgen deprivation has been accumulated by the group at Ann Arbor.[56] These investigators have two nonrandomized groups of patients,

TABLE 6.
Percent Deviation of Prostate Acid Phosphatase Above and Below Mean Over 48 Hours*

Mean	Maximum Deviation, %		Average Deviation, %	
	Above	**Below**	**Above**	**Below**
36.5	34	26	20.4	14.4
1.91	33	25	15.2	11.1
2.8	25	46	8.3	33.5
9.5	79	49	36.8	36.3
8.4	56	50	26.1	27.0

*From Maatman TJ, Gupta MK, Montie JE, et al: *J Urol* 1984; 132:58. Used by permission.

one of whom received preoperative androgen deprivation therapy prior to radical prostatectomy and the other of whom received radical prostatectomy alone. Their most recent results demonstrate that, overall, the rate of tumors with positive margins was reduced in patients who received preoperative androgen deprivation (Table 6). However, on examining their margin-positive rates on the basis of clinical stage, no patient with stage C disease who received preoperative androgen deprivation had negative tumor margins. The fact that patients who were at lower clinical stages had a lower incidence of tumors with positive margins may reflect the fact that the lesser prostatic volume resulting from preoperative androgen deprivation increases the surgeon's ability to encompass the disease during surgical extirpation, or that the surgeon's preoperative clinical assessment was in error and these "downstaged" patients were overstaged prior to surgical intervention. A more probable explanation is that preoperative androgen deprivation confounds the ability of the pathologists to assess small-volume extraprostatic disease.

Evaluation of Impact

A clinician treating a patient with metastatic disease must attempt to provide both life to his years and years to his life. The most important parameter to be evaluated is the patient's clinical or subjective response to treatment, i.e., has his general feeling of well-being improved and is somatic pain decreased or absent? Although there are objective indicators of disease response and it may be important to monitor them, identifying them in a patient who has metastatic prostate carcinoma leads to frustration for the physician and discouragement for the patient because the treatment options for progressive disease are so limited. Nonetheless, it may be important to discuss methods for evaluating disease response and progression.

Radioisotopic Bone Scan

The isotopic bone scan is much more sensitive than bone films in determining the progression and distribution of bony disease in a patient under treatment. The bone scan may be the most sensitive way to detect an increase in the number of sites of bony disease and to pinpoint their location. As indicated following, however, it may not be an effective way to monitor a patient on a routine basis. The most important use for bone scanning may be to monitor areas of specific complaint in order to prevent pathologic fractures in long, weight-bearing bones or vertebral collapse, which could produce spinal cord compression and paralysis. There are few objective means by which to categorize subtle changes in a bone scan. An increase in the density or number of "hot spots" on the scan may reflect increased disease activity, but it also may reflect only the amount of the radioisotope injected, the scanning technique used, or the degree of patient hydration. Furthermore, a patient who has rapidly progressive disease may have completely symmetrical distribution of isotope throughout the axial and appendicular skeletons, giving the bone scan a normal appearance, when, actually, the patient has developed a "superscan." The development of a superscan is indicated by inability to visualize the kidneys on the scanning film. Most students of prostate cancer do not follow their patients with bone scans unless there is a change in the clinical presentation or in one of the serum marker proteins that indicates increased disease activity.

Serum acid phosphatase, in a patient who previously has had elevated levels of this marker protein, is a classic indication of disease activity in response to treatment. As will be indicated following, it is not the most sensitive indicator of progressive disease, correlating with progression in only about 72% of patients, compared to prostate-specific antigen, which correlates with progression in about 84% of patients. As a biologic protein, serum acid phosphatase has a diurnal variation and may fluctuate as much as 50% above or below the mean as determined by either radioimmunoassay or enzymatic assay (Fig 20). These fluctuations make it imperative

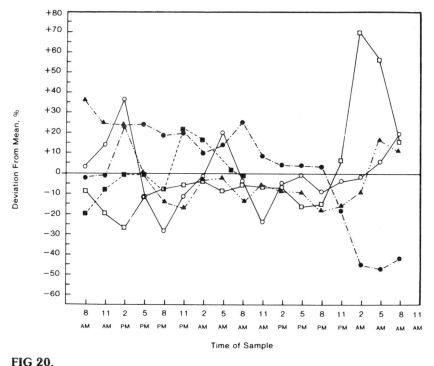

FIG 20.
Fluctuations in serum acid phosphatase level at three intervals over 24-hour periods in patients with demonstrated metastatic disease. Note the wide fluctuation about the mean in serum acid phosphatase level in patients wtih prostatic cancer. (From Brenckman WD: *JAMA* 1981; 245:2501. Used by permission.)

that the physician establish a trend in a patient's serum acid phosphatase levels before assuming that any specific observation represents either disease progression or response to treatment.

Prostate-Specific Antigen

Prostate-specific antigen may be the most sensitive indicator of disease activity or response to treatment. Rapid changes in this antigen can be seen after the initiation of androgen deprivation therapy. Normalization of previously elevated levels of prostate-specific antigen obviously are the most important response parameter. However, very few patients achieve complete normalization of previously elevated levels. Monitoring levels of this antigen gives the clinician the opportunity to detect disease activity, often months before the patient demonstrates other clinical evidence of it (Fig 21). Unfortunately, this also presents the physician with the therapeutic dilemma of seeking additional treatment when none may be available.

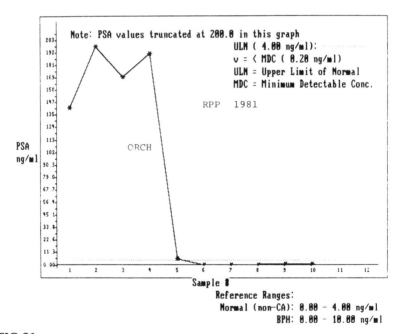

FIG 21.
This patient appeared with elevation of his prostate-specific antigen *(PSA)* level above 135 ng/mL after radical prostatectomy *(RPP)*. He was totally asymptomatic and remained so for about 1 year, at which time he underwent orchiectomy *(orch)*, with subsequent normalization of the elevated PSA level. *BPH* = benign prostatic hypertrophy.

Guidelines for Using Flutamide in the Management of Patients With Prostatic Carcinoma

The theoretical disadvantage of flutamide as monotherapy is that patients treated with this agent experience no decrease in luteinizing hormone drive of the Leydig cells and may maintain or increase their serum testosterone levels. It has been hypothesized that this increase may override the ability of the antiandrogen to block the androgen effect at a cellular level. Our own experience in using flutamide as monotherapy supports this observation, although we must state that not all patients respond in this manner. As indicated by the patient outlines on Figure 22, patient A was treated with flutamide when metastatic disease was identified and serum prostatic antigen began to rise (see Fig 22). Flutamide produced a transient decrease in prostate-specific antigen that was maintained for about 18 months before the level again began to rise. At point B, secondary androgen ablation was achieved by orchiectomy. Note the marked reduction in

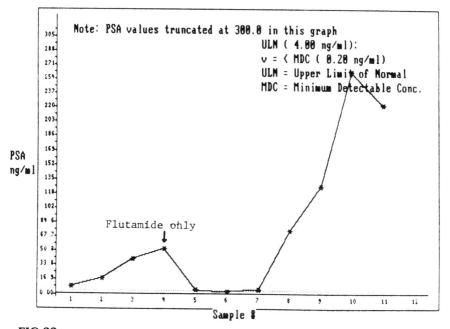

FIG 22.
This patient began to have a progressive increase in serum prostate-specific antigen *(PSA)* level. He was treated with flutamide at sample 4 and the PSA level subsequently normalized. By sample 8, however, his PSA level had begun to rise again. Orchiectomy was performed at the time of sample 10, with subsequent diminution in the PSA level.

prostate-specific antigen that correlated with a clinical improvement in the patient's disease process.

These observations do not argue against the use of flutamide as mono-therapy, they only caution that, when a patient being treated with this agent alone begins to show progression of his disease, serum testosterone must be monitored and secondary androgen deprivation initiated. In each patient in whom this has been observed and treatment initiated, an appropriate secondary clinical response has been obtained (Fig 23). No patient appears to have been disadvantaged by the initial use of flutamide as a primary therapy.

Flutamide also appears to be a safe and reasonably effective second-line therapy for patients for whom previous monotherapy has failed. Despite the fact that no overall disease response was identified in the randomized trial in which patients who initially received the luteinizing hormone ana-logue leuprolide were crossed over to flutamide at the time of progression, the gross data analysis may have obscured the subtle impact that can be

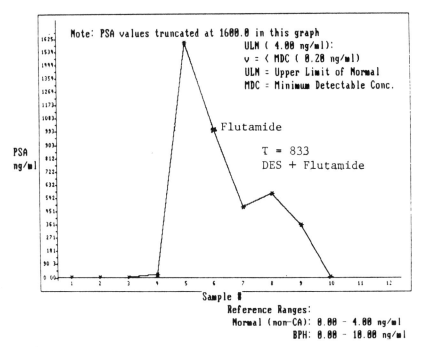

FIG 23.
This patient was treated initially with Eulixin and had a good clinical response and a good serum prostate-specific antigen *(PSA)* response. At the time of sample 8, however, he was noted to have an increase in PSA level and diethylstilbestrol *(DES)* was added. The testosterone *(T)* level at that time was 833 ng/dL. Upon initiation of DES, his T decreased to anorchid levels; by the time sample 10 was obtained, his PSA had decreased to normal levels. *BPH* = benign prostatic hyper-trophy.

achieved in approximately 30% of patients through the secondary use of flutamide.

Please note the records in Figure 24. Patient A originally received orchiectomy and spot radiation therapy for extended disease with a specific painful area. Over the next several years, he had a good clinical response. However, at point B, he began to have an increase in disease response activity and flutamide was added to his therapy (see Fig 24). Note that there was an excellent biochemical and clinical response that was maintained for about 7 months. This response has been observed in many patients. Flutamide seems to be a very safe drug. A similar effect probably would have been achieved with high-dose prednisone. However, in an elderly population, prednisone has the potential to change fluid balance characteristics, enhance salt retention, and alter glucose processing in such a way that patients will develop clinical diabetes mellitus.

Androgen Deprivation as a Surgical Adjunct in Node-Positive Prostatic Carcinoma

The use of androgen deprivation as an adjunct to surgical extirpation in patients with node-positive disease has provoked significant controversy.[57]

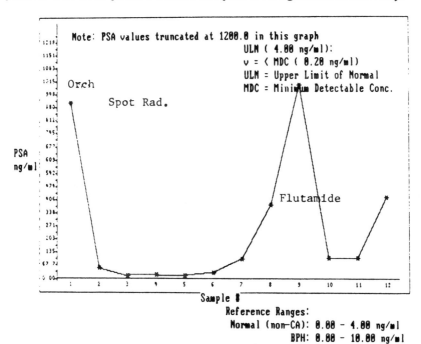

FIG 24.
Please see text for clinical course. *Orch* = orchiectomy; *spot rad* = spot radiation; *BPH* = benign prostatic hypertrophy; *PSA* = prostate-specific antigen.

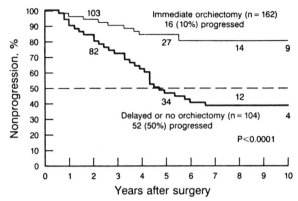

FIG 25.
Kaplan-Meier curves of nonprogression compare immediate orchiectomy with delayed (on progression only) or no immediate orchiectomy in 266 patients with stage D1 prostate cancer who had undergone bilateral pelvic lymphadenectomy. Numbers represent patients under observation at that time. (From Zincke H: *Urology* 1989; 33(suppl):31. Used by permission.)

Advocates of the combined treatment of lymphadenectomy, radical prostatectomy, and immediate androgen deprivation point with enthusiasm to the decreased progression rate seen in patients who receive early androgen deprivation. In a series published by the Mayo Clinic, 266 patients followed from 1 to 20 years (mean, 4.7 years) produced a nonrandomized population of 161 patients who had immediate adjuvant orchiectomy at the time of node dissection and radical prostatectomy. There was a highly significant ($P < .0001$) decrease in progression as compared with the 104

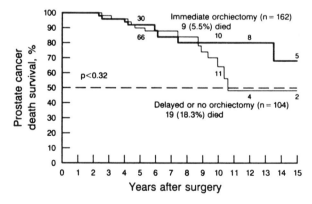

FIG 26.
Kaplan-Meier curves of cause-specific (prostate cancer) survival in 266 patients compare immediate orchiectomy with delayed (on progression only) or no immediate orchiectomy. Numbers represent patients under observation at that time. (From Zincke H: *Urology* 1989; 33(suppl):31. Used by permission.)

patients who underwent no immediate orchiectomy, but received node dissection and radical prostatectomy only (Fig 25).

Although immediate adjuvant orchiectomy delayed progression, however, examination of the survival rates of patients treated with immediate androgen deprivation and those treated with delayed androgen deprivation shows no statistically demonstrated advantage of either early or delayed treatment (Fig 26).

An even more convincing argument that early and delayed orchiectomy are equivalent in impact is afforded by a study of early vs. delayed orchiectomy in patients with diploid vs. nondiploid tumors. Examining cause-specific survival as a function of androgen deprivation and ploidy pattern in 91 patients with stage D1 prostatic carcinoma, it can be seen that diploid patients who undergo early orchiectomy and those who do not have equivalent survival rates, whereas nondiploid patients do equivalently poorly whether they are treated early or late (Fig 27). It must be concluded that adjunctive orchiectomy at the time of node dissection and radical prostatectomy provides no significant survival advantage in patients with node-positive disease. These observations by the investigators from The Mayo Clinic strongly argue that early and delayed androgen deprivation are equivalent in efficacy, and that the dominant therapeutic impact is provided by androgen deprivation and not by lymphadenectomy and radical prostatectomy.

The accrued data demonstrate that androgen deprivation can provide

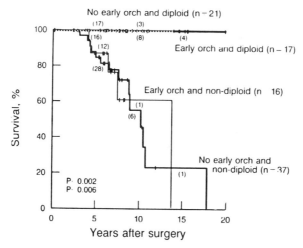

FIG 27.
Kaplan-Meier curves for cause-specific survival according to hormonal treatment and ploidy pattern in 91 patients with stage D1 prostate cancer (follow-up 5 years or more) who had undergone bilateral pelvic lymphadenectomy and radical retropubic prostatectomy. Numbers within parentheses represent patients under observation at that time. *Vertical bars* represent censored cases. *Orch* = orchiectomy. (From Zincke H: *Urology* 1989; 33(suppl):31. Used by permission.)

significant disease control. When used as an adjunctive therapy, the dominant disease control effect always seems to be provided by the androgen deprivation, obscuring evaluation of the primary treatment. The relative benefit of combination therapy over monotherapy doubtless will be debated for many years.

References

1. Birke G, Franksson C, Planton LO: Estrogen therapy in carcinoma of prostate. *Acta Chir Scand* 1955; 109:1–10.
2. Blackard CE, Byar DP, Jordan WP: Orchiectomy for advanced prostatic carcinoma—a reevaluation. *Urology* 1973; 1:533–560.
3. Huggins C: *Anti-Androgenic Treatment of Prostatic Carcinoma in Man: Approaches to Tumor Chemotherapy.* Washington, DC, American Association for the Advancement of Science, 1947.
4. Huggins C, Stevens RE, Hodges CV: Studies on prostatic cancer: The effects of castration on advanced carcinoma of the prostate gland. *Arch Surg* 1941; 43:219–223.
5. Anderson KM, Liao S: Selective retention of dihydrotestosterone by prostatic nuclei. *Nature* 1968; 219:277–279.
6. Bruchovsky N: Comparison of the metabolites formed in the rat prostate following the in vivo administration of seven natural androgens. *Endocrinology* 1971; 89:1212–1222.
7. Bruchovsky N, Wilson JD: The conversion of testosterone to 5-alpha-androstan-17-beta-ol-3-one by rat prostate in vivo and in vitro. *J Biol Chem* 1968; 243:2012–2021.
8. Mainwaring WIP, Irving R: The use of deoxyribonucleic acid-cellulose chromatography and isoelectric focusing for the characterization and partial purification of steroid-receptor complexes. *Biochem J* 1973; 134:113–127.
9. Wilson JD, Gloyna RE: The intranuclear metabolism of testosterone in the accessory organs of reproduction. *Recent Prog Horm Res* 1970; 26:309–336.
10. Coffey DS: The biochemistry and physiology of the prostate and seminal vesicles, in *Campbell's Urology,* 5th ed. Philadelphia, Saunders, 1986, pp 233–274.
11. Clark J, O'Malley B: Mechanisms of steroid hormone action, in Wilson JD, Foster DW (eds): *Williams Textbook of Endocrinology.* Philadelphia, Saunders, 1985.
12. Barrack ER: The nuclear matrix of the prostate contains acceptor sites for nuclear matrix: Steroid hormone binding. *Recent Prog Horm Res* 1982; 38:133.
13. Walsh PC, Siiteri PK: Suppression of plasma androgens by spironolactone in castrated men with carcinoma of the prostate. *J Urol* 1975; 114:254–256.
14. Vermeulen A, Verdonck L: Studies of the binding of the testosterone to human plasma. *Steroids* 1968; 11:609–635.
15. Robinson MRG, Thomas BS: Effect of hormonal therapy on plasma testosterone levels in prostatic carcinoma. *BMJ* 1971; 4:391–394.
16. Shearer RJ, Hendry WF, Sommerville IF, et al: Plasma testosterone: An accurate monitor of hormone treatment in prostatic cancer. *Br J Urol* 1973; 45:668–677.
17. Doering CH, Kraemer HC, Brodie KH, et al: A cycle of plasma testosterone in the human male. *J Clin Endocrinol Metab* 1975; 40:492.

18. Harman TM, Tsitouras PD: Reproductive hormones in aging men. I. Measurement of sex steroids, basal luteinizing hormone and Leydig cell response to human chorionic gonadotropin. *J Clin Endocrinol Metab* 1980; 51:35.

19. Sparrow D, Bosse R, Rowe JW: The influence of age, alcohol consumption and body build on gonadal function in men. *J Clin Endocrinol Metab* 1980; 51:508.

20. Mackler MA, Liberti JP, Smith MJV, et al: The effect of orchiectomy and various doses of stilbestrol on plasma testosterone levels in patients wtih carcinoma of the prostate. *Invest Urol* 1972; 9:423–425.

21. Young HH Jr, Kent JR: Plasma testosterone levels in patients with prostatic carcinoma before and after treatment. *J Urol* 1968; 99:788–792.

22. Kent JR, Bischoff AJ, Arduino LJ, et al: Estrogen dosage and suppression of testosterone levels in patients with prostatic carcinoma. *J Urol* 1973; 109:858–860.

23. McClinton S, Moffat LEF, Ludbrook A: The cost of bilateral orchiectomy as a treatment for prostatic carcinoma. *Br J Urol* 1989; 63:309–312.

24. Shimazaki J, Horaguchi T, Oki Y, et al: Properties of testosterone 5-reductase of purified nuclear fraction from ventral prostate of rats. *Endocrinol Jpn* 1971; 18:179–187.

25. Yanaihara T, Troen P, Troen BR, et al: Studies of the human testis. III. Effect of estrogen on testosterone formation in human testis in vitro. *J Clin Endocrinol Metab* 1972; 34:968–973.

26. Harper ME, Fahmy AR, Pierrepoint CG, et al: The effect of some stilbestrol compounds on DNA polymerase from human prostatic tissue. *Steroids* 1970; 15:89–103.

27. Aro J, Haapianinen R, and the Finnprostate Group: Comparison of endocrine and radiation therapy for locally advanced prostatic cancer. *Eur Urol* 1988; 15:182–186.

28. Henriksson P, Edhag O, Eriksson A, et al: Patients at high risk of cardiovascular complications in oestrogen treatment of prostatic cancer. *Br J Urol* 1989; 63:186–190.

29. Glode, Max: *Proceedings of the 13th International Congress on Chemotherapy* 1983; 242:49.

30. Murphy GP, Beckley S, Brady MF, et al: Treatment of newly diagnosed metastatic prostate carcinoma patients with chemotherapy agents in combination with hormone versus hormones alone. *Cancer* 1983; 51:1264–1272.

31. Goldman AS: Further studies of steroidal inhibitors of delta 5,3-betahydroxysteroid dehydrogenase and delta 5-delta 4,3-ketosteroid isomerase in Pseudomonas testosteroni and in bovine adrenals. *J Clin Endocrinol* 1968; 28:1539–1546.

32. Worgul TJ, Santen RJ, Smojlik E, et al: Clinical and biochemical effect of aminoglutethimide in the treatment of advanced prostatic carcinoma. *J Urol* 1983; 129:51–55.

33. Schoonees R, Schalch DS, Murphy GP: The hormonal effects of antiandrogen (SH-714) treatment in man. *Invest Urol* 1971; 8:635–639.

34. Smith RB, Walsh PC, Goodwin WE: Cyproterone acetate in the treatment of advanced carcinoma of the prostate. *J Urol* 1973; 110:106–108.

35. Pont A, Williams PL, Loose DS, et al: Ketaconazole blocks adrenal steroid synthesis. *Ann Intern Med* 1982; 97:370–372.

36. Pont A, Williams PL, Azhar S, et al: Ketoconazole blocks testosterone synthesis. *Arch Intern Med* 1982; 142:2137–2140.

37. Tachtenberg J: Ketaconazole therapy in advanced prostatic cancer. *J Urol* 1984; 132:61–63.
38. Foote JE, Crawford DE: Combined hormonal therapy in the management of adenocarcinoma of the prostate. *Probl Urol* 1990; 4:473.
39. Scott WW, Menon W, Walsh PC: Hormonal therapy of prostatic cancer. *Cancer* 1980; 45:1929.
40. Neri R, Florance K, Koziol P, et al: A biological profile of a nonsteroidal anti-androgen Sch-13521 (4-nitro-3-trifluoromethylisobutyranilide). *Endocrinology* 1972; 91:427–437.
41. Walsh PC, Korenman SG: Mechanism of androgenic action: Effect of specific intracellular inhibitors. *J Urol* 1971; 105:850–857.
42. Geller J, Vazakas G, Fruchtman B, et al: The effect of cyproterone acetate on advanced carcinoma of the prostate. *Surg Gynecol Obstet* 1968; 127: 748–758.
43. Sogani PC, Vagaiwala MR, Whitmore WF: Experience with flutamide in patients with advanced prostatic cancer without prior endocrine therapy. *Cancer* 1984; 54:744–750.
44. Stoliar B, Albert DJ: SCH-13521 in the treatment of advanced carcinoma of the prostate. *J Urol* 1974; 111:803–807.
45. Smith JA: New methods of endocrine management of prostatic cancer. *J Urol* 1987; 137:1.
46. Glick JH, Wein A, Padavic K, et al: Phase II trial of tamoxifen in metastatic carcinoma of the prostate. *Cancer* 1982; 49:1367–1372.
47. Spremulli E, DeSimone P, Durant J: A phase II study of Nolvadex: Tamoxifen citrate in the treatment of advanced prostatic adenocarcinoma. *Am J Clin Oncol* 1982; 5:149–153.
48. Luthy I, Labrie F: Development of androgen resistance in mouse mammary tumor cells can be prevented by the antiandrogen flutamide. *Prostate* 1987; 10:89.
49. Crawford ED: A controlled trial of leuprolide with and without flutamide in prostatic carcinoma. *N Engl J Med* 1989; 321:419–424.
50. Bailar JC, Byar DP: Estrogen treatment for cancer of the prostate. Early results with 3 doses of diethylstilbestrol and placebo. *Cancer* 1970; 26:257–261.
51. Byar DP: The Veterans Administration Cooperative Urological Research Group's studies of cancer of the prostate. *Cancer* 1973; 32:1126–1130.
52. Byar DP, Corle DK: The Veterans Administration Cooperative Urological Research Group's randomized trial of radical prostatectomy for stages I and II prostate cancer. *Urology* 1981; 17:7–11.
53. Veterans Administration Cooperative Urological Research Group: Treatment and survival of patients with cancer of the prostate. *Surg Gynecol Obstet* 1967; 124:1011–1017.
54. Zagars GK, Johnson DE, von Eschenbach AC, et al: Adjuvant estrogen following radiation therapy for stage C adenocarcinoma of the prostate: Long term results of a prospective randomized study. *Int J Radiat Oncol Biol Phys* 1988; 14:1085–1091.
55. Scott WW, Boyd H: Current cancer concepts: Hormone control and surgery. *JAMA* 1969; 210:1078.
56. Maatman TJ, Gupta MK, Montie JE: The role of serum prostatic acid phosphatase as a tumor marker in men with advanced adenocarcinoma of the prostate. *J Urol* 1984; 132:58.
57. Zincke H: Extended experience with surgical treatment of stage D1 adenocarcinoma of prostate. *Urology* 1989; 33(suppl):27.

Hyperthermia for Prostate Disease

Peter M. Knapp, M.D.

Methodist Hospital of Indiana; Assistant Clinical Professor, Department of
Urology, Indiana University School of Medicine, Indianapolis, Indiana

Yoram I. Siegel, M.D.

Research Fellow, Methodist Hospital of Indiana; Institute for Kidney Stone
Disease, Indianapolis, Indiana

Over the past decade, our understanding of benign prostatic hyperplasia
(BPH) has expanded greatly. Extensive investigation of prostate growth
and the dynamics of bladder outlet obstruction has increased our compre-
hension of BPH pathophysiology. Increased research activity also has led
to the development of new treatment modalities. Transurethral resection of
the prostate (TURP) has been the standard of therapy for decades. However, the costs of TURP and the morbidity of surgery has led to the exploration of other, less invasive treatment alternatives.

In recent years, prostatic hyperthermia has been studied as a treatment
alternative in the management of bladder outlet obstruction secondary to
BPH. Although hyperthermia is not likely to replace TURP, it may offer an
effective, minimally invasive, office-based treatment option that expands
the available treatment armamentarium.

Historical Perspective

The use of heat as a therapeutic tool can be traced to the ancients, who
observed that high fevers or hot water baths relieved many ailments. The
first scientific report of the therapeutic effect of heat is attributed to Busch
in 1866. He reported the spontaneous regression of a histologically confirmed sarcoma after a severe febrile episode caused by erysipelas.[1] Other
publications followed, reporting the effect of increased body temperature
on tumor growth by incidental febrile episodes[2, 3] or deliberate administration of bacteria.[4] Observation of the biologic effect of heat on tumor cells
led to the application of hyperthermia as adjunctive therapy in combination with chemotherapy[5, 6] and radiation therapy[7] in the treatment of solid
tumors. Yerushalmi and colleagues first used hyperthermia in treating disorders of the prostate in 1982.[8] Initial trials were performed using a transrectal approach to deliver controlled heat to the prostate. Initial treatment
were performed on patients with advanced cancer of the prostate that

failed to respond to other forms of therapy. Many patients experienced reduction in obstructive voiding symptoms and pelvic pain, and a decrease
in the size of the prostate on transrectal ultrasound.[8–10] The encouraging
results with relief of obstructive symptoms stimulated the investigators to
explore the role of hyperthermia in the treatment of BPH.

Currently, several forms of heat therapy are being tested worldwide. Interstitial temperatures of 40° C to 90° C can be achieved using the various
energy sources, causing a wide range of tissue effects, from mild alteration
in blood flow to severe cellular necrosis and tissue death.[11]

Several hyperthermia devices are available for the treatment of prostate
diseases. The accumulated data distinguish between thermotherapy and
hyperthermia. Thermotherapy is the heating of tissue to temperatures ex-
ceeding 45° C, resulting in necrosis of normal tissue. Hyperthermia is defined as the controlled delivery of heat to achieve interstitial temperatures
of 41° C to 44° C, which do not cause destruction of normal tissue. Thermotherapy has been tested using a transurethral device, whereas hyperthermia has been applied to the treatment of prostate diseases via a transrectal approach. In the United States, the Food and Drug Administration
(FDA) is evaluating clinical protocols using thermotherapy and hyperthermia for the treatment of BPH.

The biologic effect of hyperthermia, the physics of microwave heating,
early animal studies, and current clinical trials of prostatic hyperthermia will
be presented in this chapter to examine the usefulness of this emerging
technology.

Biologic Effect of Heat

The effect of heat on biologic tissue is dependent on the temperature
achieved and the duration of the temperature elevation. Temperatures in
excess of 45° C (thermotherapy) produce severe cellular changes and necrosis in normal tissue. Temperatures in the intermediate range of 41° C to
44° C (hyperthermia) produce variable changes in normal tissue without
causing tissue necrosis. However, hyperthermia does cause cytoplasmic
swelling, hemorrhage, and necrosis in tumor cells.[10, 12]

The biologic effect of heat on normal tissue and tumors has been studied by many investigators. Song showed that hyperthermia produces vaso-
dilatation and increased blood flow in normal tissue.[13] The increased
blood flow may provide the thermal regulation needed to prevent heat injury in normal tissue.

Several theories exist to explain why tumor cells are more sensitive to
hyperthermia. Tumor blood vessels have increased vascular resistance and
lack the ability to vasodilate in response to heat. The tumor, therefore, is
unable to dissipate heat as efficiently as does normal tissue.[12–14] Poor
thermal regulation permits tissue damage at interstitial temperatures that
are well-tolerated by normal tissue. In addition to thermal regulation factors, tumor cells may have an inherent sensitivity to heat.[15, 16] Other inves-

tigators suggest an immunologic response. Histologic studies demonstrated a diffuse mononuclear infiltrate following hyperthermia in tumors.[17]

The biologic effect of hyperthermia on tumor cells has been used as primary as well as adjunctive cancer therapy. Tumor cells in the S phase are resistant to radiation therapy, but particularly sensitive to heat. The two treatments together may have a synergistic effect.[18, 19] Other investigators have used hyperthermia in combination with cytotoxic agents to enhance the therapeutic response by a direct thermal effect or possibly by increasing cell sensitivity to the drugs.[20, 21]

Most of the clinical experience with hyperthermia has been with superficial tumors. Delivery of hyperthermia to an internal organ such as the prostate was a technologic and anatomic challenge. In addition, the biologic effect of hyperthermia on normal prostate tissue and BPH was unknown. Animal studies were designed to elucidate the effect of hyperthermia on the prostate using a microwave energy source and a transrectal microwave antenna.

Physics of Microwave Heating

Hyperthermia may be achieved by the use of several energy sources. Infrared irradiation, high-frequency ultrasound, and microwave irradiation all can heat internal organs efficiently, but differ in their depth of penetration and ease of use. Microwave frequencies make up the 300- to 3,000-MHz range of the electromagnetic spectrum. Heating occurs in biologic tissue by the energy transfer of the electromagnetic wave passing through the tissue. The electromagnetic wave causes oscillation of free ions (electrons), resulting in a conversion of molecular energy into kinetic energy, which produces heat in the targeted tissue.

The temperature increase is a direct function of several parameters, including the absorption coefficient of the tissue. The absorption coefficient is determined largely by the water content of the tissue. Higher temperatures are achieved in tissue with higher water content and more absorption of the electromagnetic wave. Muscle, which has a high water content, absorbs more energy and heats more readily than do bone and fat, which have a lower water content.

Tissue penetration of the electromagnetic wave is dependent upon the frequency of the wave and the absorption coefficient of the tissue. Wave penetration is decreased with increased wave frequency and increased tissue water content. The result is that tissues with increased water content (muscle) will absorb more energy and heat more easily, but permit less penetration of the electromagnetic wave.

Selection of the proper wave frequency to use for microwave heating was determined by the wave's depth of penetration The 915-MHz frequency was chosen as the appropriate wavelength (33 cm in air and 4.7 cm in muscle).[22] In muscle, about one half of the energy is absorbed within 1.7 cm from the antenna. The principle of heating from a microwave energy source is shown in Figure 1, A. Temperature decreases as distance from the microwave antenna increases. When surface cooling is applied to the tissue in contact with the antenna, the point of maximum temperature shifts to the right (see Fig 1, B). Some transrectal devices apply cooling systems to the antenna in order to protect the rectal wall from heating. The maximum temperature is achieved in the target tissue some distance from the cooled surface of the antenna. Temperature measured in a test medium confirmed maximum temperature elevation about 1.5 cm from the antenna. As the distance increases from the maximum temperature point, the temperature slowly decreases. At 4.5 cm from the antenna, 50% of the maximum temperature increase is maintained (Fig 2).[23]

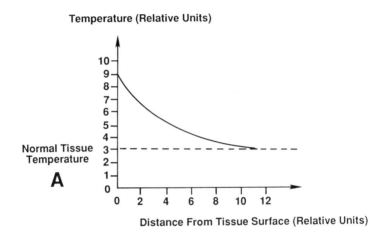

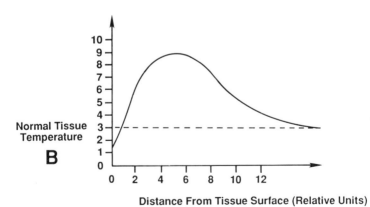

FIG 1.
Typical heating patterns due to RF radiation absorbed in a tissue. **A,** without cooling of tissue surface. **B,** with cooling of tissue surface. (From Servadio C, Leib Z, Lev A: *Urology* 1990; 35:156–163. Used by permission.)

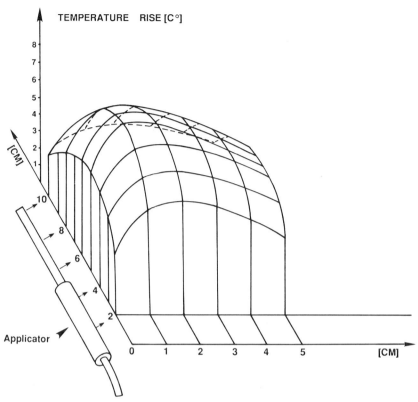

FIG 2.
Temperature distribution profile. (Courtesy of Biodan Medical Systems Division of Omilcron Scientific, Ltd. Used by permission.)

During hyperthermia administration, it is necessary to measure thermal dose to help measure thermal effect on tissue. By measuring the interstitial temperature as a function of time, an estimate of the thermal dose can be determined. The calculation of thermal equivalent dose was developed to measure the temperature, time, and energy relationship. The higher the temperature maintained over time, the higher the thermal equivalent dose value. As an example, a thermal equivalent dose of 3,600 is equivalent to heating at 43° C for 60 minutes.[24]

Animal Studies

During hyperthermia, the target tissue must be accessible within a short distance from the microwave antenna. The target tissue also must be treated preferentially while permitting minimal heating of surrounding tissue. To treat BPH with microwave hyperthermia, a transrectal approach permitted close proximity to the prostate. The rectum also provides a cavity to accommodate a 915-MHz microwave antenna with a surface cooling system and surface temperature monitors. To test microwave heating of the prostate in dogs, a water-cooled skirt-type microwave antenna operating at 915 MHz was constructed in a rectal applicator. The applicator was inserted into the rectum and the antenna was directed toward the prostate. A maximum of 40 W of power was used to heat the prostate. Cool water (20° C) from an external cooling device was circulated through the surface of the applicator to cool the rectal wall circumferentially.[25]

Temperatures were measured by specially designed copper-constantan thermocouples placed perpendicular to the electromagnetic wave polarization to prevent artifactual heating. The measurements were confirmed with a Luxtron Fluoroptic Unit (Luxtron, Mountain View, Calif) which is unaffected by electromagnetic radiation. There was no significant temperature deviation (±2° C) measured between the two types of thermometers.[26] Thermocouples were placed on the rectal applicator to monitor rectal wall temperature constantly. Additional thermocouples were placed in the prostatic urethra through a specially designed urethral catheter in order to monitor prostatic urethral temperatures constantly.[25, 26]

The dog studies were conducted to determine the temperature distribution within the prostate and to evaluate the biochemical and histologic effects of hyperthermia on prostate tissue over time.

Temperature Mapping in Dogs

Using the aforementioned technique, Servadio and coworkers[26] studied six dogs to measure intraprostatic temperature. The dogs were anesthetized and a urethral catheter was inserted into the bladder to monitor prostatic urethral temperatures. The water-cooled, 915-MHz microwave applicator then was inserted into the rectum. The prostate was exposed surgically and 3 to 4 additional thermocouples were placed directly into the prostate to measure interstitial temperatures. Two typical temperature curves are shown in Figure 3. The effect of using an applicator with surface cooling is demonstrated by lower temperatures in the rectal wall nearer to the applicator. The maximum temperature is reached deep inside the prostate, 1.5 cm away from the rectal wall. The rate of temperature decrease beyond the maximum temperature is 1.1° C/cm, demonstrating substantial heating deeper into the prostate. A calculated prostatic temperature can be determined from prostatic urethral temperature measurement, prostatic height, and rectal wall thickness.

Histologic Changes

The histologic effect of hyperthermia on the dog prostate was reported by Servadio and Leib in two separate studies.[25, 26] The investigators studied the relationship of temperature and duration of heating on the histologic changes.

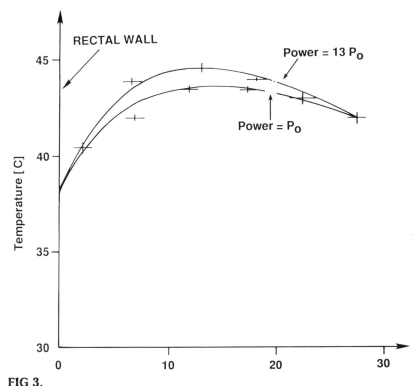

FIG 3.
Temperature profile in canine prostate. (From Servadio C, Leib Z, Lev A: *Urology* 1990; 35:156–163. Used by permission.)

Leib studied 20 dogs treated with hyperthermia at different temperatures for varying lengths of time (Table 1).[25] One dog served as a control subject, undergoing insertion of the rectal microwave applicator for 90 minutes, but with no microwave power applied. All of the dogs were killed at the end of the treatment sequence or 1 week following treatment. The histologic findings at autopsy are detailed in Table 1.

Group A demonstrated that low temperatures (40° C) applied for long periods of time (10 hours) produce focal interstitial lymphocytic and polymorphonuclear infiltrates. Group B revealed that prostate heating to 42.5° C for 1.5 hours causes diffuse mononuclear infiltrate and edema. No evidence of tissue necrosis was found in any of the 4 dogs in this group. Dogs in group C demonstrated that a temperature of 42.5° C can cause prostatic urethral and interstitial necrosis when heating time is prolonged to 5 hours. Groups D and E revealed severe necrosis at 44.5° C when heat was applied for 1.5 or 5 hours. Interestingly, dogs in group F which were treated for only 15 minutes at high temperatures (47° C), demonstrated no significant tissue change.

The following results were reported: (1) All dogs in each group demon-

TABLE 1.
Hyperthermia Treatment Program and Histologic Changes in Dogs*

Group	Number of Dogs	Temperature Range (±0.5° C)	Treatment Length	Number of Sessions	Histologic Findings
A	2	40.0	10 hr	1	Focal interstitial lymphocytic and polymorphonuclear infiltration
B	4	42.5	1.5 hr	6	Diffuse mononuclear infiltrate and edema
C	4	42.5	5 hr	2	Severe interstitial mononuclear infiltrate and focal necrosis
D	4	44.5	1.5 hr	6	Necrosis of prostatic urethra with hemorrhage and inflammatory infiltration and necrosis in prostatic interstitium
E	4	44.5	5 hr	2	Necrosis of prostatic urethra with hemorrhage and inflammatory infiltration and necrosis in prostatic interstitium
F	1	47.0	15 min	1	No significant change
G	1	Control group: probe placed, no heat applied			

*From Leib Z: *Prostate* 1986; 8:93. Used by permission.

strated the same histologic effect, whether the animal was killed following a treatment session or 1 week later. (2) All heating treatments caused inflammatory infiltrates in the interstitium and polymorphonuclear infiltration in the glandular element of the prostate. (3) The localized venous and lymphatic congestion (edema) present in the rectal wall was seen in treated dogs as well as in the control group, in which no power was applied. These changes, therefore, are due to placement of the rectal applicator and are not caused by heating. (4) The prostate can be heated repeatedly to 42.5° C for 1.5 hours without causing any tissue damage. (5) The tissue change seen are both time- and temperature-dependent.

Biochemical Changes

Before and after each treatment session, Servadio[26] measured serum chemistries, enzymes, and electrolytes. Comparison of pretreatment and posttreatment levels was performed at the end of the study.

Changes were seen in creatine phosphokinase (CPK) and serum glutamic oxaloacetic transaminase (SGOT) levels following treatment. The SGOT level was increased in dogs treated at 42.5° C for 1.5 hours. It increased further in dogs treated with a temperature of 42.5° C for 5 hours and in those treated with 44.5° C for 1.5 hours. The CPK level also increased in the same respective groups that experienced an increase in the SGOT level. Elevation in these levels reflects the degree of tissue damage demonstrated histologically in each group.[26]

Experience in Benign Prostatic Hypertrophy

Over the past several years, the study of hyperthermia in the treatment of prostate disease has advanced. Following initial trials in men with prostate cancer, efforts were made to develop a clinically useful and safe device with which to administer hyperthermia. The previously described in vitro and animal studies led to the development of a hyperthermia system that includes (1) a 100-W microwave generator operating at 915 MHz; (2) a cooling system to provide circulating cool water at 20° C; (3) a rectal applicator that contains the directional microwave antenna, circulating cool water to cool the adjacent rectal wall, and surface thermocouples to monitor rectal wall temperature continuously; (4) a specially designed urethral catheter containing thermocouples to monitor prostatic urethral temperatures; and (5) a computerized control system to regulate power delivery, water cooling, and temperature measurements.[24]

Treatment is initiated by placement of the urethral catheter with thermocouples located in the prostatic urethra. The water-cooled, 915-MHz microwave applicator is inserted into the rectum (Fig 4). Temperatures in the rectum and prostatic urethra, and a calculated intraprostatic temperature are monitored continuously throughout the treatment session. The power of the microwave generator is regulated to maintain prostatic temperatures safely at 43° C to 43.5° C without raising rectal temperatures.

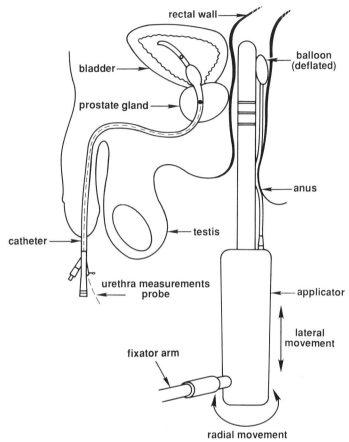

FIG 4.
Applicator in rectum and catheter in urethra.

Using this hyperthermia device, several clinical trials have been performed examining interstitial heating of the prostate and the biochemical and histologic effects of prostatic hyperthermia.

Interstitial Temperature Measurements

Actual temperature measurements in the prostatic gland during hyperthermia heating are crucially important for treatment control and safety. Using in vitro and animal models, a temperature pattern was established that represents temperature dissipation as a function of distance from the applicator[26] (see Figs 2 and 3). Based on these data, it was possible to calculate the prostatic temperature from the temperature measured in the prostatic urethra during the treatment. The calculated prostate temperature is derived from prostatic urethral temperature in relation to prostatic height and rectal wall thickness. Transrectal ultrasound is used to measure prostate height and rectal wall thickness prior to treatment.

Temperature dissipation along the prostatic urethra was studied by Siegel and Lindner.[27] Using a special thermometry system in 20 patients, six individual points were measured along the prostatic urethra starting 10 mm from the bladder neck and continuing in 5-mm intervals distally. The temperature profile revealed a single maximum temperature located at the thermocouple positioned 25 mm from the bladder neck. The current clinically used urethral catheter has three thermocouples located 20, 25, and 30 mm from the bladder neck to measure actual urethral temperatures during transrectal hyperthermia treatment.

The accuracy of the calculated prostate temperature was determined by Newman and Knapp.[28] Interstitial temperatures were measured to determine the temperature distribution in the prostate during transrectal hyperthermia treatment. The directly measured interstitial temperatures were correlated with the measured prostatic urethral temperature and the calculated prostate temperature to verify their accuracy. Interstitial temperature probes were inserted into the prostate at various locations. An attempt was made to insert the probes into areas of the prostate that would generate a representative thermal map.

Under local anesthesia with the patient in dorsal lithotomy position, a 17-gauge ultrasound needle was inserted into the desired lobe and positioned in the prostate. The location of the needle tip within the prostate was confirmed with transrectal ultrasound. The temperature probe was inserted through the needle, and the needle was removed.

Interstitial temperature measurements were performed in ten patients with symptomatic BPH who were undergoing hyperthermia treatment. The prostate height ranged from 27 to 51 mm, with an average prostate height of 38.4 mm. Rectal wall thickness ranged from 3 to 5 mm. All hyperthermia treatments were carried out using the Biodan Prostathermer (Biodan Medical Systems, Ltd, Rehovot, Israel).

The location of interstitial temperature measurements in the prostate are shown in Figure 5. The measured interstitial temperatures confirm that the entire prostate is heated above normal body temperature by transrectal microwave hyperthermia treatment. A temperature gradient in the prostate also can be mapped. The area of greatest temperature increase is in the posterior portion of the prostate between the urethra and the rectal wall. The calculated prostate temperature accurately predicts ($\pm 1°$ C) the maximum interstitial temperature measured in this area. The periurethral area also is heated into the hyperthermia temperature range. Periurethral interstitial temperatures closely approximate ($\pm 1°$ C) the intraurethral temperature measured in the Foley catheter. Temperatures outside the prostate in the periprostatic fat were measured as the temperature probes were withdrawn during treatment. The periprostatic temperatures were near normal body temperature, indicating that the periprostatic tissue was not heated significantly.

The interstitial temperature findings in the human prostate closely corre-

Coronal Section   **Sagittal Section**

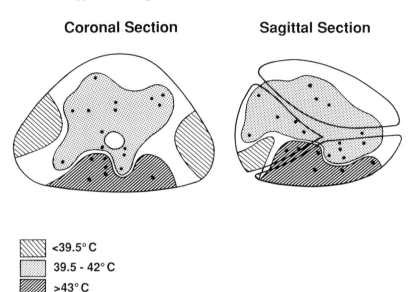

    <39.5° C

    39.5 - 42° C

    >43° C

FIG 5.
Interstitial temperature map in human prostate.

lated with previous findings in dogs (see Fig 3) and in vitro (see Figs 1 and 2). It also was observed that the amount of power necessary to heat the prostate was not consistent from one treatment to another or throughout the course of one individual treatment. It is necessary, therefore, to measure intraurethral temperature throughout each treatment to determine accurately the amount of power necessary to heat the prostate and to ensure adequate heating and prevent overheating.

Histologic Changes

The histologic effect of local hyperthermia on BPH has been studied using fine quantitative morphometric analysis. Morphometric analysis provides information on the relative volume of various tissue components in a tissue specimen. Morphometric methods were applied to determine the fibrous, muscular, vascular, and glandular components of normal and hyperplastic prostate glands.[29]

In order to evaluate the heat effect on prostate tissue, morphometric analysis was performed on operative specimens. The specimens were obtained from 13 patients in whom hyperthermia treatment had failed. Prostate tissue from 9 patients who underwent prostatectomy with no previous hyperthermia treatment served as controls. The volume fractions of the fibrous, muscular, vascular, and glandular components of the two groups are listed in Table 2.[30] The volume fraction of fibrous tissue was less and the volume fraction of muscular tissue was more in the hyperthermia-treated group. Since the specimens were obtained from patients in whom hyperthermia treatment had failed, it is unclear if the measured difference

TABLE 2.
The Volume Fractions of the Tissue Components Calculated as a Percent of the Total Tissue Volume*

Tissue Component	Control Group (n = 9)	Patients With Hyperthermia Failure (n = 13)
Fibrous (%)	46.85 ± .98	37.07 ± .72†
Muscle (%)	7.17 ± .32	14.55 ± .39†
Vascular (%)	3.04 ± .17	3.11 ± .14
Glandular (%)	18.77 ± .54	18.62 ± .45

*From Siegel YI: Br J Urol 1991; 68:383. Used by permission.
†p < .001.

is a result of the heat effect or may be identifying a tissue fraction group that can be expected to do poorly with hyperthermia treatment. No difference in the glandular component was noted between the two groups, suggesting no effect of hyperthermia on the glandular element of BPH in patients in whom this treatment is not effective.

Further fine morphometric studies were performed to measure successful treatment response using specific staining methods. Three immunohistochemical markers were studied: alpha smooth muscle actin, desmin, and vimentin. These cytoskeletal proteins have been shown to represent reliable discrimination markers to differentiate smooth muscle cells and fibroblast cells. Alpha smooth muscle actin and desmin are found in smooth muscle cells, whereas vimentin is found primarily in fibroblasts. Prostate specimens were obtained from 11 patients by random transrectal needle biopsies from each lobe of the prostate 10 days before and 3 months after the completion of hyperthermia treatment. For each component, randomized sampling methods were used. For each patient, 36 sample areas were studied. A significant increase (P < .04) in the area ratio of vimentin was observed 3 months after hyperthermia treatment (Table 3).[31] There was an increase in the actin and desmin elements, but these changes were not statistically significant.

These preliminary results demonstrate an increased amount of fibroblast marker following hyperthermia treatment, suggesting that heat may serve as an inductive stimulus for fibrous tissue differentiation. Further investigation is necessary to confirm these findings and to study their clinical significance.

Biochemical Changes

The biochemical effect of hyperthermia in the treatment of BPH was studied by measuring prostate-specific antigen (PSA) levels in patients under-

TABLE 3.
Immunohistochemical Changes in the Prostate Gland Following Transrectal Hyperthermia*

Area Ratio	ASM ± SE	DES ± SE	VIM ± SE
Before treatment (%)	43 ± 3	16 ± 5	9 ± 3†
After treatment (%)	52 ± 7	25 ± 5	25 ± 9

*ASM = alpha smooth muscle actin; DES = desmin; VIM = vimentin; SE = standard error.
†P < .04.

going transrectal hyperthermia treatment. PSA is a glycoprotein present in the epithelial cells of prostatic ducts and in seminal plasma. Elevation of the serum PSA level has been associated with prostate diseases, including cancer, BPH, and prostatitis.[32] An increased PSA level also has been reported following vigorous prostate massage, cystoscopy, and prostate needle biopsy.[33] Therefore, PSA level was used as an indicator for prostate injury following hyperthermia treatment by Lindner and associates.[33] PSA levels were drawn before and immediately following transrectal hyperthermia treatment in 18 patients with BPH. Ninety treatment sessions were performed.

The mean presession PSA level was 3.44 (±2.9) ng/mL and the mean posttreatment PSA level was 3.53 (±2.8) ng/mL. No significant difference was observed between pretreatment and immediate posttreatment serum PSA levels.

To determine if a delayed increase in the PSA level could occur, it also was measured every 3 to 4 days during the 3-week treatment course. No significant increase in the PSA level after treatment was observed.[33] The stable PSA level recorded following treatment suggests that no significant tissue damage occurs with transrectal hyperthermia treatment.

Clinical Studies

The number of clinical trials reported in the literature is increasing steadily. To date, more than 1,200 treated patients have been reported, with the longest follow-up period being more than 6 years.

As mentioned previously, the first human trials of transrectal hyperthermia treatment were reported by Servadio and Yerushalmi.[8, 9] The authors independently reported relief of obstructive voiding symptoms, improvement in urinary flow rate, and reduction of residual urine in patients with prostate cancer. Some catheter-dependent patients were able to void and no longer required an indwelling catheter. Servadio also reported a reduction in prostate size as measured on transrectal prostate ultrasound in patients with prostate cancer.

The initial success achieved in relieving obstructive voiding symptoms in patients with prostate cancer led investigators to begin clinical trials in patients with obstructive BPH who were poor operative risks. Lindner and colleagues treated six poor-risk patients in urinary retention with transrectal hyperthermia using a Model 99-D Prostathermer (Biodan Medical Systems, Ltd, Rehovot, Israel).[34] Patients were treated with 1-hour sessions twice weekly for 5 to 10 sessions. Five of the six patients were relieved of their catheter and remained catheter-free at 6 months. The mean posttreatment urinary flow rate was 18 mL/sec.

The first multicenter clinical trial using transrectal hyperthermia treatment was conducted in Israel and reported in 1989.[35] One hundred and forty patients with severe obstructive symptoms were treated. The study included patients with BPH, prostate cancer and prostatitis and used different protocols and additional treatments. The mean peak flow increased from 10.1 mL/sec to 11.9 mL/sec at 6 months. The mean residual urine volume decreased from 180 mL pretreatment to 90 mL at 6 months. The symptom score also improved in the majority of patients. Various treatment protocols were evaluated. The number, frequency, and duration of treatments were compared. The best results were seen in patients treated for 10 1-hour sessions performed twice weekly for 5 weeks.

Additional series in the literature reported success in patients with symptomatic BPH using transrectal hyperthermia treatment.[36] However, concern remained regarding the efficacy of this technique in patients with symptomatic BPH. Questions also persisted concerning a possible placebo effect of the treatment. It was suggested that frequent catheterizations for 1 hour may relieve obstructive symptoms in some patients without application of heat. It also was proposed that frequent placement of a rectal applicator may massage the prostate and reduce the obstructive effect.

In 1990, Lindner and colleagues examined the effect of temperature levels during hyperthermia treatment in a series of patients randomized to low-temperature ($<41°$ C) and high-temperature ($42.5°$ C $\pm$ $1°$ C) treatment.[37] All 72 patients were catheter-dependent and had not responded to previous voiding trials during treatment with phenoxybenzamine. A temperature effect was demonstrated, as only 9 of 27 patients (33%) treated at the lower temperature were catheter-free following treatment; 27 of 45 patients (60%) treated at the higher temperature became catheter-free.

Zerbib and coworkers reported the first prospective, placebo-controlled, randomized trial of hyperthermia treatment in 1992.[38] Sixty-eight patients with symptomatic BPH were randomized to two groups. Group I consisted of 38 patients treated to a temperature of $42°$ C ($\pm.5°$ C) for a 1-hour session weekly for 5 weeks. Group II consisted of 30 patients subjected to 5 1-hour weekly sessions with placement of the urethral catheter and rectal applicator without application of microwave power. Prostatic temperatures remained $37°$ C ($\pm.5°$ C) in the latter group. Patients were reevaluated 3 months following completion of the sessions. The mean peak flow rate in the treated group improved from 8.1 to 11.2 mL/sec, whereas no change was observed in the placebo group (8.2 mL/sec to 8.5 mL/sec). Residual urine levels decreased from 110 mL to 67 mL in the treated group, but no change was observed in the placebo group (99 to 100 mL). Symptom score (scale 6 to 38) improved in both groups, from 16.7 to 23 in the treated group and from 19.4 to 23.6 in the placebo group. The patients were categorized as responders and nonresponders. Objective responders were defined as patients with a residual urine level less than 50 mL and peak flow improvement greater than 3 mL/sec. Using the objective response criteria, 20 of 38 treated patients (52%) responded; only 5 of 30 patients (16%) in the placebo group responded. Subjective responders were those patients with a greater than five-point increase in subjective score and patient satisfaction with the treatment. Subjective response was reported in 24 of 38 patients (63%) in the treatment group and in 10 of 30 (30%) in the placebo group. Although some symptomatic improvement was seen in the placebo group, objective improvement was significantly better in the treatment group. These are the first data from a randomized, controlled trial to demonstrate an objective effect of hyperthermia treatment when compared to placebo.

More recent clinical trials have been reported in patients with obstructive BPH. The first long-term results in the United States were reported by Knapp and Newman.[39] Patients were evaluated with the Madsen-Iversen scoring system, uroflowmetry, residual urine level measurement, and pressure-flow urodynamic evaluation. Twenty-one patients were treated with six 1-hour treatment sessions in 3 weeks using a Model 99-D Prostathermer. Follow-up studies were performed at 3, 6, and 18 months.

Twenty of 21 patients were unavailable for follow-up at 18 months. Seven of 20 patients (35%) did not respond to treatment and required TURP. All treatment failures were found in the first 9 months of follow-up. Thirteen of 20 patients were evaluated at 18 months (Table 4). The mean symptom score improved from 16.8 pretreatment to 8.3 at 18 months post-treatment (Fig 6, A). All 13 patients experienced a reduction in symptom score. The mean residual urine level decreased from 250 to 96 mL (see Fig 6, B). Twelve of 13 patients had a reduction in residual urine level and 9 of 13 patients had residual urine levels of 100 or less at 18 months. The mean peak urinary flow rate increased from 9.5 mL/sec to 11.7 mL/sec (see Fig 6, C). Nine of 13 patients experienced an increase in the peak flow rate. The decreases in symptom score and residual urine level were statistically significant, with P values less than .0001 and .03, respectively (see Table 4).

Pressure-flow studies were performed before treatment and at 3 and 6 months following treatment. Pretreatment pressure-flow studies demonstrated voiding contractions in 17 of 20 patients studied. Three patients were unable to develop a voiding contraction under test conditions. Sixteen patients demonstrated an elevated bladder neck opening pressure greater than 40 cm H_2O. At 6 months, pressure-flow results were available for 12 of 20 patients (Table 5). Four patients had failed to respond to therapy, undergone TURP, and were not studied. One patient refused to undergo a pressure-flow examination. Mean bladder neck opening pressure

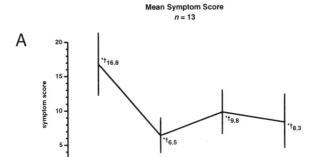

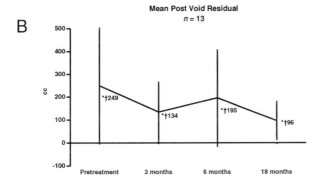

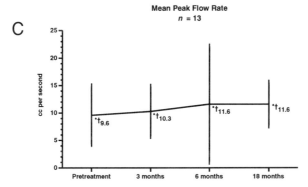

FIG 6.
Long-term follow-up. **A,** mean symptom score. *P < .0001 (statistically significant). †Vertical bars represents standard deviation. **B,** mean postvoid residual. *P < .03 (statistically significant). †Vertical bars represent standard deviation. **C,** mean peak flow rate. *P = .27. †Vertical bars represent standard deviation.

TABLE 4.
Transrectal Hyperthermia Treatment Results (18-Month Follow-up, n = 13)

Measured Parameter	Mean	STD*	Range	P Value
Symptom score				
Pretreatment	16.8	4.2	11–27	<.0001
18-Month follow-up	8.3	3.7	2–15	
Residual urine level (mL)				
Pretreatment	249	243	40–1,000	<0.03
18-Month follow-up	96	73	0–250	
Flow rate (mL/sec)				
Pretreatment	9.6	5.3	0–20	.27
18-Month follow-up	11.6	3.9	7–20	

*STD = standard deviation.

was unchanged (56 cm H_2O) at 6 months. However, 5 patients demonstrated a decrease in opening pressure associated with increases in peak flow rate of 1 to 6 mL/sec (Fig 7), suggesting a reduction of bladder outlet obstruction.

Patients ultimately were classified as improved or failed. Improved patients had a decreased symptom score, a decreased residual urine level, and an increased or unchanged peak flow rate. Patients were considered to have failed treatment if they had an increase in residual urine level or a decrease in peak flow rate, regardless of any change in their symptom score (Table 6). Overall, 13 of 20 patients (65%) were considered to be improved and to require no further treatment. Seven of 20 patients (35%) were considered to have failed treatment and were recommended for TURP. The best results were seen in patients with a pretreatment residual

TABLE 5.
Opening Pressure Results (6-Month Follow-up, n = 12)

Time of Measurement	Mean	STD*	Range
Pretreatment (cm H_2O)	56.7	18.8	20–90
18-Month follow-up (cm H_2O)	56.5	23.3	20–100

*STD = standard deviation.

Opening Pressure

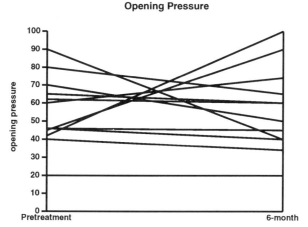

FIG 7.
Bladder neck opening pressure.

urine level less than 200 mL and in those with lateral lobe hypertrophy alone. Nine of 12 patients (74%) with a residual urine level less than 200 mL improved. Eight of 10 patients (80%) with lateral lobe hypertrophy alone improved. The study demonstrates that transrectal hyperthermia treatment was effective in relieving symptomatic BPH in some patients.

Watson and colleagues also demonstrated clinical efficacy of hyperthermia in the treatment of symptomatic BPH.[40] Thirty-six patients with obstructive BPH were treated with two different transrectal hyperthermia devices. The mean peak flow rate improved from 7.3 to 11 mL/sec with one device and from 7.8 to 10.3 mL/sec with the second device. The mean residual urine level decreased from 159 to 60 mL with the first device and

---

TABLE 6.
Clinical Results—18 Months

Status	Number of Patients (%)	Recommendation
Improved (decrease in symptom score; decreased residual urine; increase or no change in peak flow rate)	13/20 (65)	No further treatment
Failed (increase in postvoid residual or decrease in peak flow rate; increase or decrease in symptom score)	7/20 (35)	Transurethral resection of the prostate

from 112 to 38 mL with the second device. The mean symptom score (Madsen-Iversen) decreased from 14 to 7 and from 15 to 9 using the respective devices. Follow-up was a maximum of 12 months. In the follow-up period, 32 of 36 patients (88%) were considered improved and were not referred for TURP.

Complications

Complications following transrectal hyperthermia treatment have been minimal. Most patients have tolerated the treatment sessions well. A collaborative study of 435 patients was reported by Lindner and associates evaluating the complication rate associated with transrectal hyperthermia treatment.[41] Twenty-nine complications were reported in 27 patients (Table 7). Urinary tract infection (7 patients) and hematuria (6 patients) were the most common problems encountered.

In the initial studies done in patients with prostate cancer, Servadio reported two cases of rectoprostatic fistula.[9] One case was in a patient with a previous history of prostatic abscess and the other was in a patient with extensive extracapsular prostate cancer and prostatitis. Exclusion criteria have been developed since to exclude patients with a history of rectal pathology from treatment with transrectal hyperthermia. No subsequent cases of rectoprostatic fistula have been reported.

TABLE 7.
Complications of Hyperthermia Treatment in 435 Patients With Benign Prostatic Hyperplasia*

Complication	Number of Patients (%)
Hematuria	6 (1.4)
Urinary tract infection	7 (1.6)
Epididymitis	2 (0.4)
Chest pain	3 (0.7)
Rectal pain	4 (0.9)
Cold sweat	5 (1.1)
Urinary retention	2 (0.4)
Total	29 (6.6)

*From Lindner A, Siegel YI, Saranga R, et al: *J Urol* 1990; 144:1390–1392. Used by permission.

Future Prospects

Hyperthermia has been shown to be a safe and efficacious treatment of symptomatic BPH, with improvements noted in symptom scores, residual urine levels, and, in some cases, flow rate. Expanded clinical experience may help identify those patients who are best suited for hyperthermia treatment. Future investigations are needed to elucidate its mechanism of action, determine its effect in combination with medical therapy, and explore its role in the treatment of other prostatic diseases.

Mechanism of Action

Hyperthermia treatment reduces prostate size when applied to patients with prostate cancer. However, no significant change in prostate size has been reported using this treatment in patients with BPH. Hyperthermia may, however, reduce other components of bladder outlet obstruction without affecting prostate size or configuration.

Thermotherapy (temperature >45° C), on the other hand, does cause tissue necrosis in BPH. Damage to prostate tissue is demonstrated several millimeters into the adenoma. However, the short-term clinical results of thermotherapy with tissue necrosis are very similar to the clinical results of hyperthermia treatment without tissue necrosis.[39, 40, 42] The mechanism of action of heat in relieving bladder outlet obstruction may not be due to tissue damage, but rather to a change in the dynamic component of bladder outlet obstruction.

The dynamic component of bladder outlet obstruction may be reduced by hyperthermia treatment through alteration in neurologic activity in the prostate. The reduction in irritative and obstructive symptoms with improvement in urinary flow rate and residual urine level are similar to the effect of alpha receptor blockade. Heat may affect alpha receptor activity in the prostate or prostatic urethra, thus reducing outlet resistance.

Some investigators suggest that hyperthermia treatment may change the dynamic component of bladder outlet obstruction by alteration of the stromal elements of BPH.[31, 32] Hyperthermia may promote differentiation of fibroblasts, thus changing the structural components of the stromal tissue. Hyperthermia has been shown to increase significantly the amount of vimentin in prostate tissue. Increases in the amount of actin and desmin were noted also, but these changes were not statistically significant. Actin and desmin are immunohistochemical markers found in smooth muscle, whereas vimentin is a marker found primarily in fibroblasts. By inducing the differentiation of fibroblasts into noncontractile elements, hyperthermia may reduce the dynamic component of prostatic obstruction. Hormonelike polypeptides, termed tissue growth factors, are known to be capable of influencing differentiation of fibroblasts to various contractile and noncontractile tissue elements.[43] The effect of hyperthermia on fibroblast differentiation may be direct or possibly mediated through tissue growth factors.

A better understanding of the effect of heat on BPH may help select particular patient groups who are likely to benefit from hyperthermia treatment. It also may allow investigators to alter current treatment protocols to decrease the number of treatments necessary to achieve a clinical result. However, further in vitro and in vivo studies will be necessary to identify the actual mechanism of action and to determine the significance of the early morphometric studies.

Combined Therapy

The use of transrectal hyperthermia treatment in combination with medical therapy may have an additive effect. Hyperthermia therapy and an antiandrogen, cyproterone acetate, have been used in combination in previous trials. Lindner reported improved results with hyperthermia treatment when it was used in combination with cyproterone acetate.[37] Monthly injection of luteinizing hormone releasing hormone analogues combined with hyperthermia treatment may cause similar results. However, similar to cyproterone acetate, luteinizing hormone releasing hormone analogues would not be suitable for use in potent men. Hyperthermia treatment in combination with 5-α-reductase inhibitors may have an additive effect similar to that seen with antiandrogens, without the side effect of impotence.

Selected alpha-1 receptor blockade has resulted in the relief of symptomatic bladder outlet obstruction and improvements in urinary flow rate.[44] The use of alpha blockers in conjunction with hyperthermia treatments has not been reported, but may demonstrate an additive effect.

Combined hyperthermia treatment and medical therapy may prove to be an effective method to improve the results of minimally invasive outpatient therapy for BPH. Further study in placebo-controlled, randomized trials is needed.

Hyperthermia Treatment in Other Prostate Disease

The symptomatic improvement seen following hyperthermia treatment in patients with BPH led some investigators to attempt treatment of abacterial prostatitis with hyperthermia. In an uncontrolled study, Servadio treated 45 men who had abacterial prostatitis and reported partial or complete relief of irritative symptoms in 32 patients (71%) followed for a mean of 38.5 months.[45] Lindner reported partial or complete relief of irritative symptoms in 24 of 29 men (82%) followed for a mean of 18 months.[46] The use of hyperthermia treatment in patients with abacterial prostatitis potentially represents a safe, easily applied, outpatient treatment for a disease process that is notoriously difficult to remedy.

The use of hyperthermia treatment in the relief of obstructive symptoms in patients with prostate cancer has been discussed previously. Hyperthermia treatment also may be used as adjunctive therapy together with radiation in the treatment of prostate cancer. The potentiating effect of heat in combination with radiation therapy is well-documented in other tumors.[18, 19, 21, 47] Tumor cells in the S phase are particularly sensitive to heat, but usually are insensitive to radiation. However, S-phase cells can be radiosensitized by applying heat with radiation.[48] The effect of hyper-thermia treatment on prostate cancer cell lines has been studied by Kaver and coworkers.[49] The growth and survival of human prostate cancer cell lines were inhibited by the application of heat at 43° C for 1 and 2 hours. The effect was dependent on temperature and duration of exposure. The role of heat in potentiating the effect of radiation therapy in the treatment of prostate cancer remains to be studied. Randomized trials using hyper-thermia treatment in combination with radiation therapy may be helpful in defining its role. The use of hyperthermia treatment with interstitial radiation also may be beneficial.

Evaluation of Results

The outcome assessment of hyperthermia and other treatment alternatives for BPH is difficult. Reports differ in symptom score used and type of objective data obtained. Patient assessment and symptom scoring are affected by the degree of discomfort or inconvenience experienced by each patient. Some patients complain bitterly about mild changes in their voiding pattern, whereas others minimize rather severe obstructive problems. In addition, correlation of symptom score, urinary flow rate, and residual urine level often is poor.

There has been a need to develop uniform symptom scoring systems that objectively represent the patient and physician evaluation, including an assessment of the impact of obstructive symptoms on the patient's quality of life. Future study of the assessment of quality of life is necessary to improve our understanding of treatment results. The American Urological Association recently has developed a new symptom scoring system that includes a quality of life assessment. A detailed presentation of this scoring system can be found in another chapter of this publication.

Summary

Transrectal hyperthermia treatment has been demonstrated to be a safe and effective method to heat the prostate. Intraprostatic temperatures of 43.5° C can be achieved while maintaining cooling of surrounding tissue and the rectal wall. Randomized, controlled studies have demonstrated objective improvement in patients with symptomatic BPH when compared to placebo-treated control subjects.[38] Treatment with low and high temperature has demonstrated that clinical improvement is temperature-dependent.[37] Hyperthermia in the treatment of BPH has demonstrated long-term clinical improvement in symptom scores and urodynamic parameters without causing tissue damage or necrosis.

The place of hyperthermia in the treatment of symptomatic BPH is still being defined. Randomized, controlled studies comparing various BPH treatment alternatives are necessary to determine the place of all alternative treatment modalities in the urologist's treatment armamentarium. Future clinical trials and histochemical studies may help determine which patients are best suited for hyperthermia treatment. Further investigation also is necessary to understand the mechanism of action and explore other applications of hyperthermia in the treatment of prostate disease.

References

1. Busch W: Über den Einfluss Welchen Heftigere Erysipels Zuweilen auf Organisiente Neubildungen Ausuben. *Verhandl Naturh Preuss Rhein Westphal* 1866; 23:28–30.
2. Bruns P: Die Heilwirkung des Erysipels auf Geschwulste. *Beitr Klin Chir* 1877; 3:443–466.
3. Rohdenburg GL: Fluctuations in the growth of malignant tumors in man, with special reference to spontaneous recession. *J Cancer Res* 1918; 3:193–225.
4. Coley WB: The treatment of malignant tumors by repeated inoculations of erysipelas—with a report of ten original cases. *Am J Med Sci* 1893; 105:487–511.
5. Woodhall B, Pickrill KL, Georgiade NG, et al: Effect of hyperthermia upon cancer chemotherapy: Application to external cancer of head and face structures. *Ann Surg* 1960; 151:750–759.
6. Shingleton WW, Bryan FA, O'Quinn WL, et al: Selective heating and cooling of tissue in cancer chemotherapy. *Ann Surg* 1962; 156:408–416.
7. Astrahan MA, Norman A: A localized current field hyperthermia system for use with 192-iridium interstitial implants. *Med Phys* 1982; 9:419–424.
8. Yerushalmi A, Servadio C, Leib Z, et al: Local hyperthermia for treatment of carcinoma of the prostate: A preliminary report. *Prostate* 1982; 3:623–630.
9. Servadio C, Leib Z: Hyperthermia in the treatment of prostate cancer. *Prostate* 1984; 5:205–211.
10. Servadio C: Local hyperthermia for the treatment of prostatic disease; in Fitzpatrick JM, Krane RJ (eds): *The Prostate.* New York, Churchill Livingstone, 1989.
11. Castaneda F, Banno J, Brady T: Experimental prostatic hyperthermia. *J Endourol* 1991; 5:123–127.
12. Blute ML, Lewis RW: Local microwave hyperthermia as a treatment alternative for benign prostatic hyperplasia. *J Androl* 1991; 12:429–434.
13. Song CW: Effect of hyperthermia on vascular functions of normal tissues and experimental tumors. *J Natl Cancer Inst* 1978; 60:711–713.
14. Shibata HR, MacLean LD: Blood flow to tumors. *Prog Clin Cancer* 1966; 2:33–47.
15. Chen TT, Heidelberger C: Quantitative studies on the malignant transformation of mouse prostate cells by carcinogenic hydrocarbons *in vitro*. *Int J Cancer* 1969; 4:166–182.
16. Giovanella BC, Stehlin JS, Morgan AC: Selective lethal effect of supranormal temperatures on human neoplastic cells. *Cancer Res* 1976; 36:3944–3962.
17. Janiak M, Szmigielski S: Alteration of the immune reactions by whole body and local microwave hyperthermia in normal and tumor bearing animals: Review of own 1976-1980 experiments. *Br J Cancer* 1982; 45:122–120.
18. Gerweck LE: Lethal response of cells to radiation or hyperthermia under acute or chronic hypoxic conditions. *Radiat Res* 1977; 70:612–632.
19. Kim SH, Kim JH, Hahn EW: The radiosensitization of hypoxic tumor cells by hyperthermia. *Radiology* 1975; 114:727–728.

20. Hahn GM: Hyperthermia and drugs: Potential for therapy. *Cancer Res* 1979; 39:2263–2268.
21. Har-Keder I, Blechan NM: Experimental and clinical aspects of hyperthermia applied to the treatment of cancer with special reference to the role of ultrasonic and microwave heating, in Lett JT (ed): *Advances in Radiation Biology.* New York, Academic Press, 1976, pp 229–266.
22. Hunt JW: Application of microwave, ultrasound, and radiofrequency heating (monograph 61). Third International Symposium: Cancer Therapy, Hyperthermia Drugs, and Radiation.
23. Biodan Medical Systems, Ltd. *Prostathermer™ Hyperthermia System.* Investigational Device Exemption Application to the FDA, May 31, 1988.
24. Lindner A, Golomb J, Siegel Y, et al: Local hyperthermia of the prostate gland for the treatment of benign prostatic hypertrophy and urinary retention. *Br J Urol* 1987; 60:567.
25. Leib Z, Rothem A, Lev A, et al: Histopathological observations in the canine prostate treated by local microwave hyperthermia. *Prostate* 1986; 8:92–102.
26. Servadio C, Leib Z, Lev A: Local hyperthermia to canine prostate: A pilot study. *Urology* 1990; 35:156–163.
27. Siegel YI, Lindner A: Temperature profile mapping in the prostatic urethra during hyperthermia treatment (abstract). *Eur Urol* 1990; 18:516A.
28. Newman DM, Knapp PK: Interstitial temperature mapping in the human prostate during transrectal hyperthermia treatment for BPH (abstract). *J Endourol* 1990; 4:S135.
29. Siegel YI, Zaidel L, Hammel I, et al: Morphometric evaluation of benign prostatic hyperplasia. *Eur Urol* 1990; 18:71–73.
30. Siegel YI, Zaidel L, Hammel I, et al: Histopathology of benign prostatic hyperplasia after failure of hyperthermia treatment. *Br J Urol* 1991; 68:383–386.
31. Siegel YI, Lindner A, Zaidel L: Immunohistochemical changes in the prostate gland following rectal hyperthermia (abstract). J Urol 1992; 147:345A.
32. Stamey TA, Yang N, Hay AR, et al: Prostate specific antigen as a serum marker for adenocarcinoma of the prostate. *N Engl J Med* 1987; 317:909.
33. Lindner A, Siegel YI, Korczak D: Serum prostate specific antigen levels during hyperthermia treatment of benign prostatic hyperplasia. *J Urol* 1990; 144:1388–1389.
34. Lindner A, Golomb J, Siegel YI, et al: Local hyperthermia of the prostate gland for the treatment of benign prostatic hypertrophy and urinary retention: A preliminary report. *Br J Urol* 1987; 60:567–571.
35. Servadio C, Lindner A, Lev A, et al: Further observations on the effect of local hyperthermia on benign enlargement of the prostate. *World J Urol* 1989; 6:204–208.
36. Saranga R, Matzkin H, Braf Z: Local microwave hyperthermia in the treatment of benign prostatic hypertrophy. *Br J Urol* 1990; 65:349–353.
37. Lindner A, Braf Z, Lev A, et al: Local hyperthermia of the prostate gland for the treatment of benign prostatic hypertrophy and urinary retention. *Br J Urol* 1990; 65:201–203.
38. Zerbib M, Steg A, Conquy S, et al: Localized hyperthermia v sham procedure in obstructive benign hyperplasia of the prostate: Prospective randomized study. *J Urol* 1992; 147:1048.
39. Knapp PM, Newman DM: Long-term efficacy of transrectal hyperthermia in the treatment of obstructive BPH. Presented at Society for Minimally Invasive Therapy Meeting, Boston, Massachusetts, November 1991.

40. Watson GM, Perlmutter AP, Shah TK, et al: Heat treatment for severe, symptomatic prostatic outflow obstruction. *World J Urol* 9:7–11.
41. Lindner A, Siegel YI, Saranga R, et al: Complications in hyperthermia treatment of benign prostatic hyperplasia. *J Urol* 1990; 144:1390–1392.
42. Carter S, Patel A, Reddy P, et al: Single-session transurethral microwave thermotherapy for the treatment of benign prostatic obstruction. *J Endourol* 1991; 5:137–145.
43. Sappino AP, Schürch W, Gabbian G: Differentiation repertoire of fibroblastic cells: Expression of cytoskeletal proteins as marker of phenotypic modulations. *Lab Invest* 1990; 63:144–161.
44. Donnell R, Lepor H: Alpha-blockade for benign prostatic hyperplasia. *J Endourol* 1991; 5:83–87.
45. Servadio C, Leib Z: Chronic abacterial prostatitis and hyperthermia: A possible new treatment? *Br J Urol* 1991; 67:308–311.
46. Lindner A, Siegel YI, Korczak D: Local hyperthermia treatment of chronic abacterial prostatitis (abstract). *J Endourol* 1991; 5:S103.
47. Corry PM, Barlogie P, Tilchen EJ, et al: Ultrasound induced hyperthermia for the treatment of human superficial tumors. *Int J Radiat Oncol Biol Phys* 1982; 8:1125.
48. Gerweck LE, Gillette EL, Dewey WC: Effect of heat and radiation on synchronous Chinese hamster cells; killing and repair. *Radiat Res* 1975; 64:611.
49. Kaver I, Ware JL, Koontz WW: The effect of hyperthermia on human prostatic carcinoma cell lines: Evaluation *in vitro*. *J Urol* 1989; 141:1025.

Index

We've read
236,287
journal
articles
(so you don't have to).

The Year Books–
The best from 236,287 journal articles.

At Mosby, we subscribe to more than 950 medical and allied health journals from every corner of the globe. We read them all, tirelessly scanning for anything that relates to your field.

We send everything we find related to a given specialty to the distinguished editors of the **Year Book** in that area, and they pick out the best, the articles they feel every practitioner in that specialty should be aware of.

For the 1993 **Year Books** we surveyed a total of 236,287 articles and found hundreds of articles related to your field. Our expert editors reviewed these and chose the best, the developments you don't want to miss.

The best articles–condensed and organized.

Not only do you get the past year's most important articles in your field, you get them in a format that makes them easy to use.

Every article that the editors pick is condensed into a concise, outlined abstract, a summary of the article's most important points highlighted with bold paragraph headings. So you can quickly scan for exactly what you need.

Personal commentary from the experts.

If that was it, if all our editors did was identify the year's best articles, the **Year Book** would still be a great reference to have. (Can you think of an easier way to keep up with all the developments that are shaping your field?)

But following each article, the editors also write concise commentaries telling whether or not the study in question is a reliable one, whether a new technique is effective, or whether a particular trend you've heard about merits your immediate attention.

No other abstracting service offers this expert advice to help you decide how the year's advances will affect the way you practice.

No matter how many journals you subscribe to, the Year Book can help.

When you subscribe to a **Year Book**, we'll also send you an automatic notice of future volumes about two months before they publish. If you do not want the **Year Book**, this convenient advance notice makes it easy for you to let us know. And if you elect to receive the new **Year Book**, you need do nothing. We will send it upon publication.

No worry. No wasted motion. And, of course, every **Year Book** is yours to examine FREE of charge for thirty days.